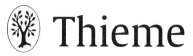

CT of the Head and Spine

Norbert Hosten, M.D.
Professor
Director Radiology
Klinikum Ernst-Moritz-Arndt
Universität
Greifswald, Germany

Thomas Liebig, M.D.
Supervising Physician
Klinik für Neuroradiologie
International Neuroscience Institute
Hanover, Germany

847 illustrations

Thieme
Stuttgart · New York

Library of Congress Cataloging-in-Publication Data

Hosten, Norbert.
  [Computertomographie von Kopf und Wirbel-säule. English]
  CT of the head and spine / Norbert Hosten, Thomas Liebig.
    p. ; cm.
  Includes bibliographical references and index.
  ISBN 1-58890-039-8–ISBN 3131267119
  1. Head—Tomography. 2. Spine—Tomography. I. Liebig, Thomas. II. Title.
  [DNLM: 1. Brain—radiography. 2. Head—radiography. 3. Spine—radiography. 4. Tomography, X-Ray Computed. WL 141 H831c 2001a]
RC936 .H6713 2001
617.5'107572–dc21   2001041519

Translated by Terry C. Telger, Fort Worth, TX, USA

This book is an authorized translation of the German edition published and copyrighted 2000 by Georg Thieme Verlag, Stuttgart, Germany. Title of the German edition: Computertomographie von Kopf und Wirbelsäule.

The front cover images are 3D-visualizations of standard CT-datasets that were obtained from a CBYON system using histogram optimized volume rendering techniques (CBYON, Inc. 2275 E Bayshore, Suite 101, Palo Alto, CA 94303, USA).

© 2002 Georg Thieme Verlag
Rüdigerstrasse 14, 70469 Stuttgart, Germany
Thieme New York, 333 Seventh Avenue,
New York, N.Y. 10001 USA

Typesetting by primustype Robert Hurler GmbH
73274 Notzingen, Germany

Printed in Germany by Druckhaus Götz, Ludwigsburg

ISBN 3-13-126711-9 (GTV)
ISBN 1-58890-039-8 (TNY)   1 2 3 4 5

Foreword

The present book, written by my colleagues Prof. Norbert Hosten and Dr. Thomas Liebig, differs from previous general accounts of computed tomography of the head and spine in that it correlates computed tomography (CT) with the now-established modality of magnetic resonance imaging (MRI). This correlation is evident throughout the text, even when it is not explicitly stated.

At a time when radiologists need to make a selection from the various imaging procedures available and choose the one that will be of greatest benefit to the patient, it is helpful to have a comprehensive reference work that continually highlights the complementary roles of CT and MRI.

I am pleased that our institution has produced scientists who are so familiar with modern radiographic and sectional imaging techniques that they are able to present CT of the head and spine against the background of other imaging modalities. Among its many strengths, the book is an excellent work for teaching purposes, and I hope it will be widely read and used.

Prof. Roland Felix

Preface

Astounding technical advances in recent years have again led to substantial improvements in the imaging quality of computed tomography (CT). These improvements, in turn, have led to progress in advanced imaging evaluations of the neurocranium, facial skeleton, spinal column, and spinal canal, which were the original focus of CT examinations during the latter half of the 1970s. Faster scanning equipment allows shorter examination times, thinner slices, and contrast-enhanced studies that could not have been anticipated 10 years ago. These technical advances prompted the authors to produce a comprehensive and up-to-date reference work on CT imaging of the head and spine.

In embarking on this project, we found that the tremendous capabilities of magnetic resonance imaging (MRI) in this field have not led to any loss of interest in CT. Indeed, as the depth of the diagnostic information provided by MRI has increased, it has stimulated even greater interest in CT, which is almost always the initial imaging procedure. With the advent of modern imaging-guided therapeutic techniques, this relatively low-cost study, which can be used in virtually all patients, has received fresh impetus for further development.

Prof. Felix, the quality of whose teaching in both the clinical and scientific fields has earned our immense respect, gave us the opportunity to acquire practical and theoretical experience in head and spine imaging. His reports dealing with temperature-related effects on diagnosis and treatment, and on the methodology and clinical aspects of hyperthermia, have made a significant contribution to the diagnostic aspects of imaging-guided therapeutic procedures, in particular.

We would like to express special thanks to Prof. Dietel, Director of the Department of Pathology at the Charité Hospital in Berlin, for his kind permission to publish photographs of specimens from the hospital's teaching collection.

We are grateful to Prof. von Deimling, Director of the Department of Neuropathology, for providing the documentation for several histological examinations.

We would also like to acknowledge the role played by professional conferences in neurosurgery, neuropathology, and neuroradiology in advancing our understanding of the diseases covered in this book.

Our thanks go to Mrs. Heimann and Mrs. Naujok of the Film and Graphics Department at the Charité Hospital for the patience with which they prepared the graphics for the book, and we are grateful to Mrs. Rösel and Mrs. Kuzmik of the photographic section of the Department of Radiology for the great care and patience with which they processed the photographic materials. Mrs. Fiebelkorn checked the language of the whole of the original German version for errors.

We would also like to acknowledge the help of the CT team in the Radiology Department and Outpatient Department in meeting our special requirements with regard to documentation and postprocessing. Dr. Rosenthal helped the authors by explaining certain issues from the neurosurgeon's perspective.

Finally, we are grateful to our wives for their patience and their constructive criticism.

The book would not have been possible without the energetic commitment shown by Dr. Pilgrim of Thieme Medical Publishers.

Greifswald　　　　　　　　　　　　*Norbert Hosten*
Hanover, Fall 2001　　　　　　　　*Thomas Liebig*

Contents

Computed Tomography of the Head

1 Fundamentals 15

2 Craniocerebral Trauma 39

3 Cerebrovascular Diseases 61

4 Inflammatory Diseases 99

5 Intracranial Tumors

6 Degenerative and Demyelinating Diseases

7 Congenital Brain Diseases 213

8 Postoperative Findings and Follow-Up 226

9 Facial Skeleton and Skull Base 229

Computed Tomography of the Spine

13 Intraspinal Masses   367

14 Inflammatory Diseases   411

Index   425

Computed Tomography
of the Head

Anatomy of the Head

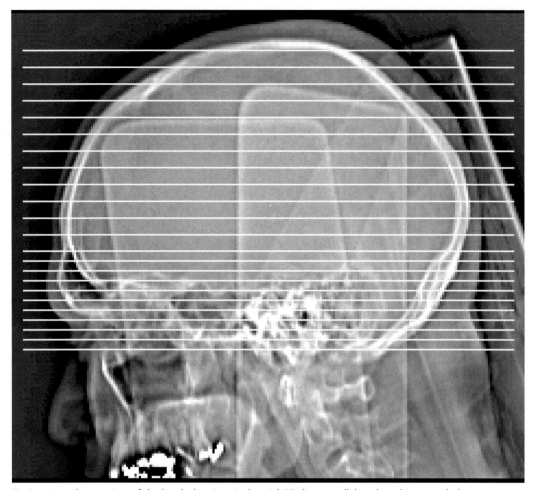

Fig. **1a**   Lateral scout view of the head, showing single axial CT slices parallel to the orbitomeatal plane.

The pages that follow illustrate the sectional anatomy of the head as it appears on modern computed-tomographic images in standard axial and temporal lobe projections. Only anatomic details that are consistently visualized and are relevant to routine image interpretation are labeled in the figures. Functional systems such as the dural sinuses are discussed more fully in subsequent chapters if they are important for understanding the relationship between clinical and radiologic findings.

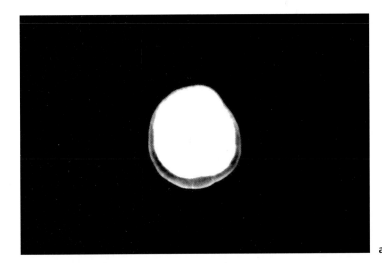

a

Fig. **1b–u** Axial noncontrast CT scans, single-slice technique. The slice thickness is 8 mm for supratentorial scans and 5 mm for infratentorial scans. Key anatomic structures are labeled.

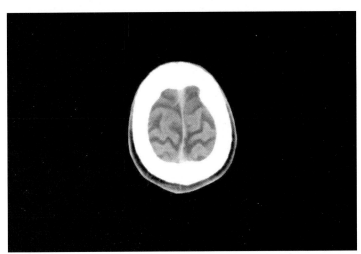

b

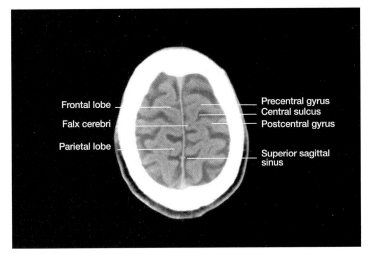

Frontal lobe

Falx cerebri

Parietal lobe

Precentral gyrus
Central sulcus
Postcentral gyrus

Superior sagittal sinus

c

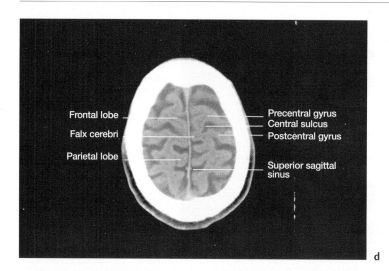

Frontal lobe

Falx cerebri

Parietal lobe

Precentral gyrus
Central sulcus
Postcentral gyrus

Superior sagittal sinus

d

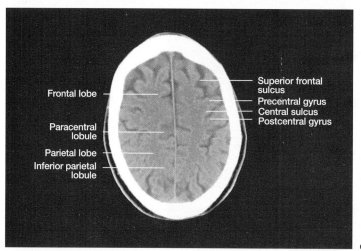

Frontal lobe

Paracentral lobule

Parietal lobe

Inferior parietal lobule

Superior frontal sulcus
Precentral gyrus
Central sulcus
Postcentral gyrus

e

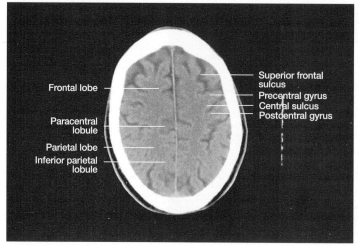

Frontal lobe

Paracentral lobule

Parietal lobe

Inferior parietal lobule

Superior frontal sulcus
Precentral gyrus
Central sulcus
Postcentral gyrus

f

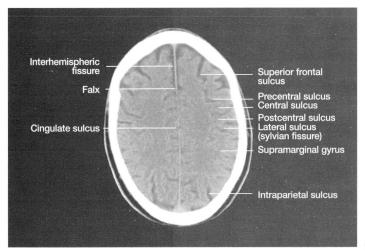

Interhemispheric fissure

Falx

Cingulate sulcus

Superior frontal sulcus

Precentral sulcus
Central sulcus

Postcentral sulcus
Lateral sulcus (sylvian fissure)

Supramarginal gyrus

Intraparietal sulcus

g

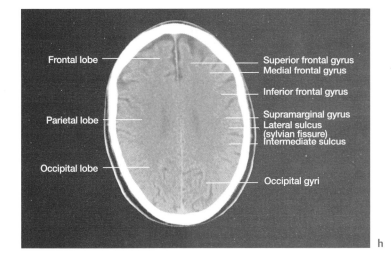

Frontal lobe

Parietal lobe

Occipital lobe

Superior frontal gyrus
Medial frontal gyrus

Inferior frontal gyrus

Supramarginal gyrus
Lateral sulcus (sylvian fissure)
Intermediate sulcus

Occipital gyri

h

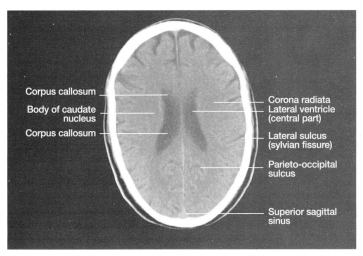

Corpus callosum

Body of caudate nucleus

Corpus callosum

Corona radiata
Lateral ventricle (central part)

Lateral sulcus (sylvian fissure)

Parieto-occipital sulcus

Superior sagittal sinus

i

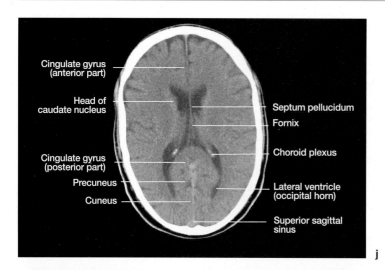

Cingulate gyrus (anterior part)

Head of caudate nucleus

Cingulate gyrus (posterior part)

Precuneus

Cuneus

Septum pellucidum

Fornix

Choroid plexus

Lateral ventricle (occipital horn)

Superior sagittal sinus

j

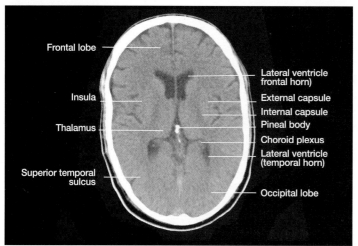

Frontal lobe

Insula

Thalamus

Superior temporal sulcus

Lateral ventricle frontal horn)

External capsule

Internal capsule

Pineal body

Choroid plexus

Lateral ventricle (temporal horn)

Occipital lobe

k

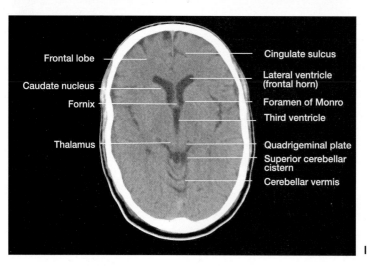

Frontal lobe

Caudate nucleus

Fornix

Thalamus

Cingulate sulcus

Lateral ventricle (frontal horn)

Foramen of Monro

Third ventricle

Quadrigeminal plate

Superior cerebellar cistern

Cerebellar vermis

l

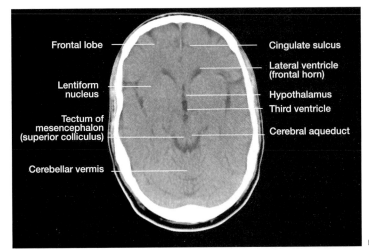

Frontal lobe

Cingulate sulcus

Lateral ventricle
(frontal horn)

Lentiform
nucleus

Hypothalamus

Third ventricle

Tectum of
mesencephalon
(superior colliculus)

Cerebral aqueduct

Cerebellar vermis

m

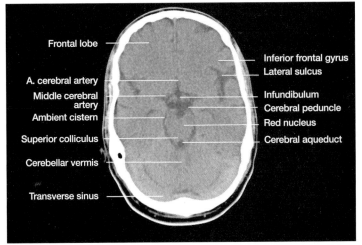

Frontal lobe

Inferior frontal gyrus

Lateral sulcus

A. cerebral artery

Middle cerebral
artery

Infundibulum

Cerebral peduncle

Ambient cistern

Red nucleus

Superior colliculus

Cerebral aqueduct

Cerebellar vermis

Transverse sinus

n

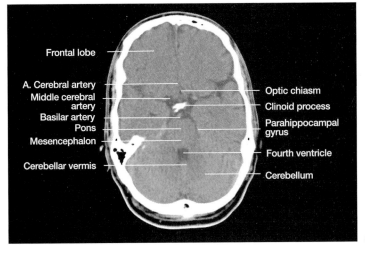

Frontal lobe

A. Cerebral artery

Middle cerebral
artery

Optic chiasm

Basilar artery

Clinoid process

Pons

Parahippocampal
gyrus

Mesencephalon

Cerebellar vermis

Fourth ventricle

Cerebellum

o

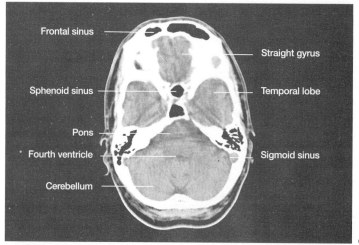

Frontal lobe — Frontal sinus

Temporal lobe — Pituitary
Basilar artery — Clinoid process

Mastoid air cells — Tentorium
Superior cerebellar peduncle — Sigmoid sinus
Cerebellar vermis — Cerebellum

p

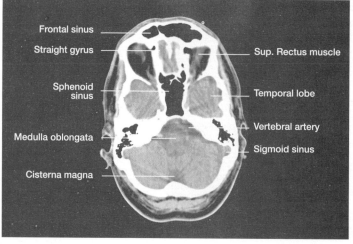

Frontal sinus — Straight gyrus

Sphenoid sinus — Temporal lobe

Pons
Fourth ventricle — Sigmoid sinus
Cerebellum

q

Frontal sinus
Straight gyrus — Sup. Rectus muscle

Sphenoid sinus — Temporal lobe

Medulla oblongata — Vertebral artery
Sigmoid sinus

Cisterna magna

r

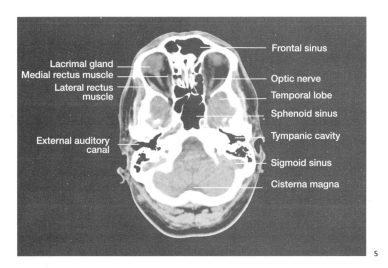

Lacrimal gland
Medial rectus muscle
Lateral rectus muscle

External auditory canal

Frontal sinus
Optic nerve
Temporal lobe
Sphenoid sinus
Tympanic cavity
Sigmoid sinus
Cisterna magna

s

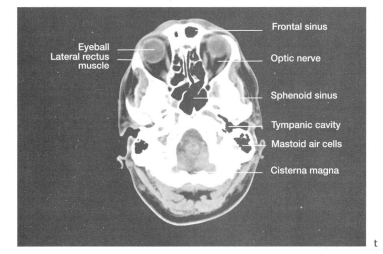

Eyeball
Lateral rectus muscle

Frontal sinus
Optic nerve
Sphenoid sinus
Tympanic cavity
Mastoid air cells
Cisterna magna

t

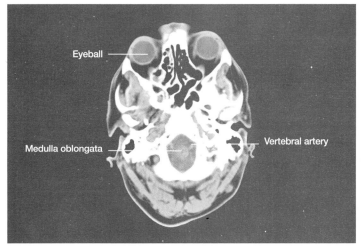

Eyeball

Medulla oblongata

Vertebral artery

u

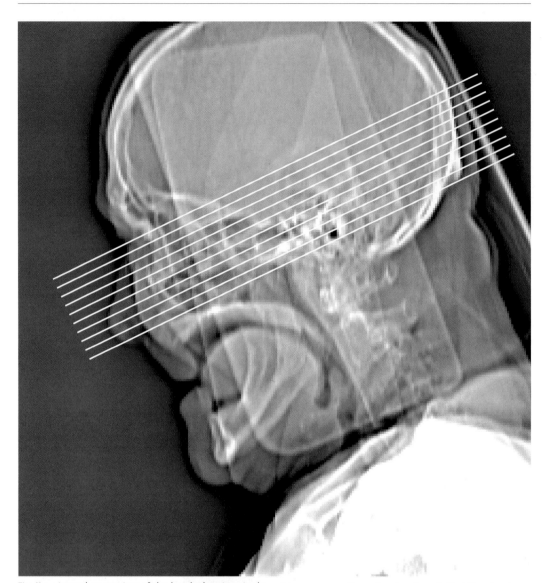

Fig. **II a** Lateral scout view of the head, showing single axial CT slices parallel to the sylvian fissure. This temporal lobe projection is useful for evaluating temporomesial structures such as the amygdaloid body and hippocampus. Its main advantage is that the structures of the brain stem and midbrain are less obscured by the beam-hardening artifacts that develop between the very radiodense petrous pyramids.

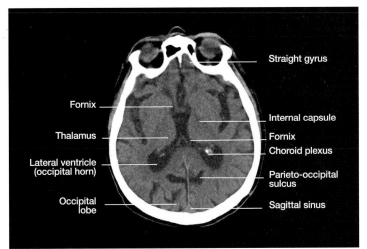

Straight gyrus

Fornix

Internal capsule

Thalamus

Fornix

Choroid plexus

Lateral ventricle
(occipital horn)

Parieto-occipital
sulcus

Occipital
lobe

Sagittal sinus

b

Fig. **II b–i** Axial 5-mm CT slices through the middle and posterior cranial fossae in the temporal lobe projection (IE, approximately parallel to the sylvian fissure). Key anatomic structures are labeled in the images.

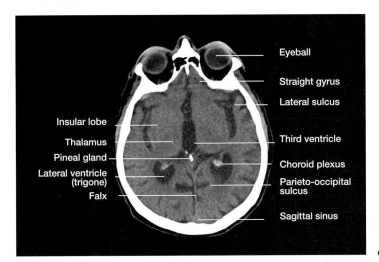

Eyeball

Straight gyrus

Lateral sulcus

Insular lobe

Thalamus

Third ventricle

Pineal gland

Lateral ventricle
(trigone)

Choroid plexus

Parieto-occipital
sulcus

Falx

Sagittal sinus

c

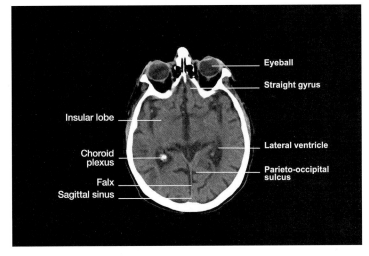

Eyeball

Straight gyrus

Insular lobe

Choroid
plexus

Lateral ventricle

Parieto-occipital
sulcus

Falx

Sagittal sinus

d

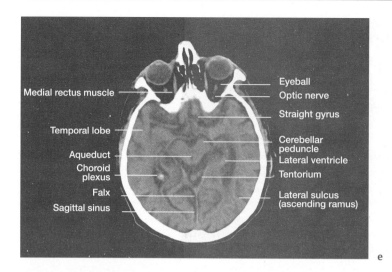

Medial rectus muscle

Temporal lobe

Aqueduct

Choroid plexus

Falx

Sagittal sinus

Eyeball

Optic nerve

Straight gyrus

Cerebellar peduncle

Lateral ventricle

Tentorium

Lateral sulcus (ascending ramus)

e

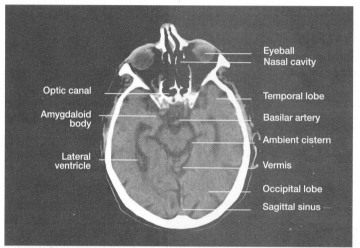

Optic canal

Amygdaloid body

Lateral ventricle

Eyeball

Nasal cavity

Temporal lobe

Basilar artery

Ambient cistern

Vermis

Occipital lobe

Sagittal sinus

f

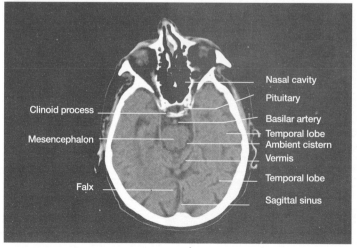

Clinoid process

Mesencephalon

Falx

Nasal cavity

Pituitary

Basilar artery

Temporal lobe

Ambient cistern

Vermis

Temporal lobe

Sagittal sinus

g

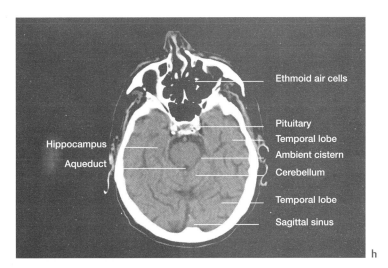

Ethmoid air cells

Pituitary

Hippocampus

Temporal lobe

Aqueduct

Ambient cistern

Cerebellum

Temporal lobe

Sagittal sinus

h

Maxillary sinus

Nasal septum

Sphenoid
sinus

Temporal lobe

Basilar artery

Pons

Pedunculo-
cerebellar cistern

Fourth ventricle

Cerebellum

Occipital lobe

i

1 Fundamentals

This chapter presents an overview of the most common cerebral findings that are noted in computed tomography (CT) examinations for central nervous system (CNS) trauma and other emergency indications. The contents of the chapter are geared toward the beginner who has no prior experience with cerebral CT.

Clinical Aspects

For many years the brain, enclosed within the cranial vault, was *terra incognita* for radiologists. The cranial bone encompassing the brain attenuated roentgen rays so strongly that density differences in the brain tissues could not be appreciated on radiographs. The bony skull precludes using a technique similar to mammography, for example, in which tissues with slightly different radiographic densities can be differentiated by imaging them with low-kilovoltage roentgen rays. Standard radiographic films of the brain were only able to detect lesions that differed markedly in attenuation from the cranial bone, such as calcifications (choroid plexus, pituitary) and air.

The introduction of air ventriculography and pneumoencephalography made it possible to detect intracranial masses indirectly by their compressive effect on the air-filled ventricular system. This was followed by cerebral angiography, in which iodinated contrast medium was instilled to opacify the intracranial vessels, and intracranial masses could be detected on the basis of direct or indirect roentgen signs.

Computed tomography, developed by the English physicist Hounsfield in the early 1970 s, used advances in computer technology to *register the density differences of brain tissues inside the cranial vault* (Fig. 1.1). CT revolutionized neuroradiology by providing a nonin-

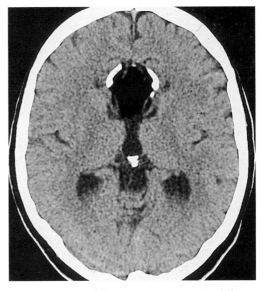

Fig. 1.**1** Density differences. Tissues with different radiographic densities are assigned different shades of gray on the computed tomography (CT) image. In the example shown, a corpus callosum lipoma situated on the midline has the lowest CT density aside from air (fat has a negative attenuation value and appears black). Calcium at the periphery of the lipoma and the cranial vault have the highest density and appear white. The cerebrospinal fluid (CSF) in the ventricular system has relatively low density. Gray matter has a slightly higher density than white matter. Typical attenuation values in Hounsfield units are:

- Air   −1000
- Fat   −100
- CSF   0–10
- White matter   30–35
- Gray matter   40–45
- Calcium, bone   approx. 1000

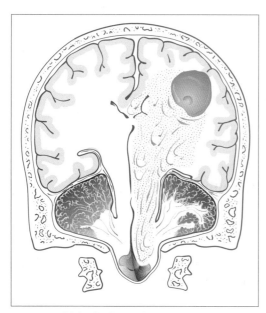

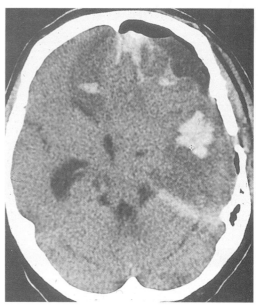

Fig. 1.2 Subfalcial, descending transtentorial, and descending tonsillar herniation. The schematic drawing illustrates the displacement of brain tissue that occurs in different types of cerebral herniation.

Fig. 1.3 Subfalcial and descending transtentorial herniation. Typical CT appearance of subfalcial and descending transtentorial herniation resulting from head trauma. In this postoperative patient, foci of extensive intracerebral hemorrhage are visible in the left frontal and temporal areas, accompanied by intracranial free air. There is a pronounced midline shift, with displacement of the supratentorial ventricular system toward the right side. Right frontal lobe hypodensity may result from anterior cerebral artery compression. Portions of the medial temporal lobe are herniated, obliterating parts of the ambient cistern.

vasive means of visualizing soft-tissue structures inside the skull.

The importance of CT in intracranial diagnosis is based on the fact that even a slight increase in intracranial volume can lead to brain herniation and death. On the other hand, invasive diagnostic procedures such as those used in the abdomen (exploratory laparotomy) cannot be safely used for intracranial diagnosis.

Increased intracranial volume can have various causes:

- Intracerebral hemorrhage
- Mass lesions
- Edema

A volume increase that would have no deleterious effects within the chest or abdominal cavity can be devastating inside the cranial cavity.

Increased intracranial volume and pressure tend to produce the following effects on intracranial structures (Fig. 1.2):

- Herniation of the medial temporal lobe (uncus, hippocampus) into the tentorial incisure (Fig. 1.3). This leads to:

– Compression of the ipsilateral oculomotor nerve with mydriasis.
– Compression of the contralateral cerebral peduncle.
– Displacement of the upper brain stem laterally and inferiorly.
– Compression of the upper midbrain against the tentorium, with possible compression of the posterior cerebral artery.
- Herniation of the cingulate gyrus under the free edge of the falx toward the contralateral side.
- Herniation of cerebellar tonsils into the foramen magnum.

Brain herniation may be caused by a circumscribed mass or by a general rise in intracranial pressure. If the calvarium is intact, the foramen

Tab.**1** Checklist for analyzing cerebral computed tomography scans

- Correct slice thickness?
- Artifacts?
- Scalp normal?
- Visible hematoma?
- Facial soft tissues?
- Discontinuities or displaced fragments in the calvarium?
- Hyperdense subdural or epidural blood bordering the calvarium?
- Sulci visible over all brain areas?
- Effacement of sulci by an underlying mass?
- Individual sulci hyperdense due to subarachnoid hemorrhage?
- Dural sinuses opacified after contrast administration with no filling defects?
- White matter free of circumscribed hyperdensities or hypodensities?
- Ventricular system uncompressed and approximately symmetrical with no midline shift?
- Contrast administration necessary? (for white-matter edema, suspicion of inflammatory brain disease, suspicion of metastases, suspicion of dural sinus thrombosis)

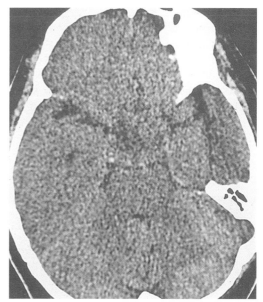

Fig. 1.**4** **Beam-hardening artifact.** Beam-hardening artifacts from the inner surface of the calvarium are a frequent problem in the CT diagnosis of intracranial hemorrhage. These artifacts make it particularly difficult to evaluate the middle cranial fossa (petrous bone), the posterior cranial fossa, and specific structures such as the internal occipital protuberance. In the case shown, the beam-hardening artifact appears as hypodense and hyperdense streaks in the middle fossa, stretching between the sphenoid wing and the petrous bone on the left side.

magnum provides the only outlet for relieving the pressure through extracranial tissue displacement. The compartmentalization of the cranial cavity by the hard, relatively rigid falx and by the tentorium tends to prevent the intracranial displacement of brain tissue into other compartments. The high mortality from unrelieved herniation results from direct compression injury of the displaced structures or indirect tissue damage due to ischemia.

The pathologic changes that are essential in emergency diagnosis involve the white and gray matter of the brain and the intracranial cerebrospinal fluid (CSF) spaces.

Attention should be given to the following changes:

- Density changes.
- Masses.
- Disruptions of the blood–brain barrier, which can be visualized by the intravenous administration of contrast medium.

As in the interpretation of radiographic films of other organ systems (chest, etc.), the beginner should get used to conducting a systematic image analysis in which the anatomic structures are progressively identified and evaluated from the outside in, or from the inside out. This makes it easier to detect abnormalities. An outside-in method of analyzing CT scans is given in Table 1.**1**.

Before interpreting a scan, the examiner should perform a brief quality control by asking the following questions:

- Is the calvarium completely imaged?
- Was a smaller slice thickness used for infratentorial scans than for supratentorial scans (e.g., 4 mm vs. 8 mm)?
- Are motion artifacts present? (If beam-hardening artifacts are increased due to motion (Fig. 1.**4**), they are easily mistaken for hematomas.)

- Is the window setting correct? (The white and gray matter should show contrasting densities. Gross errors result from using the wrong reconstruction algorithm. This can be difficult to recognize, especially in the early morning hours. Improper algorithm selection can invalidate the results of head examinations in small children.)

Errors of interpretation can have other causes as well:

- Incorrect positioning of the patient within the scanner (Fig. **1.5**).
- Equipment malfunction (Fig. **1.6**).
- Defects in the developing machine (Fig. **1.7**).

In all trauma patients, the *scalp* is examined first for any circumscribed expansion that would indicate an extracranial hematoma (Fig. **1.8**).

Of course, any patient who has lost consciousness may have fallen and struck the

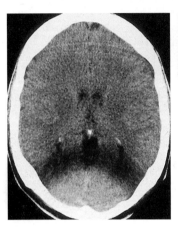 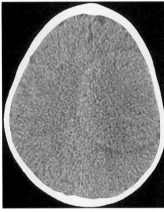 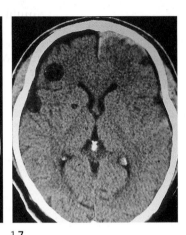

1.5   1.6   1.7

Figs. 1.5–1.7 **Artifacts caused by faulty positioning.** Figure **1.5** illustrates the importance of correctly positioning the patient in the aperture of the CT gantry. The trauma patient was wearing a neck collar that made it difficult to center the head in the aperture. The eccentric position leads to shadowing of occipital brain structures.

Figure **1.6** illustrates a circular ring artifact, which can have various technical causes such as detector malfunction. While most ring artifacts are easily recognized as such, a few can mimic an intracerebral mass. Development errors in Fig. **1.7** mimic round lesions in the frontal white matter and basal ganglia on the right side.

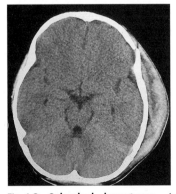

Fig. 1.8 **Subgaleal hematoma.** An extensive extracranial hematoma has developed over a fracture in the left frontoparietal calvarium.

head. The soft tissues of the facial skeleton and the periorbital soft tissues are frequent sites of hematoma formation. These findings should not be overlooked, as they may warrant additional views (e.g., direct coronal CT scans).

The *cranial bones* should be examined for gross displacement due to fractures. The cranial bones cannot be accurately evaluated on CT images acquired with an 8-mm slice thickness and a soft-tissue window. Presumed fractures are difficult to distinguish from cranial sutures, especially for the novice and especially in the occipital region, but sutures are usually distinguished by their symmetrical placement on opposite sides of the skull (Fig. **1.9**).

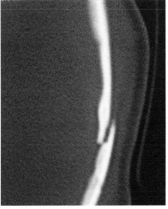 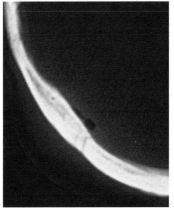 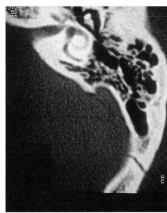

Fig. 1.**9** **Differentiation of cranial sutures and fractures. a** The discontinuity in the calvarium caused by a fracture is distinguished from a cranial suture by the relative displacement of the bone ends. **b** Intracranial air bordering on a discontinuity also indicates a fracture. **c** Sutures are distinguished by their anatomic location, the absence of bone displacement, and the presence of cortical bone separating the medullary cavity from the gap.

The area adjacent to a skull fracture should always be scrutinized for (epidural) hematoma, just as the area bordering a hematoma should be examined for a fracture. Lytic lesions of the calvarium are frequently missed, especially when solitary (e.g., eosinophilic granuloma), but multiple lytic areas due to metastases (e.g., intracerebral metastases from breast cancer) may also be overlooked.

Proceeding to the cranial contents, the radiologist should look for acute *subdural* and *epidural hematomas,* which appear as hyperdense crescents distributed along the inner surface of the calvarium. When narrow, these collections are easily missed on CT scans. This is particularly true if the patient's head was tilted to one side during the examination, resulting in asymmetry of the CT slices. Concavity (subdural) or convexity of the hematoma (epidural, Figs. 1.**10,** 1.**11**) is helpful but is not always a reliable differentiating sign.

One useful distinguishing feature is the fact that epidural hematomas stop at cranial sutures, where the dura is firmly adherent to the inner table of the skull, whereas subdural hematomas may cross the suture lines. If unen-

Fig. 1.**10** **Differentiation between subdural and epidural hematoma. a** Subdural hematoma appears as a hyperdense mass distributed along the inner table of the skull. It typically has a concave medial border and extends across cranial sutures. This hematoma overlies the left frontotemporal convexity and crosses the coronal suture. **b** Schematic drawing of epidural hematoma that appears as a more localized, biconvex hyperdense mass. The dura itself is not depicted.

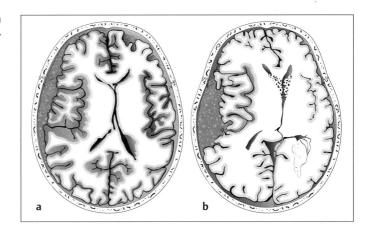

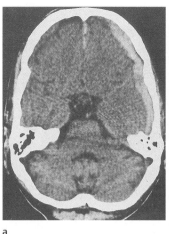 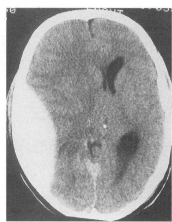

Fig. 1.**11 Differentiation of subdural and epidural hematoma** (see Fig. 1.**10**). **a** Left frontotemporal hematoma crossing the coronal suture. **b** A significant mass effect (midline shift) is often present. **c** What is your diagnosis based on the information in this newspaper article (from the Sydney *Daily Telegraph* of 14 July 1998, p. 2)?

a   b

Doctor Knows the Right Drill
By Chris Hamilton

A BRITISH doctor has been hailed as a hero after saving a man's life in the Australian outback by performing brain surgery with a rusty drill found in a school tool shed.

Steve Hindley, 42, was on just the second day of his job as the only doctor in Ravensthorpe, in the south of Western Australia, when Australian Rules footballer Hayden McGlinn was brought in to the tiny hospital. The 23-year-old had collapsed after hitting his head in a collision with another player.

As his condition worsened Dr Hindley realised he had to act quickly to relieve pressure on the brain from a blood clot. With no facilities to perform the intricate neurosurgery he had to improvise with a manual brace-and-bit drill normally used for woodwork.

After a frantic search the player's team mates and friends managed to find a drill in the school shed and after sterilising it and consulting with neuro-surgeons at Perth's Sir Charles Gairdner Hospital, Dr Hindley carried out the delicate operation.

Mr McGlinn is now in a stable condition at the Perth hospital where spokeswoman Priscilla Fouracres said he owed his life to the British doctor.

c

hanced CT cannot confirm or exclude a subdural hematoma, scanning should be repeated after intravenous contrast administration. This will increase the density difference between the brain parenchyma and hematoma, because the brain tissue enhances after contrast administration (especially the superficial pial vessels) while the hematoma does not. The most important indirect signs are subtle, because an epidural collection sufficient to cause a midline shift of 2 cm or more should be plainly visible on the scan. The "rabbit ear sign" has been described for frontal subdural hematomas: while the frontal horns of the lateral ventricles normally point forward, the mass effect from a unilateral subdural hematoma can displace the tip of one frontal horn posteriorly, creating a "rabbit ear" pattern. However, some authors refer to this sign in cases of bilateral straightening of the frontal horn, usually secondary to bilateral chronic subdural hematoma.

The *sulci* on the cerebral surface are evaluated not just in themselves but also as a potential indicator of intracerebral masses (Fig. 1.**12**).

An acute infarction of the middle cerebral artery (MCA), even when complete, may be manifested only by effacement of the cortical sulci in the corresponding territory on one side (Fig. 1.**12 b**). Analysis of the CT scan should include evaluating the width of all the sulci, and therefore the entire brain surface should be surveyed in all planes. Widening of individual

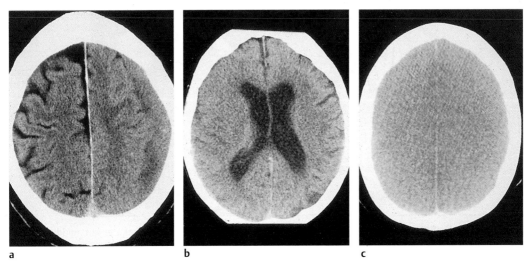

a   b   c

Fig. 1.**12** **Effacement of cortical sulci as evidence of a cerebral mass.** Subdural hematomas may be approximately isodense to the adjacent brain, especially when several weeks old. The left superior parietal hematoma in **a** is isodense, and is manifested chiefly by the effacement of cortical sulci, which are well defined on the right side. The left-sided subdural effusion shows a heterogeneous density, probably due to loculation. **a** Chronic left subdural hematoma. **b** Acute infarction of the right middle cerebral artery. **c** Bilateral brain edema.

sulci may result from an old infarct or from a small aneurysm that has led to local cortical atrophy due to microhemorrhages. The widths of the extra-axial CSF spaces over different portions of the brain should be compared with one another and with the width of the ventricles. Normal width of the extra-axial CSF spaces accompanied by ventricular enlargement may indicate a rare case of normal-pressure hydrocephalus and distinguish it from other causes of brain atrophy, which may be associated with widening of the sylvian fissures.

A CT hallmark of subarachnoid hemorrhage is hyperdense sulci (Fig. 1.**13**). These "white" sulci contrast with the majority of the cortical sulci, which are hypodense to the adjacent brain parenchyma and appear dark.

Subarachnoid hemorrhage is most commonly found in the region of the basal cisterns, known as the pentagon. Normally the basal cisterns are hypodense to brain, as they are filled with CSF. Subarachnoid hemorrhage reverses this pattern, and the pentagon becomes hyperdense (Fig. 1.**14**).

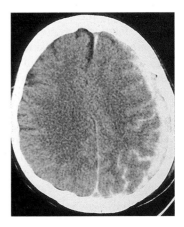

Fig. 1.**13** **Subarachnoid hemorrhage in the extra-axial cerebrospinal fluid spaces.** Individual sulci show a reversal from hypodensity to hyperdensity as a result of the subarachnoid hemorrhage.

Like intraparenchymal hemorrhage, a subarachnoid hemorrhage—especially if caused by a ruptured aneurysm—can rupture into the ventricular system and spread as far as the

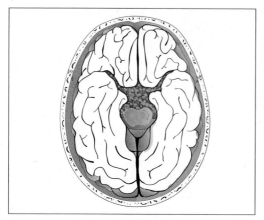

a

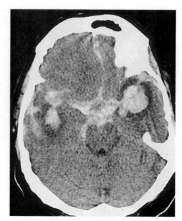

b

Fig. 1.**14 a, b   Density reversal in the pentagon caused by subarachnoid hemorrhage.** In this illustrative case of subarachnoid hemorrhage, the pentagon and frontal interhemispheric fissure appear hyperdense. The rounded hyperdense structure located approxi- mately at the bifurcation of the left middle cerebral artery is an aneurysm. Perifocal edema is apparent. Blood is also visible over the right hemisphere in this very extensive hemorrhage.

fourth ventricle. This commonly results in hydrocephalus with pressure cones. The basal cisterns are a frequent site of occurrence of subarachnoid hemorrhage from a bleeding aneurysm in the circle of Willis. The topographic relationships are shown in Fig. 1.**15**.

Care should be taken not to overlook thrombosis in acute examinations of the dural sinuses. Because the dense triangle sign is usually the only suggestive sign of dural sinus thrombosis on noncontrast CT scans, the lesion is likely to be missed unless the radiologist considers the diagnosis beforehand and actively looks for the lesion on contrast-enhanced scans. Plain scans may, however, show changes caused by occasional venous infarction. Intralesional hemorrhages and infarcts show a roughly symmetrical arrangement on both sides of the midline (Fig. 1.**16**).

The hallmark of dural sinus thrombosis on contrast-enhanced scans is the "empty triangle sign" or "delta sign," a triangular nonenhancing area caused by intraluminal thrombus and found most often in the superior sagittal sinus (Fig. 1.**17**).

Collateral venous pathways ("cord sign") may also be visible in the superior parietal region after contrast administration. These veins are located on the cerebral surface. The CT diagnosis is made difficult by frequent congenital anomalies in the size and location of the dural sinuses. On the whole, unenhanced T2-weighted magnetic resonance (MR) images are the most reliable non-invasive method for detecting dural sinus thrombus.

The *gyri* themselves may show evidence of hemorrhage (Fig. 1.**18**). Cortical infarcts are a possible cause, but herpes encephalitis can produce similar changes in the medial temporal lobe and should always be considered in the evaluation of inflammatory brain disease. In typical cases, the changes occupy a temporomesial location near the sylvian fissure (Fig. 1.**19**).

More or less pronounced changes may be found on noncontrast scans, but peripheral enhancement is seen after intravenous contrast administration. In all cases in which a diagnosis of herpes encephalitis is being considered, contrast-enhanced MR images should be obtained if the CT scans are negative.

Changes in the cerebral *white matter* may be hyperdense or hypodense (Table 1.**2**).

A classic hypertensive intracerebral hemorrhage (Fig. 1.**20**) appears as a hyperdense area in the basal ganglia region with a rounded,

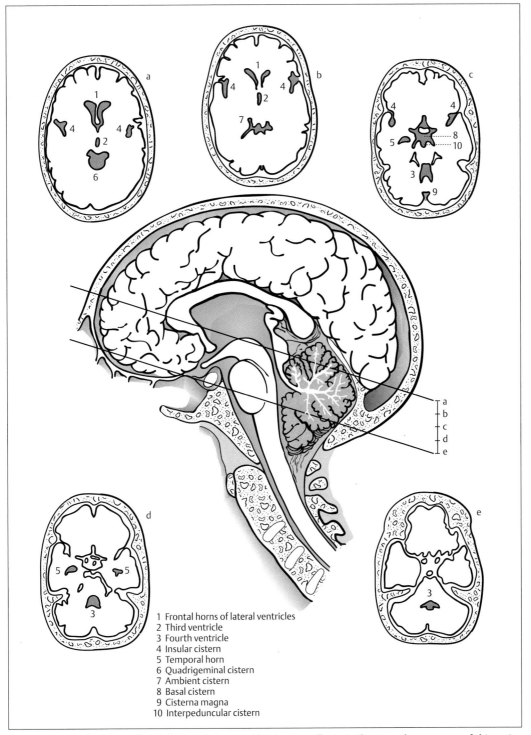

1 Frontal horns of lateral ventricles
2 Third ventricle
3 Fourth ventricle
4 Insular cistern
5 Temporal horn
6 Quadrigeminal cistern
7 Ambient cistern
8 Basal cistern
9 Cisterna magna
10 Interpeduncular cistern

Fig. 1.**15** **Normal topography of the basal cisterns.** The drawings illustrate the normal appearance of this region on axial CT slices, the location of which is shown on the sagittal diagram.

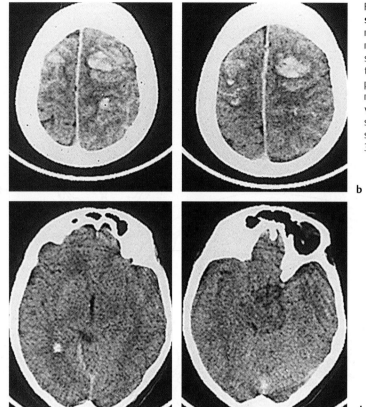

Fig. 1.**16** **Dural sinus thrombosis.** This diagnosis is frequently missed on CT scans. In pronounced cases, even noncontrast scans will demonstrate the infarction as roughly symmetrical hyperdensities on both sides of the midline. Additional signs (cortical venous stasis on postcontrast scans, filling defect within the sinus) are shown in Figs. 3.**49**–3.**53**.

a

b

c

d

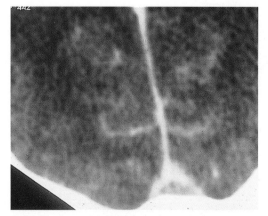

Fig. 1.**17** **Empty triangle sign.** The scan after contrast administration shows a triangular nonenhancing area within the sinus. This sign is visible only if adequate window settings are used (W: 350–400, C: 50).

oval, or occasionally whorled configuration. It has smooth margins, and may be surrounded by hypodense edema. Rupture of the hemorrhage into the ventricular system is not uncommon, in which case blood is found in the lateral ventricles and sometimes in the subarachnoid space.

Intracerebral hemorrhages can have atypical sites of occurrence such as the high parietal region, but may be present in all parts of the brain. These atypical hemorrhages may result from:

- Bleeding in tumors
- Bleeding from arteriovenous malformations
- Vasculopathies

Whenever an atypical intracerebral hemorrhage is found, contrast-enhanced scans

Fig. 1.**18 Cardiogenic emboli.** Cardiogenic emboli resulting from atrial fibrillation have produced a typical cortical hemorrhage, manifested by cortical enhancement. **a** Cortical hemorrhage (noncontrast CT). **b** Cortical enhancement (postcontrast CT).

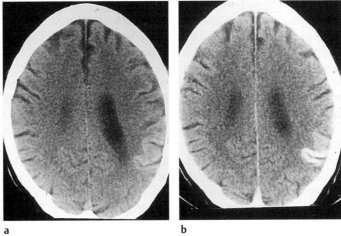

a   b

Fig. 1.**19 a, b Herpes encephalitis.** This disease typically starts in the mesial part of the temporal lobes and may present with gyral enhancement or bleeding within gyri. Frequently, however, the CT findings are somewhat nonspecific, as in the case shown, and magnetic resonance imaging is needed to detect morphologic changes. Unexplained impairment of consciousness combined with a temporal lesion on CT should always raise suspicion of herpes encephalitis.

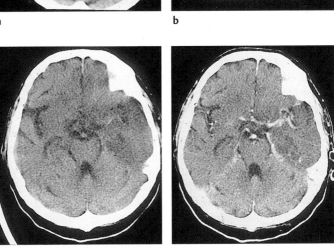

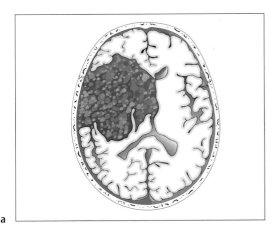

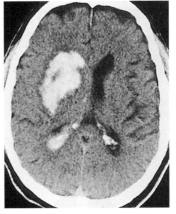

a   b

Fig. 1.**20 a, b Hypertensive hemorrhage.** Hypertensive intracerebral hemorrhage is distinguished from other types of hemorrhage by its sites of predilection (basal ganglia, thalamus, or pons) and by a history of hypertension. The illustration shows an extensive hemorrhage causing ventricular compression on the right side. The hemorrhage has ruptured into the ventricular system, producing a small crescent-shaped collection in the right occipital horn.

should be obtained. If the postcontrast examination shows no evidence of a tumor (enhancement past the boundaries of the hemorrhage) or an arteriovenous malformation (enhancing mass of tangled vessels, except with cavernoma), it will be necessary to proceed with additional studies—usually magnetic resonance imaging (MRI) and angiography. It should be noted that even in the subacute stage of a hemorrhage, postcontrast CT may show a somewhat ill-defined ring of enhancement surrounding the actual hemorrhage at a distance of several millimeters.

White-matter edema (Fig. 1.21) accompanies most pathologic processes that involve the white matter. It is most pronounced in cerebral metastases. Because the gray matter is much less susceptible to edema than the white matter, the edema tends to form a digitate pattern. Occasionally, the low-density edematous area may contain a somewhat less hypodense lesion that becomes more distinct after contrast administration. Postcontrast scans should be obtained whenever white-matter edema is diagnosed. Differentiation from an enhancing brain tumor is generally unnecessary in acute examinations. The difficult question of whether a lesion is a low-grade glioma or an infarct can be resolved by repeating the scan on the following

day and, if necessary, by obtaining MR images. Even then, it is often essential to perform stereotactic biopsy and establish a histologic diagnosis.

The most frequent diagnosis in acute cerebral CT examinations is cerebral infarction. If CT findings are normal, the study is still helpful for excluding intracranial hemorrhage.

What positive findings are encountered in stroke patients?

The early signs of brain infarction that are demonstrable by MRI (vascular and meningeal enhancement) are usually not visible on CT scans. The early CT signs of infarction are as follows:

- Loss of definition of the basal ganglia and loss of the gray matter–white matter interface at the insula (Fig. 1.**22**).
- Hyperdense vascular segments (thrombotic occlusion), often involving the MCA (Fig. 1.**23**).
- Effacement of sulci, with or without hypodensity of the adjacent brain tissue.

Given the differences in diagnostic approach, it is important to distinguish between the following types of infarction during the initial evaluation:

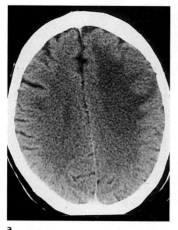 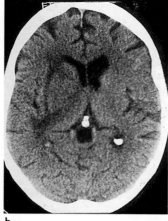

a   b

Fig. 1.**21** **CT appearance of white-matter edema.** Edema leads to decreased density of the white matter, and the affected area appears hypodense. **a** On superior scans, white-matter edema tends to form a subcortical digitate pattern as it tracks along white-matter pathways. **b** When the basal ganglia region is involved, the hypodensity conforms to the more edema-prone areas that contain exclusively white matter. In the case shown, the low-density edema demarcates the internal and external capsule on the right side.

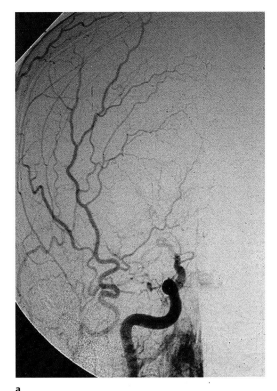

a

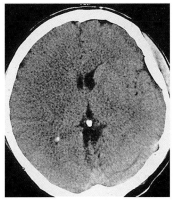

b

Fig. 1.**22** **Early signs of cerebral infarction. a** The contrast angiogram demonstrates occlusion of the internal carotid artery. Only branches of the external carotid artery and the stump of the internal carotid artery are visualized. **b** Comparison of the sides in the CT scan shows hypodensity of the lentiform nucleus, effacement of the insular cistern, and right hemispheric swelling (not an early sign).

- Thromboembolic territorial infarctions
- Hemodynamic infarctions: watershed and end-zone infarcts (Fig. 1.**24**)

Doppler ultrasonography of the cervical vessels and cerebral angiography are the best examinations in patients with hemodynamic infarctions.

The hallmark of cerebral infarction on CT scans is a hypodense area, which can range in size from a punctate lacunar infarct (Fig. 1.**25**) to a more extensive territorial infarct (Fig. 1.**26**).

In differentiating an infarct from other hypodense lesions, it is essential to know the territories of the intracranial arteries, at least for the interpretation of unenhanced scans. Besides the thromboembolic infarctions pictured above, which lead to the destruction of a vascu-

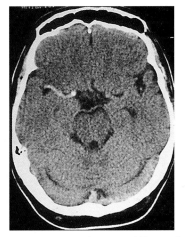

Fig. 1.**23** **Hyperdense middle cerebral artery sign.** Increased CT density of the middle cerebral artery is a characteristic feature of embolic territorial infarction.

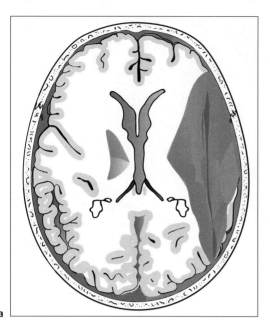

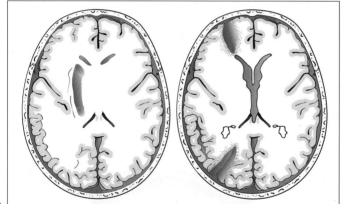

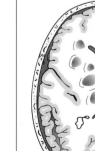

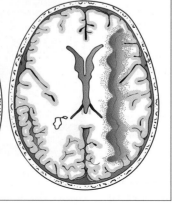

Fig. 1.**24** **Typical distribution patterns of hypodensities after stroke.**
a Thromboembolic territorial infarction.
b Hemodynamic (watershed or end-zone) infarction.
c Cerebral microangiopathy.

a

b

c

Fig. 1.**25** **Lacunar infarction.** Lacunar infarcts involv- ▷
ing the lenticulostriate branches appear as rounded hypodensities at the supraventricular level on the right
side.

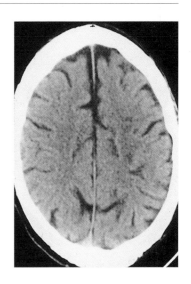

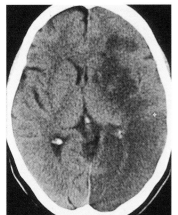

Fig. 1.**26** **Thromboembolic infarction.** The extensive hypodensity on the left side is a large territorial infarct involving the posterior
cerebral artery territory and part of
the middle cerebral artery territory
on the right side.

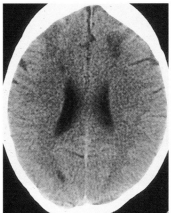

Fig. 1.**27** **Hemodynamic infarction.** Anterior watershed infarctions, like infarctions of the anterior cerebral artery, are less common than in other territories. This
scan demonstrates bilateral anterior watershed infarctions.

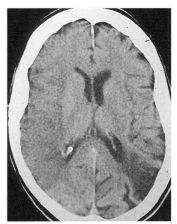

Fig. 1.**28** **Hemodynamic infarction.** An old posterior watershed
infarction appears as a wedge-
shaped hypodensity at the boundary of the middle cerebral artery
and posterior cerebral artery territories.

lar territory, it is important to be able to recognize smaller infarcts occurring in watershed
areas (Figs. 1.**27**, 1.**28**).

Contrast administration aids in the diagnosis of cerebral infarction in the following ways:

- A considerable percentage of infarctions remain isodense to uninfarcted brain tissue
throughout the acute and subacute stages.
- Gyral enhancement (Figs. 1.**29**, 1.**30**) is a useful aid for differential diagnosis.

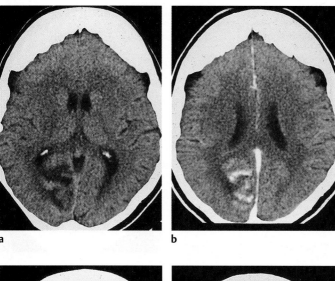

Fig. 1.**29 Posterior infarct in the luxury perfusion stage. a** The hypodense changes involve the territory of the posterior cerebral artery. There is a mass effect involving minimal displacement of the posterior falx toward the left side. The right occipital horn is slightly elevated. **b** The postcontrast scan shows moderate enhancement in the infarcted area.

a b

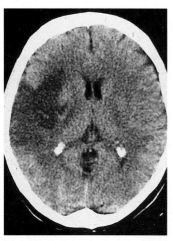 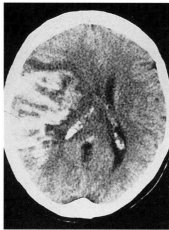

Fig. 1.**30 a, b   Gyral enhancement.** Gyral enhancement is observed in the luxury perfusion stage of cerebral infarction. It generally occurs between the third day and third week after stroke.

a b

It should be noted that gyral enhancement, which follows the tortuous course of the thin cerebral cortex, is seen only in the cerebral hemispheres. At the infratentorial level, contrast enhancement as well as the noncontrast hypodensity or hemorrhage-related hyperdensity associated with infarctions conform to the "arbor vitae" pattern of the cerebellum. This appears morphologically as a figure composed of short, concentric circular segments (Fig. 1.**31**).

Brain-stem infarcts can be detected on CT scans (Fig. 1.**32**), but small infarcts will be missed if faulty examination technique is used.

The detection of these infarcts on CT requires the use of thin slices (2 mm), intravenous contrast administration, and a gantry angulation that prevents beam-hardening artifacts from the adjacent petrous pyramids (temporal lobe projection).

The intracerebral *ventricular system* is evaluated for its size and shape. Pressure cones

Fig. 1.**31** **Infratentorial infarction.** A patchy infratentorial hypodense area in the left hemisphere is characteristic of cerebellar infarction. Hemorrhagic deposits are present in the contralateral hemisphere.

Fig. 1.**32** **Infratentorial infarction.** This scan illustrates an extensive brain-stem infarction. The brain stem appears generally hypodense, and it shows moderate expansion.

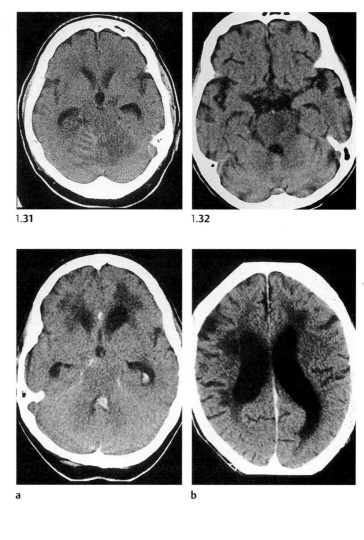

1.**31**   1.**32**

a   b

Fig. 1.**33** **Periventricular lucencies.** Unlike pressure cones, which signify increased intraventricular pressure (**a**), periventricular lucencies are of vascular origin (**b**) and show a strictly symmetrical arrangement. In **a**, the hyperdensity in the fourth ventricle is intraventricular blood. Impairment of cerebrospinal fluid (CSF) circulation leads to enlargement of the supratentorial CSF spaces, in this case involving both frontal horns and both temporal horns. The left temporal horn shows greater enlargement and contains a small hemorrhage. The perimesencephalic CSF spaces are also filled with blood. The scan in **b** shows conspicuous atherosclerotic lucencies along both frontal horns, predominantly on the left side. Note the ventriculomegaly and cortical narrowing in the right frontoparietal region.

(Fig. 1.**33a**) are hypodense areas that abut the frontal and occipital horns. They may signify an obstructive hydrocephalus and require differentiation from the periventricular lucencies that occur in chronic vascular insufficiency (leukoaraiosis). The elevated pressure in the ventricular system causes CSF to enter the interstitium of the surrounding brain parenchyma. Pressure cones are seen much less frequently on CT scans than on MR images, however. The differential diagnosis should always include vasogenic white-matter changes (periventricular lucencies, Fig. 1.**33b**), which are commonly observed in hydrocephalus ex vacuo.

As noted for the extra-axial CSF spaces, a proportional size ratio should exist between the intra-axial and extra-axial CSF spaces. Fresh blood in the ventricles forms fluid levels in the occipital horns, which will be missed unless looked for. Blood may also be found in the fourth ventricle. Calcifications of the choroid

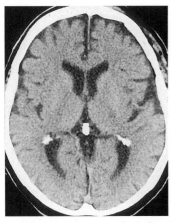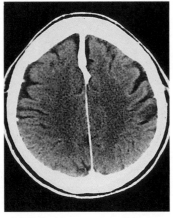

a   b

Fig. 1.**34** **Expansions and calcifications.** Calcifications of the choroid plexus and pineal body (**a**) are extremely common findings. **a** Moderate to marked enlargement of the intra-axial cerebrospinal fluid (CSF) spaces, moderate expansion of the extra-axial CSF spaces, and typical calcifications in the occipital horns and pineal body are seen here. Calcification or ossification of the falx needs to be differentiated from subdural hematomas of the interhemispheric fissure. **b** This postcontrast CT scan shows very pronounced ossification of the falx in the frontal interhemispheric fissure. This can be distinguished from interhemispheric hematoma by densitometry, since hemorrhage usually has a density of approximately 150 Hounsfield units (HU), while calcification or ossification far exceeds 1000 HU. In these cases, magnetic resonance imaging often demonstrates a central fat intensity (fatty marrow within the bone).

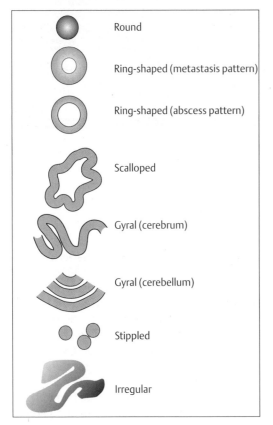

plexus and pineal body (Fig. 1.**34 a**) should not be mistaken for pathology. Both types of calcification (Fig. 1.**34 b**) are very common CT findings, as are calcifications of the falx. It should be noted that calcifications of the falx may contain fat marrow, which can produce high central signal intensity on T1-weighted MR images (Fig. 1.**35**).

Fig. 1.**35** **Terminology for patterns of contrast enhancement.**

Technical Aspects

Even in emergency CT of the head, it is crucial to follow a standard examination technique. This should include the acquisition of a lateral scout view. After the slices have been positioned parallel to the orbitomeatal reference line, the desired degree of gantry angulation is determined. The temporal lobe projection is recommended for presumed brain-stem or cerebellar lesions. After the gantry angle has been set, scan acquisition is begun. The slice thickness should be 8 or 10 mm for supratentorial scans and 4 or 5 mm for infratentorial scans.

It is crucial to review the result of the examination before the patient leaves the table.

The following are typical situations that require additional scans:

- Digitate pattern of white-matter hypodensity that may conceal a mass lesion.
- Motion artifacts in individual scans that require the repetition of selected scans.
- Uncertainties in brain-stem evaluation due to superimposed structures or beam-hardening artifacts.
- Uncertainties in the differentiation of bony structures and hemorrhages in the frontal lobes or above the petrous bones.
- Ventricular enlargement with pressure cones, raising suspicion of an infratentorial mass.

As CT technology has progressed in recent years, CT imaging of the head has undergone many refinements. Specific display modes such as the various types of CT angiography and data acquisition for image-guided therapeutic procedures will require corresponding technical capabilities of the CT scanner. At the same time, one should not underestimate the diagnostic gain that can be achieved by optimizing scan parameters such as gantry angulation, scan delay time after contrast administration, etc.

■ Patient Positioning

The *supine position* is considered standard for CT examinations of the head. The head should be comfortably supported in a padded rest. If contrast administration is proposed, the patient should be informed about potential risks and adverse effects and provide consent before the examination begins. An intravenous line should also be placed before the start of the examination. Although current scan times for head examinations are usually very short, it is still advisable to tell the patient to keep the head stationary during the examination. Any degree of head tilting in the sagittal plane will make image interpretation difficult for less experienced examiners by preventing direct side-to-side comparisons in the image slice.

Deviation from the standard supine position is necessary for the acquisition of direct coronal scans. The *prone position* is recommended in selected cases to avoid dental artifacts and to allow coronal scanning in patients who cannot hyperextend the head while supine. To avoid dental artifacts, it is often advantageous to adjust the head position after obtaining the scout view and then acquire a new scout view. The maximum gantry angulation allowed by the scanner is a consideration in this regard. Modern scanners allow up to 25° of gantry angulation in both directions, and some of the latest scanners allow up to 30°. For completeness, it should be noted that ultrafast electron-beam scanners allow table angulation of up to 25°.

The orbitomeatal line is the standard reference line for the various scan planes through the skull. This line extends from the center of the orbit in the lateral scout view to the external acoustic meatus. Routine cranial CT examinations are performed with + 10° of gantry angulation (i.e., 10° of flexion in relation to the orbitomeatal line). For examinations of the posterior fossa, + 20° is recommended to minimize beam-hardening artifacts from the petrous bones. The opposite applies to orbital imaging, which generally requires – 10° of angulation relative to the reference line. Coronal scans for orbital imaging require + 105°. A similar angle is recommended for imaging the sellar region, and + 105° or + 70° is recommended for middle ear imaging. Imaging at + 70° orients the scanning plane approximately perpendicular to the clivus.

Spiral scanning is generally not employed for routine brain examinations (stroke, trauma, screening, etc.), and simple contiguous slices are obtained. A slice thickness of 8 mm is recommended for supratentorial scans and 4 mm for infratentorial scans. A slice thickness of 2 mm is generally used for imaging the orbits and petrous temporal bone. A 1-mm slice thickness is advantageous for para-axial reconstructions, for imaging the inner ear, and for three-dimensional reconstructions. A 2-mm slice thickness is desired for survey bone-window imaging to detect fractures, for example, or to evaluate bony lesions.

There are no standard values that can be recommended for the window and center settings (Fig. 1.**36**). The settings should be adjusted so that visible contrast is obtained between the white matter and cortical gray matter in the monitor image. Incorrect kernel selection is a common error, and care should be taken to select algorithms with kernels that are appropriate for the situation. Head examinations in children require the use of special kernels to achieve acceptable contrast. Surveys at various imaging centers have shown that most operators use a kilovoltage setting in the range of 120–140 kV and a power setting between 140 and 450 mAs.

■ Techniques for Reducing Artifacts

Artifact reduction is important for imaging brain areas that are located near bone. The following areas are commonly obscured by artifacts:

- Middle fossa (the temporal lobes)
- Cerebellum in the posterior fossa

The temporal lobe projection (Figs. 1.**37**, 1.**38**) has proved effective for CT visualization of the temporal lobe. Instead of the standard + 10° of gantry angulation relative to the orbitomeatal line, the temporal lobe projection is angled approximately + 20°. The lateral scout view can be used to set the appropriate scan angle; in most cases, it is easy to determine the degree of angulation necessary to keep the beams from passing through the petrous temporal bone before traversing the middle fossa. The temporal lobe projection is also of major value for reducing artifacts in the brain-stem region. In particular, it is extremely difficult to detect a brain-stem infarction on standard axial scans with + 10° gantry angulation. Some modern scanners can reduce artifacts by adding two thinner slices to one slice of nominal thickness.

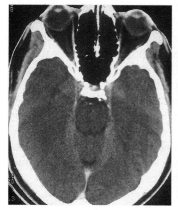 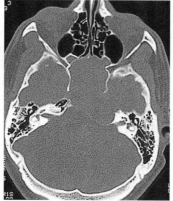

Fig. 1.36 Importance of using the correct window and center settings. a When a soft-tissue window setting is used, the interior of the nasal cavity and sphenoid sinus appear black. Both appear to be air-filled. **b** The bone-window image shows a difference in attenuation between the nasal cavity and the sphenoid sinus. The sphenoid sinus is filled with tumor tissue of fat density (cholesterol granuloma).

a

b

Contrast Administration

CT examination of the head without contrast medium can exclude various types of pathology such as intracranial hemorrhage, infarction (in many cases), and mass lesions.

However, scanning after the intravenous administration of contrast medium can provide a substantial diagnostic gain in many patients.

Aside from the modern techniques of arterial and venous cerebral CT angiography, intravenous contrast medium is administered to

Fig. 1.**37** **Gantry angulation.** Angling the gantry to the temporal lobe projection is advantageous for imaging the brain stem. **a** In a standard projection parallel to the orbitomeatal line, the brain stem is obscured by beam-hardening artifact between the petrous apices. It cannot be completely evaluated. **b** The temporal lobe projection not only gives a nonsuperimposed view of the temporal lobes but also displays the fourth ventricle and brain stem without beam-hardening artifact.

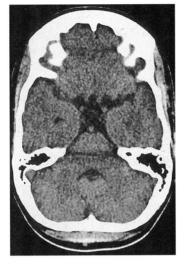 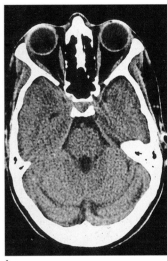

a   b

Fig. 1.**38** **Temporal lobe projection.** The temporal lobe projection is useful for detecting lesions in the posterior fossa. **a** In this example, a left-sided acoustic neuroma is markedly obscured by artifacts in a standard projection parallel to the orbitomeatal line. Expansion of the internal auditory canal is clearly demonstrated, however. **b** The temporal lobe projection gives an unobscured view of the acoustic neuroma, which appears as an enhancing mass within the left internal auditory canal.

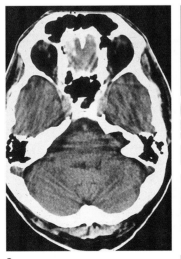 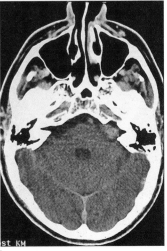

a   b

detect or exclude disruption of the blood–brain barrier. In the absence of cerebral pathology, the parenchyma shows only a minimal density increase after intravenous contrast administration. This enhancement is greater in the cerebral cortex than in the white matter because of the higher cortical perfusion. The blood–brain barrier, which is created by the specialized structure of the capillary walls, prevents contrast medium from entering the interstitium as long as the barrier is intact. Among the various types of capillaries in the human body, the capillaries in the cerebrum possess a single layer of endothelial cells with "tight junctions" and a continuous basement membrane. As a result, intravenous contrast enhancement normally occurs only in the tentorium, dura, choroid plexus, pituitary (Fig. 1.**39**), pineal body, and in the major intracranial vessels.

These structures enhance because they do not possess a blood–brain barrier. Enhancement of brain parenchyma at the supratentorial and infratentorial levels can occur only if the blood–brain barrier has become disrupted. This breakdown can result from cytotoxic or interstitial brain edema, leading to enhancement of the brain parenchyma at varying time intervals after contrast administration. The

pattern of this enhancement (e.g., gyral pattern in cerebral infarction, ring pattern with metastases, scalloped pattern with glioblastoma) provides a useful criterion for differential diagnosis. Consequently, a defect in the blood–brain barrier demonstrated by contrast extravasation or enhancement is considered important evidence for the presence of a brain lesion.

Today, it is standard practice to use nonionic contrast media, and a moderate concentration is adequate with modern CT scanners. If an old scanner is being used, it may be possible to compensate for the reduced contrast to some extent by using a higher concentration (370 versus the usual 300 mg/mL). Regardless of the examination technique used (contiguous slices or spiral scanning), a common error when acquiring cerebral CT scans is to initiate scanning too soon after contrast administration. If very intense vascular enhancement is observed in the circle of Willis, it is likely that scanning was initiated with an inadequate postinjection delay. The timing of maximal enhancement will vary depending on the degree of disruption in the blood–brain barrier. Extreme examples are diseases such as disseminated encephalomyelitis and toxoplasmosis, in

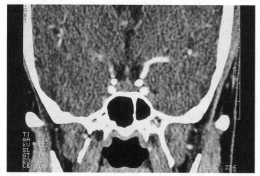
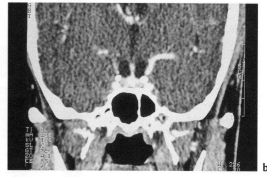

Fig. 1.39 Importance of enhancement dynamics for visualizing the pituitary and cavernous sinus.

a The coronal scan through the sella in the early dynamic phase already shows bilateral opacification of the carotid arteries. The pituitary stalk shows only minimal enhancement, and the body of the pituitary is not yet enhanced.

b The scan in a later phase shows intense enhancement of the pituitary body and stalk.
Because pituitary adenomas enhance later than the normal pituitary, they are more easily detected on scans acquired shortly after the start of contrast administration.

which enhancement cannot be adequately evaluated until two hours after the administration of a double dose. This technique, known as double dose delay (DDD), has become less important since the advent of MRI, with its higher contrast resolution.

■ Spiral CT

For both noncontrast and standard contrast-enhanced examinations of the brain, spiral CT offers the advantage of a reduction in scanning time. Spiral CT is most useful, however, for obtaining largely artifact-free data sets for three-dimensional reconstructions, CT-guided therapeutic procedures, and contrast-enhanced vascular imaging. Both the arterial and venous sides of the cerebral circulation can be imaged with spiral CT. A total dose of approximately 80 mL of radiographic contrast medium administered at a rate of 3 mL/s is recommended for both arterial and venous studies. Following contrast administration, a scan delay time of 25 s should be allowed for arterial imaging and 40 s for venous imaging. Many authors recommend a pitch of 2 for cerebrovascular imaging, in which case a 1-mm collimation is combined with a table feed of 2 mm/s. Depending on the scan length (i.e., the cranial and caudal extent of the spiral acquisition), scanning should proceed caudad from the vertex for imaging venous structures. A pitch of 1 may be used for arterial studies. The scan should start 1 cm below the sellar floor and proceed toward the vertex to image the circle of Willis. Both studies can be performed with or without a standard 10° gantry angle. A contrast concentration of 300 mg/mL may also be used for vascular imaging. In all cases, a power injector should be used for contrast administration.

■ Window Settings

In addition to the standard soft-tissue window, generous use should be made of the bone window setting for image documentation. The bone window not only permits better evaluation of the cranial bones but also facilitates the detection of intracranial air. It has major value in the diagnosis of skull fractures and dural injuries, and very fine calcifications of the brain parenchyma can often be evaluated more accurately with a bone window setting.

■ Three-Dimensional Imaging and Multiplanar Reconstructions

The quality of three-dimensional reconstructions and multiplanar reformatted images (sagittal and coronal views) is significantly improved by the use of a small slice thickness. Whenever the desired imaging volume, patient cooperativeness, and available CT scanner permit it, a slice thickness of 1 mm should be used. Larger volumes may require two or more spiral acquisitions.

■ CT Data Sets for Image-Guided Interventions

The acquisition of data sets for image-guided interventions (e.g., using neurosurgical navigation devices) is becoming increasingly important. Deviation from standard protocols is a major source of error in image-guided surgery. For example, care must be taken to conduct CT scanning with 0° of gantry angulation. There must be no shifting of individual slices within a scanning sequence (scanner commands such as "review center"). Additionally, all scan parameters must remain absolutely constant within the data set, which often consists of more than 100 slices.

■ References

Recommended for further study

Huckman MS, Russel EJ. Selecting the optimal plane for CT examination of the base of the skull. AJNR Am J Neuroradiol 1984; 5: 333–4.
● *Very brief, practical outline.*
Kleihues P, Burger PC, Scheithauer BW. Histological typing of tumors of the central nervous system. Berlin: Springer, 1993. (World Health Organization: International histological classification of tumors, 8).
● *Includes basic principles of CT diagnosis of brain tumors.*
Levy RA, Edwards WT, Meyer JR, Rosenbaum AE. Facial trauma and 3 D–reconstructive imaging: insufficiencies and correctives. AJNR Am J Neuroradiol 1992; 13: 885–92.

- *See also Zinreich SJ. 3-D reconstruction for evaluation of facial trauma [comment]. AJNR Am J Neuroradiol 1992; 13: 893–5.*
McGuckin JF, Akhtar N, Ho VT, et al. CT and MR evaluation of a wooden foreign body in an in vitro model of the orbit. AJNR Am J Neuroradiol 1996; 17: 129–33.
- *Deals with the practical difficulties of detecting wooden foreign bodies.*
Osborn AG. Diagnosis of descending transtentorial herniation by cranial computed tomography. Radiology 1977; 123: 93–6.
Osborn AG. The medial tentorium and incisure: normal and pathological anatomy. Neuroradiology 1977; 13: 109–13.
- *Both articles by Osborn use anatomic drawings and selected cases to explain the mechanism and CT features of intracranial herniation.*
Rothfus WE, Deeb ZL, Daffner R H, Prostko ER. Head-hanging CT: an alternative method for evaluating CSF rhinorrhea. AJNR Am J Neuroradiol 8 (1987) 155–156
- *Presents a simple alternative to contrast cisternography.*

Recent and basic works

Casey SO, Alberico RA, Patel M, et al. Cerebral CT venography. Radiology 1996; 198: 163–70.
Ebert DS, Heath DG, Kuszyk BS, et al. Evaluating the potential and problems of three-dimensional computed tomography measurements of arterial stenosis. J Digit Imaging 1998; 11: 151–7.
Fishman EK. High-resolution three-dimensional imaging from subsecond helical CT data sets: applications in vascular imaging. AJR Am J Roentgenol 1997; 169: 441–3.
Görzer H, Heimberger K, Schindler E. Spiral CT angiography with digital subtraction of extra- and intracranial vessels. J Comput Assist Tomogr 1994; 18: 839–41.
Johnson DW, Stringer WA, Marks MP, Yonas H, Good WF, Gur D. Stable xenon CT cerebral blood flow imaging: rationale for and role in clinical decision making. AJNR Am J Neuroradiol 1991; 12: 201–13.
- *Reviews physiologic and technical basis for clinical application of xenon CT-derived quantitative cerebral blood flow information.*
Johnson PT, Heath DG, Bliss DF, Cabral B, Fishman EK. Three-dimensional CT: real-time interactive volume rendering. AJR Am J Roentgenol 1996; 167: 581–3.
Johnson PT, Fishman EK, Duckwall JR, Calhoun PS, Heath DG. Interactive three-dimensional volume rendering of spiral CT data: current applications in the thorax. Radiographics 1998; 18: 165–87.
Kingsley DPE, Dale G, Wallis A. A simple technique for head repositioning in CT scanning. Neuroradiology 1991; 33: 243–6.
- *Simple and accurate method of repositioning the head not requiring conventional stereotactic fixation.*
Kishore PRS, Lipper MH, Becker DP. Significance of CT in head injury: correlation with intracranial pressure. AJNR Am J Neuroradiol 1981; 2: 307–11.
- *Deals with the important relationship between necessary ICP monitoring and CT findings.*
Knauth M, von Kummer R, Jansen O, Hähnel S, Dörfler A, Sartor K. Potential of CT angiography in acute ischemic stroke. AJNR Am J Neuroradiol 1997; 18: 1001–10.

Kuchiwaki H, Inao S, Furuse M, Hirai N, Misu N. Computerized tomography in the assessment of brain shifts in acute subdural hematoma. Zentralbl Neurochir 1995; 56: 5–11.
Kuszyk BS, Fishman EK. Technical aspects of CT angiography. Semin Ultrasound CT MR 1998; 19: 383–93.
Kuszyk BS, Ney DR, Fishman EK. The current state of the art in three-dimensional oncologic imaging: an overview. Int J Radiat Oncol Biol Phys 1995; 33: 1029–39.
Kuszyk BS, Heath DG, Bliss DF, Fishman EK. Skeletal 3-D CT: advantages of volume rendering over surface rendering. Skeletal Radiol 1996; 25: 207–14.
Kuszyk BS, Beauchamp NJ Jr, Fishman EK. Neurovascular applications of CT angiography. Semin Ultrasound CT MR 1998; 19: 394–404.
Latchaw RE. Neuroradiology research: the opportunities and the challenges. Radiology 1998; 209: 3–7.
Leeds NE, Kieffer SA. Evolution of diagnostic neuroradiology from 1904 to 1999. Radiology 2000; 217: 309–18.
- *Historical overview of almost 100 years of technical improvements in the last century.*
Lev MH, Farkas J, Gemmete JJ, et al. Acute stroke: improved nonenhanced CT detection—benefits of softcopy interpretation by using variable window width and center level settings. Radiology 1999; 213: 150–5.
- *This paper emphasizes the advantages of variations in window settings for the diagnosis of stroke.*
Mukherji SK. Head and neck imaging: the next 10 years. Radiology 1998; 209: 8–14.
Noguchi K, Ogawa T, Inugami A, Toyoshima H, Okudera T, Uemura K. MR of acute subarachnoid hemorrhage: a preliminary report of fluid-attenuated inversion-recovery pulse sequences. AJNR Am J Neuroradiol 1994; 15: 1940–3.
- *Includes information on the inherent drawbacks of MRI in the detection of fresh blood.*
Peeples TR, Vieco PT. Intracranial developmental venous anomalies: diagnosis using CT angiography. J Comput Assist Tomogr 1997; 21: 582–6.
Puskás Z, Schuierer G. [Determination of blood circulation time for optimizing contrast medium administration in CT angiography; in German]. Radiologe 1996; 36: 750–7.
- *Well-organized review of basic principles.*
Sanjay S, Raju S, Levine LA, Barmson RT, Jordan PF, Thrall JH. Technical cost of CT examinations. Radiology 2001; 218: 172–5.
- *Detailed cost analysis based on more than 45.000 CT examinations*
Shrier DA, Tanaka H, Numaguchi Y, et al. CT angiography in the evaluation of acute stroke. AJNR Am J Neuroradiol 1997; 18: 1011–20.
Sighvatsson V, Ericson K, Tomasson H. Optimizing contrast-enhanced cranial CT for the detection of brain metastases. Acta Radiol 1998; 39: 718–22.
- *CT as an alternative to MRI.*
Smith PA, Heath DG, Fishman EK. Virtual angioscopy using spiral CT and real-time interactive volume rendering techniques. J Comput Assist Tomogr 1998; 22: 212–4.
Vieco PT, Morin EE, Gross CE. CT angiography in the examination of patients with aneurysm clips. AJNR Am J Neuroradiol 1996; 17: 455–7.

2 Craniocerebral Trauma

Closed and Open Head Injuries

Closed Head Injuries

A head injury is classified as "closed" if it leaves the dura intact. Unlike gunshot injuries, for example, traumatic head injuries caused by a force acting over a large area (motor vehicle accidents, falls) do not penetrate the dura. Because the dura is firmly adherent to the inner table of the skull, however, it may be lacerated by a skull fracture (Fig. 1.**9 b**).

Open Head Injuries

An open head injury is one in which the dura has been breached (Fig. 1.**13 b**). These injuries are generally caused by a violent force acting on a small area, as in a gunshot injury or an impact from a sharp-pointed object. Open head injuries include *frontobasal fractures* and *temporal bone fractures with cerebrospinal fluid (CSF) leakage*. Immediate surgical treatment is a priority in open head injuries, to reduce the ever-present risk of infection.

Skull Fractures

Frequency: a common computed tomography (CT) finding in patients with head injury.

Suggestive morphologic findings: discontinuity in the bone; diploë not separated from the fracture line by cortical bone; other linear discontinuities.

Procedure: if plain skull films demonstrate a fracture, obtain thin-slice cranial CT scans to exclude intracranial hemorrhage.

Other studies: plain skull films are good for demonstrating calvarial fractures, but it is essential to detect or exclude an intracranial mass lesion.

Checklist for scan interpretation:
▶ Fracture depressed (by more than the width of the calvarium)? Burst fracture (vertex) or bending fracture?
▶ Intracranial displacement of fragments?
▶ Intracranial air signifying dural injury?
▶ Accompanying hemorrhage or contusion?

■ **Pathogenesis**

Skull fractures should not be considered in isolation, but must be viewed in connection with lesions of the brain parenchyma and other intracranial structures (blood vessels, cranial nerves). A skull fracture is commonly associated with cranial nerve lesions, vascular injuries, and dural injuries that create portals for the entry of air and microorganisms and for CSF leakage. At the same time, the inability to visualize a fracture does not exclude extensive cerebral contusions or intracranial hematomas. Generally, it is not the fracture itself that is of primary interest in head injuries (at least not a calvarial fracture) but the space-occupying or disruptive intracranial lesions that may accompany the fracture.

■ Frequency

Frequency data will vary depending on the make-up of the clinical population, but the following general guidelines may be helpful:

- Nearly one-third of head-injured patients do not have a skull fracture, including cases with a fatal outcome.
- When a skull fracture is detected, the likelihood of brain injury is increased 30-fold.

■ Clinical Manifestations

The clinical manifestations of skull fractures are as varied and diverse as the potential sites of occurrence.

- A petrous bone fracture may be manifested by bleeding from the ear or a collection of blood behind the tympanic membrane.
- Frontobasal fractures are often associated with unilateral or bilateral periocular hematomas ("monocle" or "eyeglass" hematomas).
- Fractures of the sphenoid wing may cause blindness due to rupture or infarction of the optic nerve.

- If the fracture involves the sella, avulsion of the pituitary stalk can lead to hormonal deficits.
- Fractures of the cribriform plate often result in anosmia.
- The cranial nerves most commonly involved by basal skull fractures are the trochlear nerve, trigeminal nerve (first and second divisions), facial nerve, and vestibulocochlear nerve.

■ CT Morphology

Fractures are clearly demonstrated by CT when the fracture line is perpendicular to the scanning plane (Fig. 2.1). Fractures that run along the plane of the scan may be missed.

■ Differential Diagnosis

Cranial sutures should not be mistaken for fracture lines. Differentiation is aided by noting that with a suture, the diploë is separated from the gap by cortical bone. In a fracture, however, the diploë borders directly on the fracture gap. Comparison with the opposite side also helps to identify sutures. Vascular channels generally have a visible sclerotic margin.

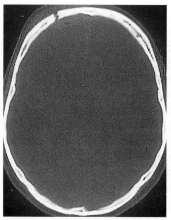 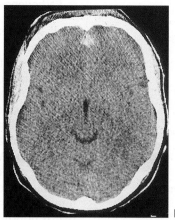

a   b

Fig. 2.**1 Spectrum of CT findings in open head injury.** Many such injuries result from a blow to the face or forehead, creating a coup–contrecoup mechanism with marked occipital lesions and less severe frontal lesions. The scans above show a discontinuity in the right anterior calvarium, consistent with a frontal skull fracture (**a**, bone window). Scanning with a soft-tissue window, just below the scan level in **a**, shows blood in the frontal interhemispheric fissure (**b**), with no other significant signs of injury. Intracranial air bordering the fracture line in panel **a** signifies an open skull fracture.

■ Follow-Up

The main role of CT in follow-up is to check for CSF leakage in patients who have sustained an open head injury. Moreover, follow-up is generally advised in patients with initially mild-appearing parenchymal injuries such as contusions and in patients with small intracranial hemorrhages, particularly if clinical deterioration cannot be inferred from the patient's neurologic status because of intoxication or other causes.

Cerebral Contusion

Frequency: a common CT finding in head-injured patients.

Suggestive morphologic findings: acute hypodense lesions, usually located in the frontal or temporal region. Hyperdense hemorrhage appears after a variable delay.

Procedure: schedule CT follow-ups postoperatively and as dictated by intracranial pressure (herniation, hemorrhage after decompression).

Other studies: magnetic resonance imaging (MRI) is more sensitive than CT in the subacute stage (especially with diffuse axonal injury and other shearing injuries; see below).

Checklist for scan interpretation:
▶ Location and extent of contusions? Hemorrhagic contusions?
▶ Associated injuries (calvarial fracture, basal skull fracture, petrous bone fracture, subdural or epidural hematoma, traumatic subarachnoid hemorrhage)?

■ Pathogenesis

Contusions are caused by acceleration or deceleration trauma to the head (Fig. 2.**2**). The lesions are characterized morphologically by edema of the brain tissue, with a variable hemorrhagic component.

The location of cerebral contusions is governed by the following principles:

● Relative differences in the acceleration and deceleration of the calvarium and brain cause forces to act over a broad area of brain tissue according to the coup–contrecoup principle: the brain tissue is first injured at the site of impact (the calvarium is accelerated toward the underlying brain) and then on the opposite side of the skull (the moving brain strikes the inner surface of the decelerating calvarium). The contrecoup lesions may be more severe than the coup lesions at the site of impact.

Fig. 2.**2 a, b Cerebral contusion.** Contusions appear on CT as patchy hypodensities. A hemorrhagic component may be absent, as in the bifrontal contusions shown here.

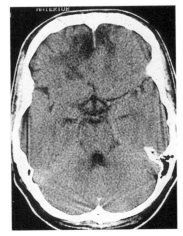
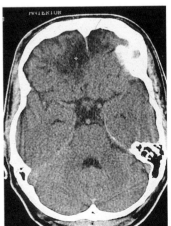

a   b

- Most contusions occur in the frontal or temporal brain (Fig. 2.**3**), presumably partially due to the rough-edged bony structures that occur in those areas. Occipital contusions are less common owing to the smooth inner surface of the occipital calvarium.
- *Shearing injuries* are also common in head-injured patients. They are caused by the shear strain that develops at the gray–white junction due to the different acceleration properties of the gray and white matter. The lesions consist of axonal injuries and the rupture of very small vessels. The corpus callosum and subcortical white matter are most commonly affected. Hemorrhage within contusions can be identified on CT scans. Although MRI can demonstrate increased T2-weighted signal intensity with much greater sensitivity, practical problems have prevented the use of this modality, at least in the early stages.

■ Frequency

Examination of trauma patients is a field for CT, and cerebral contusions are consistently detected in patients with relatively severe head trauma.

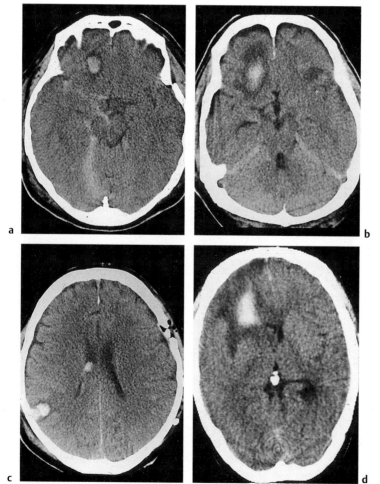

Fig. 2.**3** **Spectrum of CT findings in contusion.** These scans illustrate the typical features of hemorrhagic contusions in different patients. **a** A small hemorrhage rimmed by hypodense edema is visible in the right frontal lobe. There is associated traumatic subarachnoid bleeding in the right basal cisterns. **b** A large hemorrhagic contusion with prominent perifocal edema. **c** Coup and contrecoup lesions. A fracture is evident in the left frontoparietal calvarium, and a hemorrhagic contusion is visible on the opposite side in the area of the right parieto-occipital junction. Intraventricular blood is also present on the right side. **d** The extensive hypodensity almost filling the entire right frontal lobe is a hemorrhagic area at the center of a contusion. A small ring artifact is visible in front of the internal occipital protuberance.

■ Clinical Manifestations

Patients often show decreased vigilance at the time of CT examination. A lucid interval may have been present. Whenever CT scans are positive for cerebral contusion, it should be assumed that the patient has sustained relatively severe head trauma with at least a transitory loss of consciousness.

■ CT Morphology

Contusions appear on CT scans as hypodense areas that are located within the white matter but may also occasionally involve the cortex. As hemorrhage increases, the lesion may show varying degrees of increased density or layering.

■ Differential Diagnosis

Contusional hemorrhage, which may have a delayed onset, is not always distinguishable from hypertensive intracerebral hemorrhage.

The clinical features at the time of CT examination are not helpful for differentiating the pathogenic mechanisms. This is a particular problem if there is uncertainty as to whether trauma was the cause or result of the intracerebral hemorrhage (e.g., rupturing an aneurysm on the steering wheel of an automobile).

■ Evolution of Lesions

With passage of time, cerebral contusions lead to tissue breakdown, with the formation of parenchymal defects of variable size. This occurs even in nonhemorrhagic contusions. In some cases, however, even severe contusions may undergo almost complete resolution without causing significant cavitation.

■ Follow-Up

As noted at the start of this chapter, CT has an important role in the follow-up of contusions, especially since an enlarging contusion with increasing mass effect frequently leads to clinical deterioration.

Epidural Hematoma

Frequency: less common than subdural hematoma, but frequent in cases with extensive skull fractures in patients with head injuries.

Suggestive morphologic findings: hyperdense, biconvex mass usually bordering the calvarium in the temporoparietal area. The adherence of the dura to the cranial sutures prevents the mass from crossing the sutures.

Procedure: immediate surgical decompression.

Other studies: MRI is indicated in very rare cases (subacute epidural hematoma, hematoma near the vertex).

Checklist for scan interpretation:
▶ Report CT findings without delay.
▶ Location (temporal lobe!) and maximum diameter?
▶ Measured degree of midline shift?
▶ Associated injuries (subgaleal hematoma, calvarial fracture)?
▶ Hypodense inclusions signifying active hemorrhage?

■ Pathogenesis

Bleeding into the epidural space usually has an arterial origin, i.e., damage to the middle meningeal artery or one of its branches. A subgaleal hematoma and calvarial fracture are often found at the site of the impact. The classic causal mechanism of epidural hematoma is the rupture of a meningeal arterial branch caused by a calvarial fracture, as these vessels generally are firmly adherent to the bone. Epidural hematoma displaces the dura away from the inner table of the skull.

■ Frequency

Epidural hematomas are not uncommon in patients with head injuries.

■ Clinical Manifestations

The intracranial collection forms quickly after the trauma (with arterial bleeding), distinguishing it from the more insidious development of a subdural hematoma. Unless the epidural hematoma is evacuated without delay, the resulting mass effect can lead to brain herniation and death.

■ CT Morphology

CT demonstrates a hyperdense, biconvex, peripheral mass in direct contact with the calvarium (Fig. 2.**4**) and showing a smooth interface with the cerebral convexity.

The smooth medial border of an epidural hematoma is defined by the underlying dura. The hematoma may still appear isodense shortly after the trauma, but its density increases as clotting progresses and the plasma components are reabsorbed. Because hematomas of arterial origin develop rapidly, different stages of coagulation are not observed, and consequently the hematoma usually presents a homogeneous density. The mass effect from the hematoma almost always causes a shift of midline structures, which may be extensive. The temporoparietal location of most epidural hematomas may cause herniation of the medial temporal lobe, with displacement of the parahippocampal gyrus and uncus into the tentorial incisure.

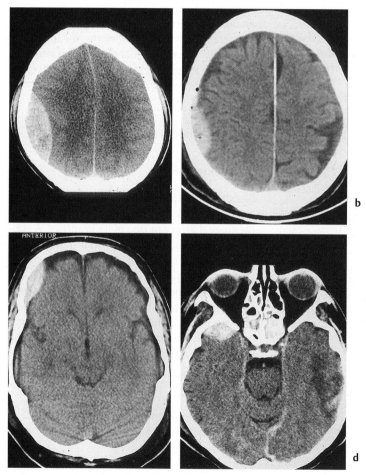

a

b

ANTERIOR

c

d

Fig. 2.**4 Epidural hemorrhage.** Epidural hematoma typically appears as a lentiform collection with a convex medial border. **a** A large parietal epidural hematoma, associated with a definite midline shift. **b** A smaller epidural hematoma. The tiny air bubbles near the hematoma often signify open head trauma with dural injury. **c** An epidural hematoma located anterior to the coronal suture. Unlike subdural hematomas, epidural hematomas do not cross cranial sutures. **d** A small epidural hematoma overlying the right temporal pole. A hematoma at this location is usually visible only in the temporal lobe projection. Contusional changes are visible on the left side.

Fig. 2.**5** **Epidural hemorrhage.**
a Careful interpretation is needed to avoid missing tiny epidural hematomas like these in the right parietal area. **b** A calvarial fracture and large subgaleal hematoma in the bone-window scan mark the location of a very small epidural hematoma.

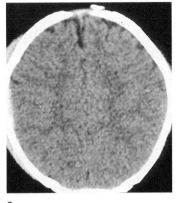

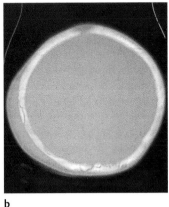

a

b

The fixation of the dura to the inner table of the skull is variable. The dura is firmly adherent to the calvarium in very young patients (Fig. 2.**5**) and in the elderly, and so epidural hematomas are less common in these age groups.

The dura is very firmly attached at the cranial sutures. If the classification of a hematoma is unclear, it is assumed to be subdural if it crosses a suture. With older hematomas, the relationship of the mass to the dura may be the only criterion available for epidural/subdural differentiation. With an epidural hematoma, the dura appears as a thin linear density between the hematoma and cerebral surface. Often this is evident on plain CT scans, and it is almost always visible after contrast administration.

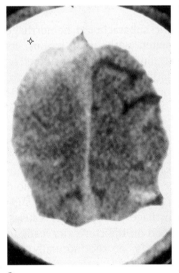

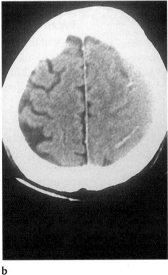

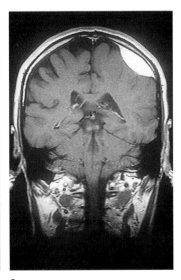

a

b

c

Fig. 2.6 A special case of an epidural hematoma located near the vertex. As noted in the text on p. ■, a blow to the vertex has special significance. Injuries to the sagittal sinus are common, and small epidural hematomas may be missed.

a This scan shows a hematoma in the right superior frontoparietal area that was classified as epidural by coronal magnetic resonance imaging (MRI). In side-to-side comparison, note the sulcal effacement and peripheral hemorrhages on the right side. Such injuries are often caused by a falling object striking the head (construction site injury, etc.).

b Same patient as in **a**.

c Coronal MRI demonstrates the now-subacute hematoma more clearly, owing to its high signal intensity. A high epidural hematoma located near the midline often requires angiographic evaluation of the dural sinuses.

Special cases of epidural hematoma are the *subacute* and *chronic forms.* These forms, which can occur in the very rare epidural hematomas caused by venous bleeding (dural sinus rupture, bleeding from a fracture line), display varying CT densities.

Infratentorial epidural hematomas are rare and take a fulminating course. Care should be taken not to overlook epidural hematomas located near the vertex (Fig. 2.**6**).

Coronal reconstructions may be necessary to demonstrate these hematomas and evaluate the adjacent bone. Their relationship to the superior sagittal sinus may require contrast angiography.

■ Differential Diagnosis

Differentiation is mainly required from subdural hematoma. The differentiating criteria are described above, although there are cases in which the usual criteria are difficult to apply, especially when findings are minimal. However, the imaging findings and an accurate localization of the mass to the epidural or subdural space are less important than the degree of mass effect and the severity and acuteness of the clinical findings in deciding whether to proceed with surgical evacuation.

Traumatic Subarachnoid Hemorrhage

Frequency: often coexists with other traumatic brain hemorrhages.

Suggestive morphologic findings: hyperdense blood on the cerebral surface, in the interhemispheric fissure (differential diagnosis: subdural hematoma), or on the tentorium.

Procedure: thin-slice CT examination with a bone window is appropriate in some cases. If the distribution of blood suggests a ruptured berry aneurysm, the lesion can be demonstrated by intravenous contrast administration.

Other studies: lumbar puncture is more sensitive for detecting subarachnoid hemorrhage. MRI has practically no role in acute diagnosis, due to its relative insensitivity to unclotted blood.

Checklist for scan interpretation:
▶ Location and extent?
▶ Follow-up: malabsorptive hydrocephalus?
▶ Blood in the ventricular system (usually non-traumatic; obstructive hydrocephalus)?

■ Pathogenesis

Traumatic subarachnoid hemorrhage may occur in isolation after a head injury or may be associated with other traumatic lesions (epidural/subdural/intracerebral hematomas, contusions, fractures).

■ Frequency

Subarachnoid hemorrhage is frequently detected in severely head-injured patients and may be accompanied by bleeding into other compartments.

■ Clinical Manifestations

Because traumatic subarachnoid hemorrhage is usually associated with other lesions, its clinical manifestations cannot be considered or evaluated in isolation. The clinical features are generally determined by the extent of cerebral contusions.

■ CT Morphology

Blood in the basal cisterns and sylvian fissure resulting from a traumatic subarachnoid hemorrhage has the same appearance as subarachnoid hemorrhage due to other causes. Subarachnoid blood on the convexity leads to increased CT density of the normally hypodense sulci (Fig. 2.**7**).

■ Differential Diagnosis

Traumatic subarachnoid hemorrhage mainly requires differentiation from subarachnoid bleeding due to a ruptured aneurysm. This type of hemorrhage is mainly located in the basal cisterns, whereas traumatic subarachnoid hemorrhage tends to be distributed

Fig. 2.**7 Traumatic sub-arachnoid hemorrhage.** This hemorrhage is often found in association with subdural or epidural hematoma. There is a copious amount of subarachnoid blood, with some of it forming pools on the convexity. An extensive subdural hematoma is also present. Its location is mainly parietal in **a** and more frontal in **b**, which also shows a small fluid–blood level.

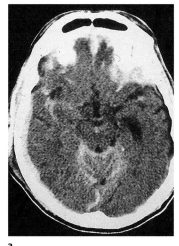 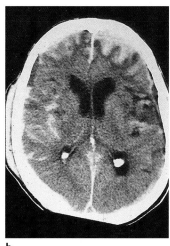

a   b

along the sulci of the frontal and parietal lobes. Reliable differentiation is sometimes difficult, however. If the findings are equivocal, angiography can be performed to detect or exclude other bleeding sources.

■ **Follow-Up**

If follow-up is not indicated for other intracranial traumatic lesions, the presence of a traumatic subarachnoid hemorrhage still warrants short-interval follow-up in patients who develop neurologic deficits. As with subarachnoid hemorrhage caused by a ruptured aneurysm, the neurologic deficits may result from regional hypoperfusion due to vasospasm.

Subdural Hematoma, Acute and Chronic

Frequency: common in the setting of head trauma, including minor injuries. Predisposing factors are expansion of the extra-axial CSF pathways and coagulation disorders.

Suggestive morphologic findings: peripheral mass abutting the calvarium and presenting a convex lateral border and a concave or ill-defined medial border. The collection is hyperdense in the acute stage, later showing decreasing density.

Procedure: surgical drainage.

Other studies: MRI can define septations in a chronic subdural hematoma.

Checklist for scan interpretation:
▶ Prominence (in centimeters), extent?
▶ Mass effect (measured midline shift)?
▶ Density of hematoma, layering? Evidence of septation?

■ **Pathogenesis**

Bounded by the dura mater and arachnoid, the subdural space can expand with considerably less resistance than the epidural space (Fig. 2.**8**).

Subdural hematomas result from venous bleeding, most commonly from the tearing of bridging veins in the subdural space. A distinction is made between acute and chronic subdural hematomas.

Acute subdural hematoma. Acute subdural hematomas have a traumatic etiology. The usual cause is a traumatic event sufficient to rupture the bridging veins in the subdural space. Atrophy and friable vessel walls, which

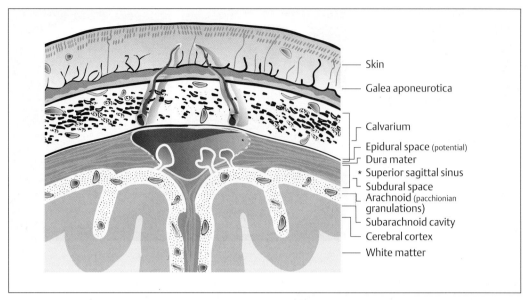

Skin
Galea aponeurotica
Calvarium
Epidural space (potential)
Dura mater
* Superior sagittal sinus
Subdural space
Arachnoid (pacchionian granulations)
Subarachnoid cavity
Cerebral cortex
White matter

Fig. 2.8 Schematic diagram of arterial vessels and venous sinuses at the cerebral surface, with associated spaces.

are predisposing factors in chronic subdural hematoma, may be absent, although every chronic subdural hematoma was once an acute subdural hematoma. Due to expansion of the extra-axial CSF spaces, severe neurologic deficits may be absent and the condition may remain clinically silent. The traumatic etiology accounts for the frequent presence of cerebral contusion. Edema of the brain tissue exacerbates the usual significant midline shift that occurs with acute subdural hematoma. If surgical drainage is withheld and the patient survives, the hematoma will progress to a chronic stage.

Chronic subdural hematoma. The factors noted above predispose to chronic subdural hematoma, which occurs mainly in older individuals. The patient may or may not recall antecedent trauma. The following circumstances account for the variable morphology of chronic subdural hematoma (see below):

- Since chronic subdural hematoma is usually caused by minor trauma, it is not accompanied by brain edema or contusions.

- Consequently, the midline shift is determined entirely by the width of the hematoma.
- As the hematoma ages, it becomes encapsulated and hypodense. Layering may be seen as blood products settle within the collection.
- Meanwhile the surrounding meninges become thicker, and septations may form within the hematoma.

■ Frequency

Subdural hematoma is a common finding in routine CT examinations, even in patients who deny a history of trauma.

■ Clinical Manifestations

With an acute subdural hematoma, the following symptoms occur:

- Impairment of consciousness
- Contralateral hemiparesis
- Ipsilateral mydriasis

With a chronic subdural hematoma, the following symptoms are predominant:

- Headache
- Dementia-like symptoms
- Unilateral deficits in some cases

These symptoms can cause the diagnosis of chronic subdural hematoma to be missed in elderly patients. Anticoagulant medication predisposes to subdural hematomas and other types of intracranial hemorrhage.

■ CT Morphology

An acute subdural hematoma typically appears on CT scans as a hyperdense mass distributed along the inner table of the skull and presenting a concave, somewhat ill-defined medial border (Fig. 2.**9**).

With a chronic subdural hematoma or an acute hematoma that evolves to a chronic stage, the collection becomes less attenuating and more isodense to brain, finally appearing as a homogeneous hypodensity. Clot formation without septation leads to sedimentation and layering, with hemosiderin-containing blood elements of high density forming a layer

Fig. 2.**9** **Subdural hematoma.** Subdural hematomas and effusions typically present a concave medial border. **a** Typical appearance of a left frontotemporal subdural hematoma. Note that the hematoma crosses the coronal suture. **b** Very small foci of subdural hemorrhage. **c** These collections, similar to those in **b**, also extend into the interhemispheric fissure on the left side. **d** Sedimentation of blood elements in older subdural hematomas often causes layering, as seen here in the left frontoparietal area. Note the higher density of the dependent portions of the hematoma. The presence of a right anterior ventricular drain underscores the chronic nature of the hematoma.

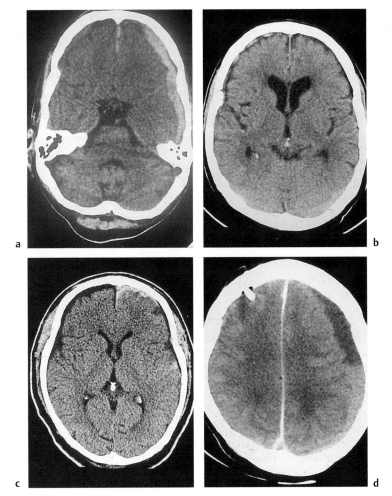

beneath acellular components of lower density. Septation by fibrin filaments and membranes can produce a heterogeneous pattern of mixed attenuation values.

Because subdural hematomas may be isodense to the brain parenchyma, there are rare situations in which additional evidence must be sought:

- If the midline is shifted (Fig. 2.**10**) but a hematoma is not seen, contrast medium can be administered to increase the density of the brain tissue. Subdural hematoma can then be identified as an area of relatively low density.
- Bilateral collections do not cause a midline shift. If the hematomas are isodense, dis-

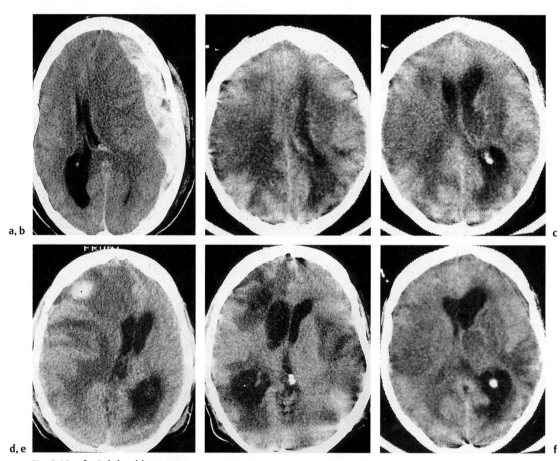

a, b

c

d, e

f

Fig. 2.**10 a–f Subdural hematoma.**

a   The mass effect of subdural hematomas in young patients can be substantial. An extensive subdural hematoma on the left side has caused a massive midline shift, with ventricular distortion.

b–d Very extensive head trauma can produce cerebral changes that are difficult to classify. Bilateral hematomas do not cause a midline shift, and there is no significant compression or displacement of the ventricular system. Patchy hypodensities with very ill-defined margins overlie both hemispheres. At

least some of the more peripheral hyperdensities are caused by motion rather than hemorrhages.

e, f With unilateral trauma causing unilateral lesions, even diffuse contusions and hemorrhages can cause extensive ventricular displacement. CT in the acute stage (**e**) shows massive displacement of the ventricular system to the left, with a large hemorrhagic contusion in the right frontoparietal area. The scan six days later (**f**) shows regression of the midline shift, but the contusions persist and additional foci are now visible on the left side.

placement of the frontal horns of the lateral ventricles may provide the only clue. This distortion is called the "rabbit ear sign," although there appears to be disagreement in the literature as to its exact configuration.

- The normally hypodense cortical sulci fill in with isodense material.

■ Differential Diagnosis

The following criteria can be applied as needed for differentiating between subdural and epidural hematomas (Fig. 2.**11**):

- Subdural hematomas can cross cranial sutures without interruption or distortion.

Fig. 2.**11 Special forms of subdural hematoma.** It is important to make an accurate classification of effusions at atypical locations, bearing in mind that subdural and subarachnoid hemorrhages, but not epidural hemorrhages, are observed in the interhemispheric fissure.

a This large right subdural hematoma has already caused a midline shift. Subdural blood is visible in the posterior falx, the layers of which are dissected. Subdural blood overlying the tentorium can also produce subtle findings.

b An irregular subdural collection overlying the tentorium on the left side.

c A subtle hemorrhagic collection delineates the right margin of the tentorium.

d This hyperdense feature is not a subdural hematoma, but the superior portion of a large arachnoid cyst that has been opacified by cisternography.

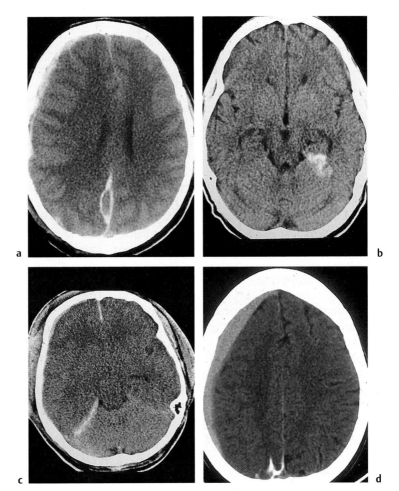

- Blood in the interhemispheric fissure or on the tentorium confirms subdural hemorrhage.
- After contrast administration, arachnoid membrane (short enhancing segments) rather than dura (linear enhancement) is defined between the hematoma and brain.

■ Follow-Up

After a subdural hematoma has been surgically evacuated, CT is recommended to confirm successful drainage. It is normal to find loculi of air retention in the subdural space at postoperative follow-up. Also, the dura often appears thickened postoperatively due to membrane formation, as described earlier.

Subdural Hygroma

Frequency: a common CT finding.

Suggestive morphologic findings: subdural mass that is isodense to CSF.

Procedure: depending on the clinical symptoms, needle aspiration (children) or open drainage with CT follow-up.

Other studies: MRI can distinguish with a reasonable degree of confidence between hygromas containing no blood breakdown products and chronic subdural hematomas.

Checklist for scan interpretation:
▶ Unilateral or bilateral?
▶ Extent? Mass effect?
▶ Homogeneous or nonhomogeneous density (bleeding within the hygroma)?

■ Pathogenesis

Subdural hygromas can have numerous causes, depending on the patient's age and prior history. They are often found with no apparent cause in children (potential explanations being intracranial hemorrhage, or inflammatory changes with a serous reaction due to entry of microorganisms into the subdural space). Hygromas can develop after ventricular drainage in both children and adults, and are frequently bilateral. Acute subdural hygroma in all age groups is believed to result from CSF leakage through an arachnoid tear (valve mechanism). Finally, subdural hygroma may result from failure of the brain to reexpand after surgical resection of a long-standing mass lesion and from excessive drainage during the implantation of a CSF shunting device.

■ Frequency

Subdural hygromas may be found at CT quite frequently, depending on the clinical population.

■ Clinical Manifestations

Subdural hygroma in infants and small children may be manifested by macrocephaly and bulging fontanels. Clinical symptoms include:

● Mental dullness
● Irritability
● Fever (if the hygroma has an inflammatory cause)

■ CT Morphology

Subdural hygroma appears as a unilateral or bilateral crescent-shaped extracerebral mass in contact with the inner table of the skull (Figs. 2.**12**, 2.**13**). The frontal and parietal regions are sites of predilection. The mass may show an approximately uniform width over all of its sagittal extent, or it may be wider at its center than at the edges. Unilateral hygromas exert a mass effect on the ventricular system that does not occur with bilateral collections. In some cases, only the frontal horns of the lateral ventricles are displaced toward the midline.

■ Differential Diagnosis

The CT features of subdural hygroma may be identical to those of a long-standing chronic ("faded") subdural hematoma, but generally a subdural hygroma can be diagnosed from the prior history (ventricular drainage, etc.) or by MRI.

■ Follow-Up

The success of drainage procedures should always be confirmed by CT.

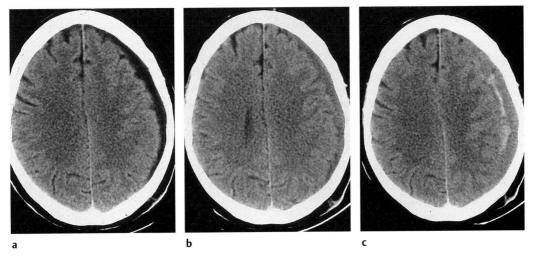

a   b   c

Fig. 2.**12**   **Evolution of a chronic subdural hygroma/ hematoma.**

a The subdural fluid collection is hypodense due to the absence of hemorrhagic elements.

b One month later, bleeding within the mass has caused increased CT density.

c Four months later, hyperdense material along the medial border of the mass indicates fresh rebleeding.

Fig. 2.**13**   **Evolution of cerebral contusion.**

a Typical appearance of a bifrontal contusion with frontal lobe hypodensities and central hemorrhagic areas.

b Six months after successful treatment, CT shows reactive expansion of the frontal horns of both lateral ventricles. The white matter of the diminished frontal lobes appears hypodense, as a sign of leukomalacia.

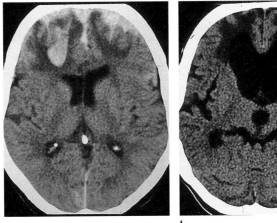

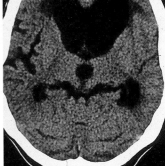

a   b

Gunshot Injuries

Frequency: depends on circumstances.

Suggestive morphologic findings: the clinical presentation suggests the correct diagnosis. Typical CT findings are a small comminuted area in the skull, a hyperdense missile track, and in driven bone fragments.

Procedure: surgical treatment (usually the missile is left in place).

Other studies: angiography is used to diagnose arterial and dural sinus injuries.

Checklist for scan interpretation:
▶ Location of bony lesion? Brain structures in missile track?
▶ Displaced bone fragments, projectile?
▶ Vascular damage?

■ CT Morphology

While CSF leakage suggests the correct diagnosis, as mentioned, CT shows string-of-beads air collections along the inner table of the skull, signifying a penetrating head injury. Air may enter the cranial cavity through a direct communication with the outside or through an air-filled paranasal sinus.

Fragmentation of the calvarium is apparent at the missile entry site and possibly also at an exit site. The missile track is marked by bone fragments and debris from the projectile. Occasionally it is hyperdense due to hemorrhage within the track.

■ Differential Diagnosis

Impalement injuries often cause gross disruption of brain tissue with intracerebral hemorrhage and subsequent infection (subdural empyema, abscess). As with a gunshot injury, gross comminution of the skull may be observed.

Other Open Brain Injuries

Frequency: less common than closed brain injuries.

Suggestive morphologic findings: intracerebral air (continuity).

Procedure: it may be necessary to investigate for dural injury (CT cisternography, CSF scintigraphy, fast T2-weighted MRI).

Other studies: functional studies are superior for detecting dural injury. Intrathecal fluorescent agents can demonstrate the leakage site intraoperatively or microscopically when a special light source is used.

Checklist for scan interpretation:
▶ Extent and location of bony and brain-tissue injuries?
▶ Intracranial air? Proximity to paranasal sinus?
▶ Mass effect due to bone fragments or air?
▶ Intraventricular hemorrhage?

■ Pathogenesis

Open brain injuries may be observed in impalement injuries, basal skull fractures, facial fractures, petrous bone fractures, other depressed skull fractures, or as a complication of surgical procedures (e.g., otolaryngologic surgery).

■ Frequency

Facial fractures are the most frequent cause of dural disruption by various mechanisms (e.g., in motor vehicle accidents).

■ Clinical Manifestations

As mentioned above, CSF leakage suggests the correct diagnosis. Suspicion is confirmed by detecting glucose in fluid nasal secretions. If necessary, radionuclide imaging (CSF scintigraphy) or fluorescent dye localization can be employed. A simple method is to acquire very thin CT slices with a bone window setting, orienting the scans perpendicular to the bone in the presumed area of injury. Occasionally this will demonstrate bony discontinuities that are associated with dural injury.

■ CT Morphology

CT scans may demonstrate the following:

- Lacerations with associated intracranial hemorrhage
- Displaced fragments, etc.
- Intracranial air

Intracranial air is often found at the rostral border of the petrous bone and along the inner table of the calvarium behind the frontal sinus. With passage of time, it should be considered that a hypodensity in the white matter of the injured lobe may be perifocal edema surrounding an abscess rather than a simple contusion. Postcontrast examination should be performed to exclude a brain abscess. When making a differential diagnosis, it should be considered that intracranial wooden foreign bodies have the same appearance as air in standard soft-tissue CT images. When higher window and center settings are used, the attenuation values will approach those of the surrounding soft tissues. Streak-like density changes within the foreign body are also characteristic of wood.

■ Differential Diagnosis

As noted earlier, intracranial air caused by CSF leakage and its replacement by air through a dural rent requires differentiation from penetrating injuries with the intracranial deposition of foreign material. While the former type of injury is associated with a moderate risk of ascending infection, the latter type is associated with a very high infection risk.

Traumatic Vascular Injuries

Frequency: rare complication of head trauma.

Suggestive morphologic findings: the location of the hemorrhage correlates with the type of vessel injured—subarachnoid with injury to a cerebral artery, subdural with injury to bridging veins, and epidural with injury to middle meningeal arterial branches.

Procedure: contrast angiography, if necessary combined with contrast-enhanced CT or MRI (dural sinuses).

Other studies: angiography is definitive.

Checklist for scan interpretation
(in addition to the criteria for trauma patients listed above):
▶ New infarction?
▶ Epidural hematoma near a dural sinus?
▶ Expansion of the ophthalmic vein or thickening of extraocular eye muscles?
▶ Need for further investigation (arterial or venous angiography)?

■ Pathogenesis

Traumatic vascular injuries include damage to the middle meningeal artery in fractures of the temporal squama, injuries of the large dural sinuses in calvarial fractures, injuries of major arteries in basal skull fractures, and traumatic fistula formation (especially a carotid–cavernous fistula). The posterior meningeal artery may be injured in fractures of the occipital squama.

■ Frequency

On the whole, injuries of major intracranial vessels are an infrequent complication of head trauma. Carotid–cavernous fistula is a separate entity that can be diagnosed clinically in patients who may or may not recall significant prior head trauma.

■ **Clinical Manifestations**

Increased intracranial pressure may be the dominant sign of vascular complications in comatose patients. By contrast, carotid–cavernous fistula presents with the classic clinical features of pulsatile exophthalmos and conjunctival vascular congestion.

■ **CT Morphology**

Lesions of the middle meningeal artery lead to epidural hematoma (see p. ■). Epidural hematoma is also the most common result of major dural sinus injury. In many cases, however, the collection cannot be localized to the epidural space, and the sinus rupture is difficult to detect even by angiography. Direct coronal CT scans or coronal reformatted images can be helpful in the diagnosis of superior sagittal sinus injury (blow to the vertex from a falling rock, etc.). Carotid–cavernous fistulae are manifested clinically by the transmission of arterial blood and pulsations to the ophthalmic vein (pulsatile exophthalmos). CT can suggest the lesion by showing unilateral enlargement of the vein, and angiography or ultrasound can confirm the diagnosis. Lesions of the cerebral supply arteries can lead to ischemic infarcts in the corresponding arterial territories.

■ **Differential Diagnosis**

Aids to the localization of specific bleeding vessels are described above. The differentiation of traumatic subarachnoid hemorrhage from that caused by a ruptured aneurysm relies in the acute stage on the CT detection of an aneurysmal outpouching using intravenous contrast enhancement and, if possible, spiral acquisition (CT angiography). Conventional angiography is added in most cases to positively exclude a vascular malformation.

Late Sequelae of Head Trauma

Frequency: CT has been largely superseded by MRI for disability assessment in patients with a history of head trauma.

Suggestive morphologic findings: parenchymal defect.

Procedure: plain CT examination. Obtain post-contrast scans if a lesion is suspected.

Other studies: MRI is more sensitive than CT for demonstrating gliosis and blood breakdown products.

Checklist for scan interpretation:
▶ Atrophy?
▶ Parenchymal defects, circumscribed atrophy?
▶ Gliosis, other residua (blood breakdown products)?
▶ Abscesses or other complications?

■ **Pathogenesis**

Typical traumatic brain lesions such as contusions, hemorrhages, and lacerations all have a common end result: a parenchymal defect due to the destruction of brain tissue. Neuronal destruction can lead to reactive gliosis. Residual hemorrhagic changes may remain visible for some time on CT scans.

■ **Frequency**

Approximately 30 % of patients with an open head injury will eventually develop epilepsy. This means that a substantial percentage of head-injured patients will require CT follow-up. The same is true of closed brain injuries, though to a lesser degree (lower incidence of epilepsy).

■ **Clinical Manifestations**

The principal late complication of head trauma is *epilepsy,* and years may pass before the first symptoms of a seizure disorder are manifested (other causes, especially mass lesions, should also be excluded in patients with a known history of head trauma). Epilepsy is considerably more common after open brain injuries than after closed injuries.

■ CT Morphology

Typical traumatic brain lesions (contusion, hemorrhage) eventually lead to tissue breakdown with the development of gliosis and parenchymal defects. One manifestation of these changes is atrophy, in which there is a reduction in brain volume without shape distortion. Posttraumatic brain atrophy may be generalized, affecting both hemispheres or one entire hemisphere, or it may be localized to one or more areas. Generally the causal relationship to trauma can be established only if serial examinations are available that cover the acute and particularly the subacute stages. MRI is better for the detection of gliosis, with CT showing no more than faint hypodensities in the white matter. An important late complication of head trauma is brain abscess, which may develop following an open head injury that has created a communication between the cranial cavity and the paranasal sinuses or petrous bone. The inadequate treatment of an unrecognized dural fistula can lead to the development of a brain abscess. An abscess located in the frontal white matter or occipital temporal lobe is consistent with this pathogenic mechanism. Another common sequel to head trauma is hydrocephalus, which may result from impaired CSF circulation due to adhesions following a subarachnoid hemorrhage or from the destruction of brain tissue due to extensive contusions (hydrocephalus ex vacuo).

■ Differential Diagnosis

A finding such as local atrophy is not a very useful criterion for differential diagnosis. To establish a causal relationship with trauma, one must at least correlate the site of the injury with the location of original brain lesions. Atrophy in the setting of a dementing syndrome of different etiology should always be considered in the differential diagnosis (see pp. 197 f). One should also consider the typical distribution patterns of focal atrophic changes that are associated with specific diseases.

■ Follow-Up

It should be noted that the radiographic features of skull fractures often do not resolve completely. This is important to consider when interpreting an isolated fracture line seen in a patient with a suspicious history (e.g., an alcoholic patient with a prior history of falls).

■ References

Recommended for further study
Open head injuries
Kelly AB, Zimmerman RD, Snow R, et al. Head trauma: comparison of MR and CT experience in 100 patients. AJNR Am J Neuroradiol 1988; 9: 699–708.
● *Although MRI plays little part in acute examinations, it is still instructive to consider the problems and weaknesses of CT.*
Klufas RA, Hsu L, Patel MR, Schwartz RB. Unusual manifestations of head trauma. AJR Am J Roentgenol 1996; 166: 675–81.
● *Compilation of highly educational cases with good image quality.*
Lloyd DA, Carty H, Patterson M, Butcher CK, Roe D. Predictive value of skull radiography for intracranial injury in children with blunt head injury. Lancet 1997; 349: 821–4.
● *Addresses the question of biplanar skull films versus cranial CT in a very large series of head-injured children.*
Teasdale G, Jennett B. Assessment of coma and impaired consciousness: a practical scale. Lancet 1974; ii: 81–4.
● *Based on the Glasgow Coma Scale.*

Skull fractures
Lipkin AF, Bryan RN, Jenkins HA. Pneumolabyrinth after temporal bone fracture: documentation by high-resolution CT. AJNR Am J Neuroradiol 1985; 6: 294–5
● *Brief review of fracture types with associated clinical features; older CT images.*
Holland BA, Brant-Zawadzki M. High-resolution CT of temporal bone trauma. AJNR Am J Neuroradiol 1984; 5: 291–5.
● *Although imaging quality has improved in the meantime, this still provides a comprehensive and well-illustrated review of the spectrum of CT findings.*

Cerebral contusion
Hesselink JR, Dowd CF, Healy ME, et al. MR imaging of brain contusions: a comparative study with CT. AJNR Am J Neuroradiol 1988; 9: 269–78.
● *Focuses on MRI and its advantages, but also discusses the effects that underlie CT contrast.*
Hymerl KP, Rumack CM, Hay TC, Strain JD, Jenny C. Comparison of intracranial computed tomographic (CT) findings in pediatric abusive and accidental head trauma. Pediatr Radiol 1997; 27: 743–7.

● *Illustrative images are well selected and expertly documented.*

Küker W, Thron A. Routine evaluation and specific investigation of head trauma. Chirurg 1996; 67: 1098–1106.

● *An overview that provides an excellent introduction.*

Mittl RL, Grossman RI, Hiehle JF, et al. Prevalence of MR evidence of diffuse axonal injury in patients with mild head injury and normal head CT findings. AJNR Am J Neuroradiol 1994; 15: 1583–9.

● *Describes the superiority of MRI over CT for detecting diffuse axonal injury after trauma.*

Epidural hematoma

Braun J, Borovich B, Guilburd JN, Zaaroor M, Feinsod M, Grushkiewicz I. Acute subdural hematoma mimicking epidural hematoma on CT. AJNR Am J Neuroradiol 1987; 8: 171–3.

● *Presents two cases with atypical findings.*

Hamilton M, Wallace C. Nonoperative management of acute epidural hematoma diagnosed by CT: the neuroradiologist's role. AJNR Am J Neuroradiol 1992; 13: 853–9.

● *With critical comments by the authors cited below; informative discussion of sites of occurrence, pathogenic mechanisms, etc.*

Sagher O, Ribas GC, Jane JA. Nonoperative management of acute epidural hematoma diagnosed by CT: the neuroradiologist's role. AJNR Am J Neuroradiol 1992; 13: 860–2.

Zimmerman RA, Bilaniuk LT. Computed tomographic staging of traumatic epidural bleeding. Radiology 1982; 144: 809–12.

● *Informative review of the stages of epidural hemorrhage.*

Traumatic subarachnoid hemorrhage

Zimmerman RD, Russel EJ, Yurberg E, Leeds NE. Falx and interhemispheric fissure on axial CT, 2: recognition and differentiation of interhemispheric subarachnoid and subdural hemorrhage. AJNR Am J Neuroradiol 1982; 3: 635–42.

● *Precise description of the differential diagnosis, as well as the complex relationships in children and in brain edema.*

Subdural hematoma

Borzone M, Altomonte M, Baldini M, Rivano C. Typical interhemispheric subdural hematoma and falx syndrome: four cases and a review of the literature. Zentralbl Neurochir 1995; 56: 51–60.

● *Illustrates several cases at this unusual location.*

Reed D, Robertson WD, Graeb DA, Lapointe JS, Nugent RA, Woodhurst WB. Acute subdural hematomas: atypical CT findings. AJNR Am J Neuroradiol 1986; 7: 417–21.

● *Describes findings and causes of acute subdural hematomas of mixed density.*

Subdural hygroma

Wilms G, Vanderschueren G, Demaerel PH, et al. CT and MR in infants with pericerebral collections and macrocephaly: benign enlargement of the subarachnoid spaces versus subdural collections. AJNR Am J Neuroradiol 1993; 14: 855–60.

Gunshot injuries

Besebski N, Jadro-Santel D, Lelavic-Koic F, et al. CT analysis of missile head injury. Neuroradiology 1995; 37: 207–11.

● *Series of 154 patients, with follow-up CT in half the cases.*

Schumacher M, Oehmichen M, König HG, Einighammer H. Intravital and postmortem CT examinations in cerebral gunshot injuries [in German]. RöFo Fortschr Geb Röntgenstr Nuklearmed 1983; 139: 58–62.

● *One of the few studies that describe forensic applications.*

Other open brain injuries

Ginsberg LE, Williams DW, Mathews VP. CT in penetrating craniocervical injury by wooden foreign bodies: reminder of a pitfall. AJNR Am J Neuroradiol 1992; 14: 892–5.

● *Describes the CT appearance of wooden foreign bodies—an important pitfall.*

Traumatic vascular injuries

Mirvis SE, Wolf AL, Numaguchi Y, Corradino G, Joslyn JN. Posttraumatic cerebral infarction diagnosed by CT: prevalence, origin, and outcome. AJNR Am J Neuroradiol 1990; 11: 355–60.

● *Describes compression syndromes caused by hematomas and their causal role in posttraumatic infarction.*

Traflet RF, Babaria AR, Bell RD, et al. Vertebral artery dissection after rapid head turning. AJNR Am J Neuroradiol 1989; 10: 650–1.

● *Deals only with angiograms and MRI, but helps direct attention to this easily missed complication.*

Late sequelae of head trauma

CT follow-up after trauma is mainly discussed indirectly in the journals belonging to the specific clinical disciplines.

Gudeman SK, Kishore PRS, Becker DP, et al. Computed tomography in the evaluation of incidence and significance of posttraumatic hydrocephalus. Radiology 1981; 141: 397–402.

● *Brief review of the pathogenesis and evolution of posttraumatic hydrocephalus.*

Küker W, Thron A. Routine evaluation and specific investigation of head trauma. Chirurg 1996; 67; 1098–1106.

● *Recommended as an introduction.*

Reider-Groswasser I, Cohen M, Costeff H, Groswasser Z. Late CT findings in brain trauma: relationship to cognitive and behavioral sequelae and to vocational outcome. AJR Am J Roentgenol 1993; 160: 147–52.

● *Correlation of atrophy and neuropsychological outcome in 32 trauma patients.*

Recent and basic works

Open head injuries

Gentry LR, Thompson B, Godersky JC. Trauma to the corpus callosum: MR features. AJNR Am J Neuroradiol 1988; 9: 1129–38.

Haydel MJ, Preston CA, Mills TJ, Luber S, Blaudeau E, DeBlieux PMC. Indications for computed tomography in patients with minor head injury. N Engl J Med 2000; 343: 100–5.

● *Excellent work on the indications of CT in patients with a normal Glasgow Coma Scale.*

Bruce DA. Imaging after head trauma: why, when and which. Childs Nerv Syst. 2000; 16(10, 11):755–9.

Lipper MH, Kishore PRS, Enas GG, et al. Computed tomography in the prediction of outcome in head injury. AJNR Am J Neuroradiol 1985; 6: 7–10.

Olson EM, Wright DL, Hoffman HT, Hoyt DB, Tien RD. Frontal sinus fractures: evaluation of CT scans in 132 patients. AJNR Am J Neuroradiol 1992; 13: 897–902.

Warren LP, Djang WT, Moon RE. Neuroimaging of scuba diving injuries to the CNS. AJNR Am J Neuroradiol 1988; 9: 933–8.

Skull fractures
Rubinstein D, Symonds D. Gas in the cavernous sinus. AJNR Am J Neuroradiol 1994; 15: 561–6.

Cerebral contusion
Zimmerman RA, Bilaniuk LT, Genneralli T. Computed tomography of shearing injuries of the cerebral white matter. Radiology 1978; 127: 393–6.
- *Despite the old images, one of the few CT studies on white-matter shearing injuries, which today are evaluated exclusively and more successfully by MRI.*

Epidural hematoma
Orrison WW, Gentry LR, Stimac GK, Tarrel RM, Espinosa MC, Cobb LC. Blinded comparison of cranial CT and MR in closed head injury. AJNR Am J Neuroradiol 1994; 15: 351–6.

Manjunath-Prasad KS, Gupta SK, Khosla VK. Chronic extradural hematoma with delayed expansion. Br J Neurosurg 1997; 11: 78–9.

Schumacher M, Oldenkott P, Pfeiffer J, Schumm F. Unusual radiologic and clinical findings in calcified chronic epidural hematomas. Neurochirurgica 1982; 25: 1–6.
- *Describes unusual calcification and ossification of epidural hematomas in three patients.*

Traumatic subarachnoid hemorrhage
Cohen RA, Kaufman RA, Myers PA, Towbin RB. Cranial computed tomography in the abused child with head injury. AJR Am J Roentgenol 1986; 146: 97–102.
- *Documents the spectrum of cranial CT findings in child abuse.*

Subdural hematoma
Aoki N, Oikawa A, Sakai T. Symptomatic subacute subdural hematoma associated with cerebral hemispheric swelling and ischemia. Neurol Res 1996; 18: 145–9.

Nussbaum ES, Wen DYK, Latchaw RE, Nelson MJ. Meningeal sarcoma mimicking an acute subdural hematoma on CT. J Comput Assist Tomogr 1995; 19: 643–5.

Wilms G, Marchal G, Geusens E, et al. Isodense subdural haematomas on CT: MRI findings. Neuroradiology 1992; 34: 497–9.

Subdural hygroma
Rupprecht T, Lauffer K, Storr U, et al. Extracerebral intracranial fluid collections in children: differentiation between benign enlargement of the subarachnoid space and subdural effusion with color Doppler imaging. Klin Pädiatr 1996; 208: 97–102.

Gunshot injuries
Hayes E, Ashenburg R, Philips D. Cerebral embolism after gunshot wounds. AJNR Am J Neuroradiol 1989; 10 (Suppl 5): S77.
- *Rare complication of gunshot injury (no. 11 buckshot).*

Wilms G, Vanderschueren G, Demaerel PH, et al. CT and MR in infants with pericerebral collections and macrocephaly: benign enlargement of the subarachnoid spaces versus subdural collections. AJNR Am J Neuroradiol 1993; 14: 855–60.

Other open brain injuries
Thong HV, McGuckin JF, Smergel EM. Intraorbital wooden foreign body: CT and MR appearance. AJNR Am J Neuroradiol 1996; 17: 134–6.
- *Describes how MRI is unrewarding in this situation.*

Traumatic vascular injuries
O'Sullivan RM, Robertson WD, Nugent RA, Berry K, Turnbull IM. Supraclinoid carotid artery dissection following unusual trauma. AJNR Am J Neuroradiol 1990; 11: 1150–2.

Segev Y, Goldstein M, Lazar M, Reider-Groswasser I. CT appearance of a traumatic cataract. AJNR Am J Neuroradiol 1994; 16: 1174–5.

Toro VE, Fravel JF, Weidman TA, et al. Posttraumatic pseudoaneurysm of the posterior meningeal artery associated with intraventricular hemorrhage. AJNR Am J Neuroradiol 1993; 14: 264–6.

Tucci JM, Maitland CG, Pcsolyar DW, Thomas JR, Black JL. Carotid–cavernous fistula due to traumatic dissection of the extracranial internal carotid artery. AJNR Am J Neuroradiol 1984; 5: 828–9.

Late sequelae of head trauma
Kraus JK, Trankle R, Kopp KH. Posttraumatic movement disorders in survivors of severe head injury. Neurology 1996; 47: 1488–92.

Lee TT, Aldana PR, Kirton OC, Green BA. Follow-up computerized tomography (CT) scans in moderate and severe head injuries: correlation with Glasgow Coma Scores (GCS), and complication rate. Acta Neurochir 1997; 139: 1042–7.

Mitchener A, Wyper DJ, Patterson J, et al. SPECT, CT and MRI in head injury: acute abnormalities followed up at six months. J Neurol Neurosurg Psychiatry 1997; 62: 633–6.

Winking M. Computer tomographic assessment of the pre- and postoperative ventricle width in patients with traumatic intracranial hematomas. Acta Neurochir 1994; 126: 128–34.

3 Cerebrovascular Diseases

Brain Infarction

Frequency: a leading indication for computed tomography (CT) examination and a very common CT diagnosis.

Suggestive morphologic findings: hyperdense middle cerebral artery (MCA); loss of definition of the basal ganglia and insular region (early sign); hypodensity with moderate mass effect in the distribution of a cerebral artery (territorial infarction with embolic occlusion); lacunar or cortical lesion; contrast enhancement at the appropriate stage of clinical evolution (third day to third week after stroke).

Procedure: early diagnosis is desirable. Exclude hemorrhage, determine whether angiography is required. Consider atypical causes (vasculitis, dissection, dural sinus thrombosis).

Other studies: CT is the modality of choice, even in special cases. Modern magnetic resonance imaging (MRI) techniques (diffusion-weighted images) allow very early diagnosis. MRI can also demonstrate the brain stem without artifacts. With the higher contrast sensitivity of MRI, even subtle foci of enhancement can be detected.

Checklist for scan interpretation:
▶ Location of suspected infarcted areas?
▶ Intracerebral hemorrhage?
▶ Age of the infarct(s)?
▶ Infarction due to microangiopathy, macroangiopathy, or other cause?
▶ Follow-up?
▶ Need for MRI or angiography?

■ Pathogenesis

A distinction is made between microangiopathic and macroangiopathic disease in the pathogenesis of brain infarction. *Microangiopathic disease* includes changes that develop in the distribution of the long medullary arteries:

- Supratentorial lacunar infarcts
- Subcortical atherosclerotic encephalopathy

Macroangiopathic disease consists of:

- Embolic territorial infarctions
- Hemodynamic (watershed and end-zone) infarctions

Territorial infarctions. Territorial infarctions result from embolism or thrombosis. The embolism may have a cardiac origin in patients with a corresponding history (atrial thrombi due to absolute arrhythmia, mitral stenosis), or emboli may be shed from the walls of large arteries supplying the brain. A classic pattern results from embolic occlusion of the main trunk of the MCA. In other cases, portions of the MCA territory may become infarcted due to the occlusion of specific branches.

Hemodynamic infarction. Hemodynamically induced infarcts may be of the watershed (border-zone) or end-zone type. They are based on a reduction in cerebral perfusion caused by occlusion or stenosis of large cervical arteries or basal cerebral arteries, leading to insufficiency in the more distal branches of the arterial tree. Each type may occur in isolation, or the two types may coexist. The anterior and posterior communicating arteries can compensate for occlusion or stenosis of individual vessels, but the circle of Willis may be unable to provide adequate collateral flow, depending on the location and extent of the flow-reducing lesions.

Lacunar infarcts. Lacunar infarcts are small infarcts located in the deep noncortical areas of the brain and brain stem. They are caused by the occlusion of peripheral branches of the large cerebral arteries: the middle cerebral artery, posterior cerebral artery, basilar artery, and less commonly the anterior cerebral artery and vertebral arteries (Fisher 1982). Lacunar infarcts are attributed to thrombosis, but most causative lesions in symptomatic patients are angiographically occult. Lacunar infarcts culminate in a parenchymal defect 3–25 mm in size that is isodense to cerebrospinal fluid (CSF).

Subcortical atherosclerotic encephalopathy. This refers to marked atherosclerotic changes found in the basal arteries of the brain. Atherosclerotic changes are also found in the long penetrating medullary arteries (medial thickening with stenoses and occlusions). By contrast, the vessels supplying the cerebral cortex show minimal histologic changes. Given the nature of the vascular changes, only isolated cortical foci are affected by ischemic necrosis. White-matter changes are pronounced, however, and consist of demyelination, axonal degeneration, and microglial proliferation.

Other causes. Besides the changes described above, which are based on atherosclerotic lesions and are the most frequent cause of brain infarction, the following additional causes should be considered:

- Dissection
- Vasospasm
- Dural sinus thrombosis

■ Frequency

Embolic infarction is considerably more common than hemodynamic infarction. Since the advent of antihypertensive therapies, hypertensive causes of cerebral blood flow disturbances (subcortical atherosclerotic encephalopathy, lacunar infarcts) have become less frequent. Supratentorial infarcts are over ten times more common than infratentorial infarcts.

■ Clinical Manifestations

The term *stroke* denotes a clinical syndrome characterized by the sudden onset of focal neurologic deficits (Fig. 3.**1**). Conditions other than ischemic brain lesions should be considered in the differential diagnosis.

Among the clinical manifestations of *hemodynamic infarction,* sensorimotor hemiparesis has been reported for end-zone infarcts. Anterior watershed infarction is characterized by hemiparesis predominantly affecting one leg, and posterior watershed infarction by homonymous lower-quadrant hemianopia.

Lacunar infarcts typically produce combinations of symptoms, and sensory deficits are common. A clinical diagnosis of homonymous hemianopia, aphasia, coma, or seizures does not support the diagnosis of a lacunar infarct—or at least, an infarction of this type cannot account for these symptoms by itself.

Lacunar infarcts most commonly occur in hypertensive individuals, and have a favorable prognosis.

In *subcortical atherosclerotic encephalopathy* (Binswanger disease), lacunar infarcts lead to sensory and motor deficits. The dementia in this condition is attributed to extensive demyelination. Binswanger disease is secondary to protracted hypertension.

■ CT Morphology

Territorial Infarctions

The most important early signs of cerebral infarction on plain CT scans are the hyperdense MCA sign (Fig. 3.**2a**) and loss of definition of the basal ganglia (Fig. 3.2 **b**).

Both signs can be observed at a time after stroke when systemic thrombolytic therapy can still be beneficial. The hyperdense MCA sign (and increased density of other vascular segments that are less often and less easily visualized) is based on an acute embolic occlusion that usually affects the MCA segment proximal to its bifurcation (M1 segment). With further evolution of the stroke, the infarcted area often becomes more clearly demarcated, due to the low density of the surrounding brain. Loss of definition of the basal ganglia affects the anterior areas. Normally, the basal ganglia are clearly delineated from the hypodense internal and external capsule by their somewhat higher attenuation. In the initial hours after a stroke, the basal ganglia become slightly less attenuating and more isodense in relation to the capsule. The entire region then shows a slight, homogeneous low density. It should be noted that loss of definition of the basal ganglia signifies an infarction of the MCA, which supplies the anterior basal ganglia. With further evolution of the territorial infarction, brain swelling in the infarcted area leads to effacement of the sulci, variable hypodensity of the brain parenchyma, and other signs of mass effect such as slight ventricular compression (Fig. 3.**3**).

If the occlusion is located near the circle of Willis and there is deficient collateral flow, the entire territory of the posterior, middle, or (less commonly) the anterior cerebral artery will be affected (Fig. 3.**4**).

If the occlusion is limited to peripheral branches, only part of the arterial territory will be affected (Fig. 3.**5 a**). Many of these infarcts are wedge-shaped. Cortical infarcts display a gyral pattern of involvement (Fig. 3.**5 b, c**).

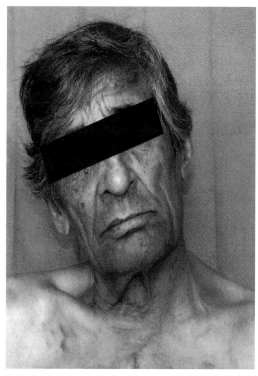

Fig. 3.**1** **Brain-stem infarction.** Involvement of the left accessory nerve is evidenced by the lateral head tilt and the effacement of the left supraclavicular fossa. There is accompanying palsy of the trapezius and sternocleidomastoid muscles.

Fig. 3.**2 a, b** **Early signs of ischemic infarction:**

a Hyperdense middle cerebral artery (MCA) sign. The MCA on one side (here the right) appears hyperdense due to fresh thrombosis. The dependent portion of the MCA territory still appears unchanged.

b Loss of definition of the right basal ganglia and insular region is noted when the sides are compared.

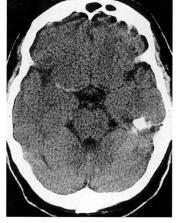
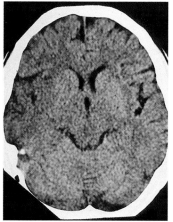

a   b

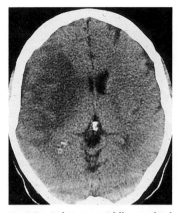

Fig. 3.**3 Subacute middle cerebral artery (MCA) infarction (territorial infarction) with ventricular compression and mass effect on the extra-axial cerebrospinal fluid spaces.** The scan already shows marked hypodensity of the infarcted brain area. The anterior basal ganglia supplied by MCA branches are also affected.

Fig. 3.**4a–f Typical CT features of territorial infarctions in one of the three major arterial territories.**
a Infarction in the territory of the anterior cerebral artery may involve a wedge-shaped area next to the anterior part of the falx in the frontal lobe.
b Another pattern consists of tissue destruction near the midline in the superior portions of the brain.
c This scan shows hemorrhage within a subacute, incomplete infarction of the left middle cerebral artery (MCA). The infarct involves the lentiform nucleus. The left ventricular system is markedly compressed and shifted across the midline.
d Infarction in the posterior cerebral artery territory in the left hemisphere.
e This scan show another posterior territory infarct that extends into medial portions of the temporal lobe.
f Multiple-territory infarction involving both the right middle and posterior cerebral arteries.

▽

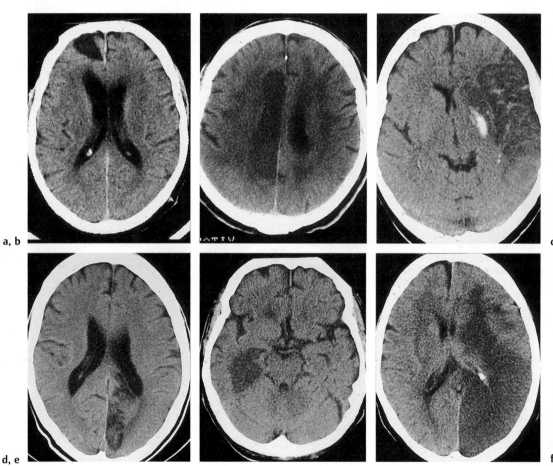

a, b

c

d, e

f

Abb. 3.**4a–f**

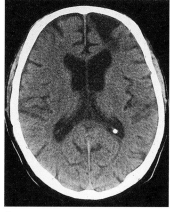
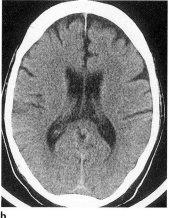
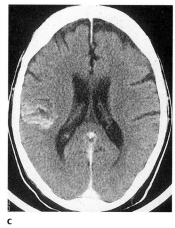

a   b   c

Fig. 3.**5 a–c** **Small territorial infarctions.** Partial involvement of the distribution of a cerebral artery results in a small territorial infarct:

a Involvement of both the cortex and white matter leads to a peripheral wedge-shaped infarct.
b, c Cortical infarcts display a typical gyral pattern (**b** plain, **c** postcontrast).

An infarct confined to the brain stem (Fig. 3.**6**) signifies that leptomeningeal collaterals are delivering adequate blood to the portions of the cortex and white matter supplied by the MCA.

These infarcts are also territorial infarcts, and should be managed accordingly.

Hemodynamic Infarctions

Hemodynamic infarctions result from a reduction in perfusion pressure caused by high-grade stenotic arterial lesions in the neck. These lesions are often bilateral and may coexist with stenoses in the circle of Willis. The resulting distal-field insufficiency can lead to an end-zone infarction (Fig. 3.**7**) or watershed infarction (Fig. 3.**8**).

Watershed infarctions can develop in any of the following areas:

- The anterior watershed area, between the territories of the anterior and middle cerebral arteries.
- The posterior watershed area, between the territories of the middle and posterior cerebral arteries.

Fig. 3.**6 a, b** **Basal ganglia infarcts.** These brain-stem infarcts in the distribution of the middle cerebral artery are not accompanied by infarction of the dependent white matter or associated cortex.

a The left lentiform nucleus is infarcted along with the posterior crus of the right internal capsule.
b Isolated infarction of the head of the left caudate nucleus. Because the penetrating medullary arteries are unaffected, lacunar infarcts are absent.

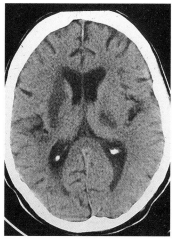
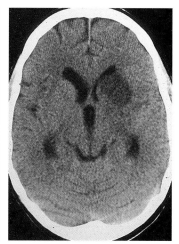

a   b

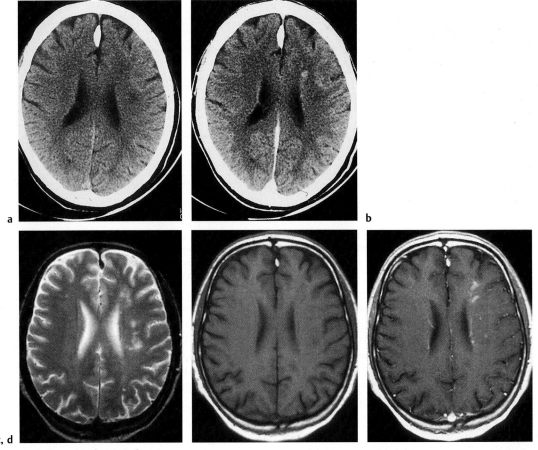

a

b

c, d

e

Fig. 3.**7 a–e** **End-zone infarction.**

a, b CT (**a** plain, **b** postcontrast) shows characteristic end-zone infarcts in the territory of the deep medullary arteries. These infarcts occur in the cen-

trum semiovale or above the ventricles and show a string-of-beads pattern in pronounced cases.

c–e The CT findings are surprisingly subtle when compared with magnetic resonance images in the same patient.

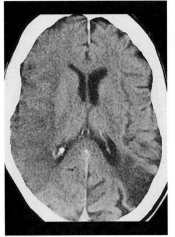

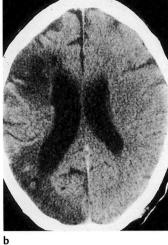

a

b

Fig. 3.**8 a, b** **Watershed infarction.** Watershed infarcts are sometimes difficult to distinguish from infarcts of the far anterior or far posterior middle cerebral artery (MCA) branches.

a Left posterior watershed infarction accompanied by a complete right MCA infarction undergoing demarcation.

b Posterior watershed infarction and partial MCA infarction on the right side.

Fig. 3.**9 a, b   Subcortical atherosclerotic encephalopathy.** This disease is characterized by lacunar infarcts of the white matter and basal ganglia and by confluent, bilateral periventricular hypodensities.

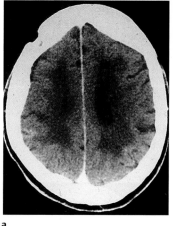 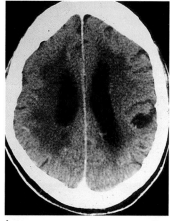

a   b

- The subcortical watershed area, between the deep and superficial branches of the middle cerebral artery.

End-zone infarcts are located in the periventricular white matter or centrum semiovale, and produce remarkably subtle changes in CT density compared with MRI.

Microangiopathy

Subcortical atherosclerotic encephalopathy (Fig. 3.**9,** Binswanger disease) is characterized by internal and external cerebral atrophy.

Ventricular enlargement in this disease is somewhat more pronounced than expansion of the subarachnoid spaces. In addition, lacunar infarcts are detected in the basal ganglia and white matter. White-matter hypodensity is usually bilateral and shows an approximately symmetrical distribution.

Evolution of CT Density Changes

Besides the morphologic CT patterns that characterize particular types of stroke, it is important to consider the density changes that are observed in the different stages.

Acute stage. Any of the following early signs may be noted on CT scans acquired during the initial hours after onset (acute stage):

- Hyperdense MCA sign (Fig. 3.**2 a**) refers to unilateral increased density of the MCA due to its occlusion by a thrombus. This sign precedes   infarction-induced   density

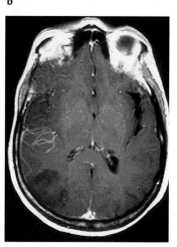

Fig. 3.**10   Intravascular and meningeal enhancement as early signs of cerebral infarction on magnetic resonance imaging (MRI).** With an extensive infarction, MRI shows linear intravascular enhancement (horizontal) in the right middle cerebral artery territory, along with meningeal enhancement in the right parietal area.

changes in the brain tissue supplied by the vessel.
- Loss of definition of the basal ganglia (Fig. 3.**2 b**) is another early CT sign of infarction.

It should be noted that the early MRI signs of brain infarction (Fig. 3.**10,** meningeal and intravascular enhancement in the infarcted area preceding T2-weighted signal enhancement) do not have a correlate on the CT scan.

The next change to occur is mild brain swelling in the infarcted area, which is manifested on CT by effacement of the overlying sulci.

These early signs are followed by the characteristic hypodensity, which is generally seen 12 hours after the stroke.

Subacute stage. In the subacute stage, the infarcted area becomes clearly demarcated as a hypodense lesion. The great majority of infarcts at this stage (approximately 80% on CT)

enhance after intravenous contrast administration (Fig. 3.**11**).

As a general rule of thumb, contrast enhancement of the infarcted area is observed from approximately the third day to the third week after stroke. The CT detection of contrast enhancement is important because a small percentage of infarcts (5–10%) are isodense to the surrounding brain. Today, however, CT detection of enhancement is of limited useful-

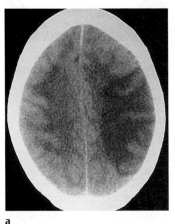
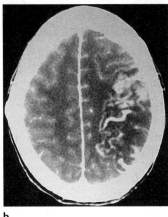

a   b

Fig. 3.**11 a, b   Marked contrast enhancement in the luxury perfusion stage of an infarction.**

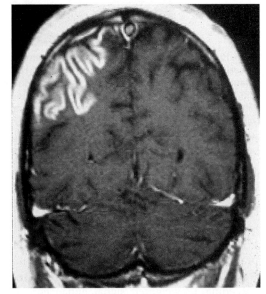

Fig. 3.**12   Gyral enhancement on magnetic resonance imaging.** Signal enhancement traces a conspicuous gyral pattern on the post-gadolinium magnetic resonance image.

ness in the differential diagnosis of hypodense lesions, and MRI is preferred for the differentiation of brain tumors. MRI is also better than CT for demonstrating gyral enhancement (Fig. 3.**12**).

The enhancement on CT scans tends to be patchy, hazy, and indistinct.

Chronic stage. Evolution to the chronic stage is marked by a hypodense parenchymal defect with attenuation values equivalent to CSF. The margins of the defect are generally well-defined (Fig. 3.**13**).

Associated Findings

Besides CT findings in the infarcted areas, one should be alert for changes that may be found in association with stroke. These include *traumatic brain injuries* that may be sustained when the stroke occurs (Fig.3.**14**).

Skull fractures and various types of *intracranial hemorrhage* may be observed. CT

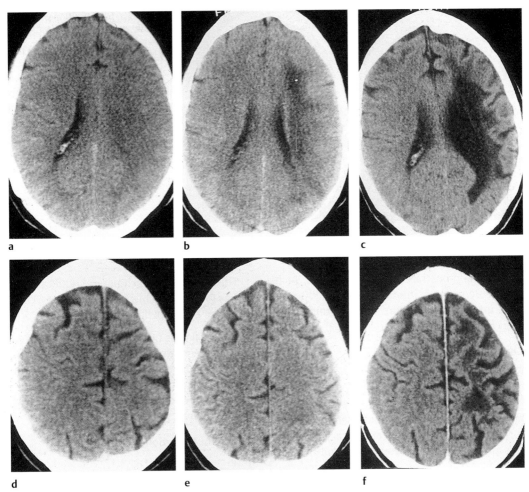

a   b   c

d   e   f

Fig. 3.**13 a–f   Cerebral infarction.** CT course of cerebral infarction, from initial brain swelling (**a, b** on two different planes) to a faint hypodensity three days after the stroke (**c, d**; same planes as in **a, b**) and—three years later—to the cavitation stage, with ventricular enlargement (**e, f**).

Fig. 3.**14 a, b   Middle cerebral artery (MCA) infarction.** These scans show an old right MCA infarction at two different levels accompanied by a fresh left-sided MCA infarction with hemorrhage in the left basal region. The subdural hematoma along the interhemispheric fissure was caused by a head injury sustained during the stroke.

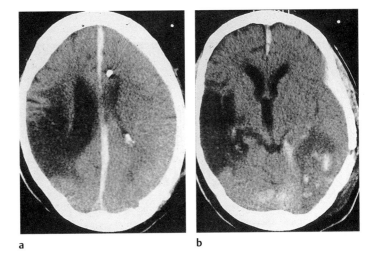

a   b

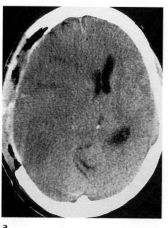

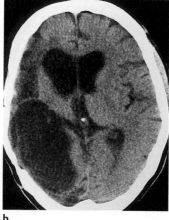

a   b

Fig. 3.**15 a, b Evolution of a middle cerebral artery (MCA) infarction.**
a A craniotomy was performed to relieve intracranial mass effect (gross ventricular displacement toward the contralateral side) following a right MCA infarction.
b Follow-up scan documents a large, CSF-isodense parenchymal defect with associated ventricular enlargement.

may also demonstrate *iatrogenic changes,* such as an emergency craniotomy performed to relieve intracranial pressure due to brain swelling (Fig. 3.**15**).

Cerebellar Infarction

Generally, the incidence of cerebellar infarction is about 10 times lower than that of cerebral infarction. Just as with supratentorial infarctions, a distinction is made between territorial infarcts (superior cerebellar artery, anterior inferior cerebellar artery, posterior inferior cerebellar artery) and watershed infarcts. CT detection of cerebellar infarction is unsatisfactory compared with MRI, due mainly to bone-related artifacts and the lack of multiplanar (especially sagittal) imaging capability.

The examination technique should be modified as follows to achieve the optimum CT visualization of cerebellar infarcts:

- Slice thickness of 2 mm
- Adequate contrast administration (Fig. 3.**16**)
- Proper gantry angulation, using the temporal lobe projection as required
- Artifact-reducing algorithms (available with modern scanners)

Brain-stem Infarction

Brain-stem infarcts (Fig. 3.**17**) can lead to typical lateral medulla oblongata "crossed" syndromes, which are known by a variety of terms (such as Weber syndrome and Wallenberg syndrome).

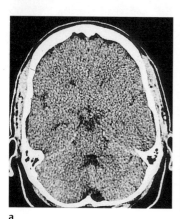

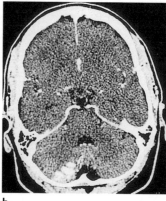

a   b

Fig. 3.**16 a, b Partial infarction in the territory of the posterior inferior cerebellar artery.**
a Plain CT demonstrates the infarct as a faint hypodensity.
b Postcontrast CT shows conspicuous enhancement of the infarcted cortical areas.

"Crossed" refers to the ipsilateral involvement of cranial nerves accompanied by a contralateral dissociated sensory deficit. Since the blood supply is subject to numerous variants, both complete and incomplete syndromes can occur. Also, it is not always easy for the first examining neurologist to differentiate supratentorial infarction from a brain-stem infarct.

CT scans are often negative for brain-stem infarcts, due in some cases to inadequate examination technique. Except in the case of large infarcts, for which imaging documentation is often a less pressing concern, scans should be acquired in the temporal lobe projection to eliminate temporal bone artifacts, and a slice thickness of 2 mm should be used.

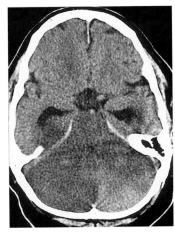

Fig. 3.**17 Cerebellar and brain-stem infarction.** CT shows marked hypodensity in addition to severe swelling.

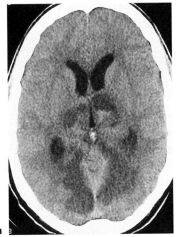

a

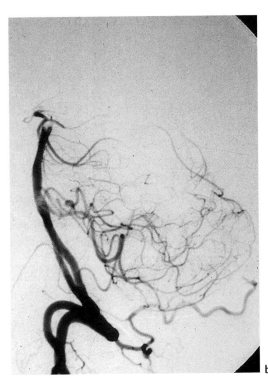

b

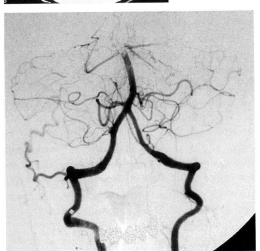

c

Fig. 3.**18 a–c Basilar artery thrombosis.**
a Typical infarcts due to basilar artery thrombosis.
b, c Angiographic cut-off sign, with opacification of the contralateral vertebral artery.

This technique can significantly reduce the need for supplementary MRI. Brain-stem infarcts typically appear as somewhat rounded hypodensities with ill-defined margins. Intravenous contrast administration does not contribute anything to the study.

Brain-stem gliomas and cavernomas have similar morphologic features but are not difficult to distinguish from infarction in routine diagnostic situations.

Infarction at the level of the pons may be a manifestation of basilar artery thrombosis (Fig. 3.**18**).

Infarction Based on Nonatherosclerotic Vascular Disease (Figs. 3.**19**–3.**22**)

A dissection or dissecting aneurysm, occurring when blood enters the vessel wall and separates its layers (Fig. 3.**19**), should be considered as a cause of brain infarction in younger patients.

A history of neck trauma accompanied by pain in the face or nuchal region suggests dissection in a carotid vessel. Suspicion is raised by Doppler localization of stenoses or occlusions past the bifurcation, although these lesions are difficult to visualize. Angiography

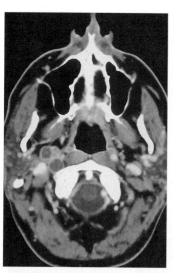
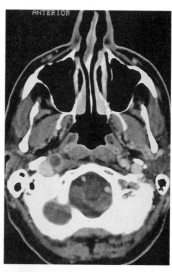

a   b

Fig. 3.19 a–c   Infarction (not shown) due to a dissecting aneurysm.
a, b The postcontrast CT of the cerebral supply arteries shows a dissecting aneurysm of the right internal carotid artery, which appears as a second lumen. This finding should not be mistaken for thrombosis.
c The coronal MRI shows aneurysmal dilatation of the vessel.

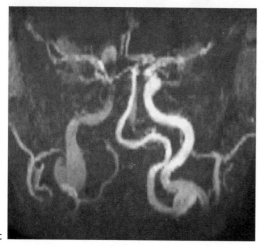

c

raises suspicion by showing tapered vessel narrowing ("peaked-hat sign"), a double-lumen sign, or consecutive sites of luminal narrowing ("string sign"). The diagnosis should not be missed, as the prognosis is favorable with anticoagulant therapy. Either an increase in vessel diameter or a reduction of the perfused lumen may be seen, depending on the entry site of the dissection in the vessel wall. Pseudoaneurysms are also seen. The differential diagnosis should include vessel wall pathology such as fibromuscular dysplasia. Air emboli (Fig. 3.**22**) lead to disseminated hypodensities at the cortical level.

Fig. 3.**20 a–d** **Infarction due to vasculitis.** Plain CT with a bone window shows only clouding of the right mastoid. Intracranial extension has led to inflammatory cerebrospinal fluid changes, and spread from the subarachnoid space has produced multiple disseminated cortical infarcts.

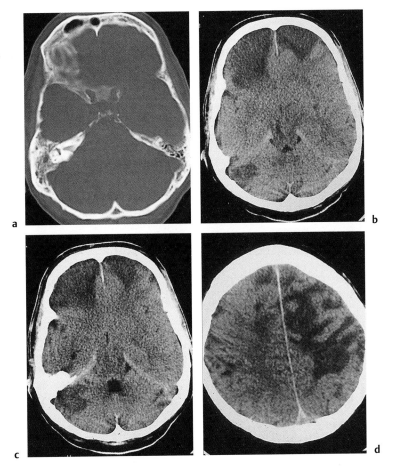

Embolism secondary to valvular endocarditis has similar features but is often associated with marked enhancement after contrast administration (Fig. 3.**23**).

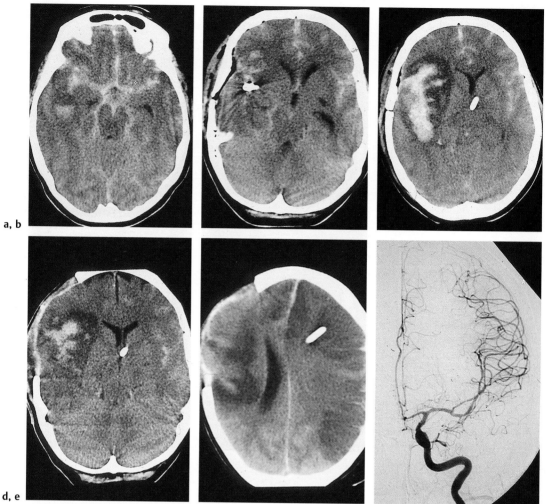

a, b

c

d, e

f

Fig. 3.**21 a–f   Infarction due to vasospasm.**
a Subarachnoid hemorrhage in a 60-year-old woman.
b The causative aneurysm was clipped on the second day.

c A scan at a higher level on the same day shows extensive hemorrhage in the sylvian fissure and adjacent parenchyma.
d Craniotomy was performed on day 6 for decompression. Note the marked perifocal edema.
e The scan on day 7 shows contralateral infarcts in the distribution of the anterior and middle cerebral arteries.
f Angiography demonstrates vasospasms at the origin of the middle cerebral artery.

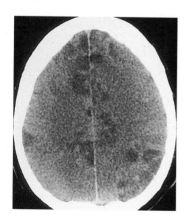

◁ Fig. 3.**22   Air emboli.** Besides a marked decrease in gray–white matter contrast (brain swelling), plain CT shows multiple disseminated hypodensities in the cerebral cortex. These lesions represent embolic cortical infarcts.

◼ Differential Diagnosis

Cerebral metastases can be almost indistinguishable from infarcts in certain cases (Fig. 3.**24**).

Noting the shape of the lesion and correlating it with the known patterns of brain infarction is the best aid to differential diagnosis. It is important to recognize hemodynamic infarcts, as these require further investigation by cerebral angiography (Fig. 3.**25 a**).

Territorial infarcts should be differentiated from low-grade brain tumors, and enhancing lesions require differentiation from higher-grade malignancies. An important criterion is whether the detected lesions conform to vascular territories. If contrast enhancement occurs, it should be determined whether the clinical onset is consistent with the period of enhancement in brain infarctions. For example, enhancement occurring three months after the onset of clinical symptoms would not support the diagnosis of a neoplasm. The pattern of contrast enhancement is also helpful in some cases: purely cortical enhancement does not occur with tumors.

When lacunae are found, a long list of differential diagnoses should be considered.

The lesions of multiple sclerosis (Fig. 3.**25 b**; see also acute disseminated encephalomyelitis) are usually bilateral, and sagittal T2-weighted MRI usually shows involvement of the corpus callosum.

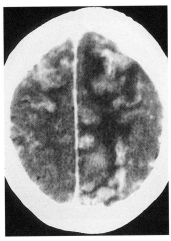

Fig. 3.**23 Septic emboli secondary to valvular endocarditis.** Postcontrast CT shows enhancing areas in the cerebral cortex that represent cortical infarcts caused by septic emboli. Hypodense perifocal edema is also apparent.

Cerebral vasculitis is a difficult differential diagnosis that should be considered in all patients with an unexplained multifocal neurologic symptom complex. Headache, personality changes, and even seizures may also occur. Diagnostic confirmation is difficult and has to rely on caliber irregularities in cerebral angiograms, nonspecific white-matter hypodensities, and biopsy findings. MR images are frequently positive even when CT scans are negative.

Pontine myelinolysis should be considered in the morphologic differential imaging diag-

Fig. 3.**24 a, b   Metastasis.**
a The hypodensity in the right occipital area might be interpreted as an infarct in the posterior cerebral artery territory.
b The postcontrast CT does not show the luxury perfusion typical of an infarction, but instead demonstrates a ring-enhancing lesion that was confirmed as a metastatic tumor.

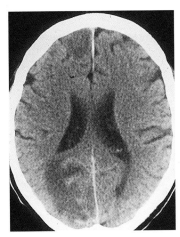

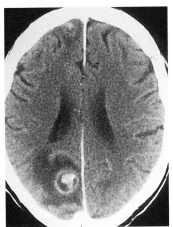

a   b

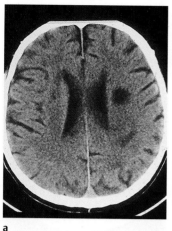

a

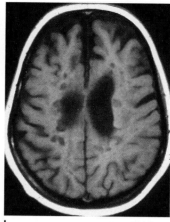

b

Fig. 3.**25 a, b Differentiation of end-zone infarction from multiple sclerosis.** If the clinical presentation is unknown, it is difficult on axial CT to distinguish end-zone infarcts in the lenticulostriate territory from the periventricular defects seen in long-standing multiple sclerosis. Generally, differential diagnosis is aided by noting involvement of the corpus callosum, which is very typical of multiple sclerosis. This is best appreciated on sagittal T2-weighted MR images.
a CT.
b Unenhanced T1-weighted MRI.

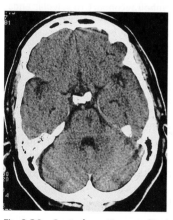

Fig. 3.**26 Central pontine myelinolysis.** This scan demonstrates the characteristic location of the hypodense lesion.

nosis of brain-stem infarcts (Fig. 3.**26**). Differentiation should be straightforward when the history and clinical presentation are known. Pontine myelinolysis is most commonly encountered in intensive-care patients with electrolyte disorders.

With bilateral lesions involving the white matter and cortex, reversible posterior leukoencephalopathy syndrome should be considered. It is seen in hypertensive crises due to various causes and is common in preeclampsia and eclampsia (Fig. 3.**27**).

■ Follow-Up

The main role of CT in follow-up is to detect secondary bleeding into the infarcted area, especially in patients who manifest neurologic deterioration.

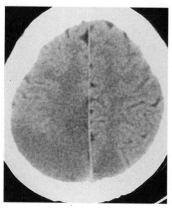

a

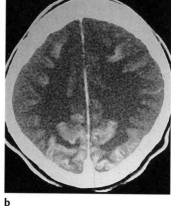

b

Fig. 3.**27 a, b Occipital lobe changes in eclampsia and cocaine abuse.**
a Eclampsia. Plain CT scan in a 21-year-old woman shows patchy bilateral occipital hypodensities in the cortex and white matter. The hypodensities extend toward the parietal lobe.
b Cocaine abuse. Plain CT in a cocaine abuser shows bilateral hyperdense hemorrhagic areas in the occipital cortex.

Hypertensive Intracerebral Hemorrhage (Figs. 3.**28**–3.**35**)

■ **Frequency:** a common CT finding.

Suggestive morphologic findings: hyperdense mass in the basal ganglia region, occasionally involving the brain stem or cerebellum.

Procedure: atypical hemorrhage requires evaluation by angiography, MRI, and follow-up.

Other studies: with an atypical hemorrhage, MRI is better for tumor detection, while angiography is better for detecting vascular malformation.

Checklist for scan interpretation:
▶ Location, extent?
▶ "Typical" appearance of hypertensive hemorrhage?
▶ Intraventricular rupture?
▶ Mass effect, edema?

■ Pathogenesis

Intracerebral hemorrhages occur more frequently in hypertensive patients. Parenchymal hemorrhages due to other causes (cerebral metastases in tumor patients, coagulation disorders) are less common.

The most frequent sites of occurrence for spontaneous hematomas are the putamen, internal capsule, and white matter. Thalamic, cerebellar, and pontine hemorrhages are less common.

■ Frequency

Intracerebral hemorrhage is a frequent CT finding, especially in high-risk patients with generalized vascular disease and poorly controlled hypertension. Hypertensive hemorrhage is the most common cause of nontraumatic intracerebral hemorrhage in adults.

■ Clinical Manifestations

A typical hemorrhage located in the basal ganglia region presents clinically as a "stroke," with hemiparesis and possible aphasia. Other cases present with the signs and symptoms of a cerebellar or brain-stem lesion. Intraventricular rupture is frequent, and the CSF is therefore often blood-tinged. The hematoma may also

rupture into the subarachnoid space, producing a subarachnoid collection that can be detected on serial CT scans.

■ CT Morphology

Typical hypertensive hemorrhages are found in the basal ganglia region on CT scans (Fig. 3.**28**). They appear as hyperdense foci surrounded by low-density edema. Cerebellar hemorrhages (Fig. 3.**29**) may result from a hemorrhagic infarct or vascular malformation. These lesions are also hyperdense but take a more dramatic course.

■ Differential Diagnosis

The main role of CT in intracerebral hemorrhage is to differentiate typical hemorrhages occurring in hypertensive patients from atypical hemorrhages. An atypical hemorrhage can have various causes:

- Neoplastic hemorrhage (Fig. 3.**30,** metastatic melanoma or hypernephroma)
- Bleeding from a vascular malformation (Fig. 3.**31**)
- Hemorrhagic infarction (Fig. 3.**32**)
- Small dural fistula (Fig. 3.**33**)

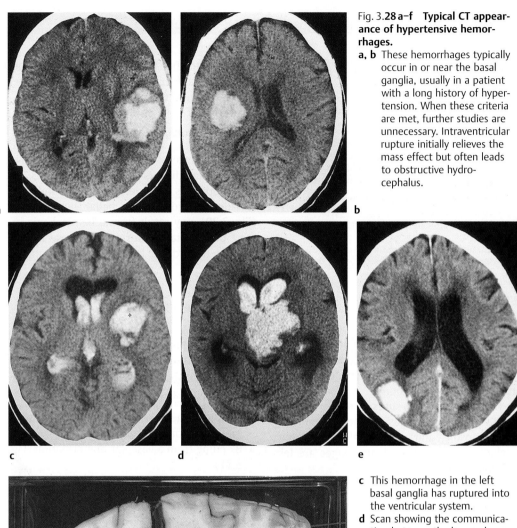

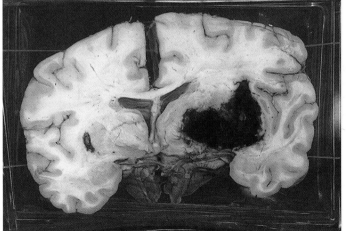

Fig. 3.**28 a–f   Typical CT appearance of hypertensive hemorrhages.**

a, b These hemorrhages typically occur in or near the basal ganglia, usually in a patient with a long history of hypertension. When these criteria are met, further studies are unnecessary. Intraventricular rupture initially relieves the mass effect but often leads to obstructive hydrocephalus.

c This hemorrhage in the left basal ganglia has ruptured into the ventricular system.

d Scan showing the communication between the hemorrhage and ventricles.

e Typical location of intracerebral hemorrhage in amyloid angiopathy.

f Typical gross appearance of hypertensive intracerebral hemorrhage in a pathologic specimen (from the pathology collection of the Charité Hospital, Berlin).

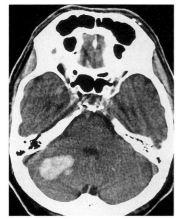

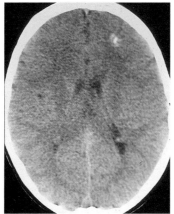

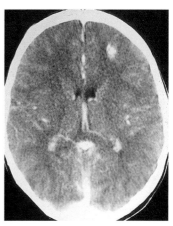

Fig. 3.**29   Cerebellar hemorrhage.** This is less common than supratentorial hemorrhages. The scan illustrates an infratentorial hemorrhage in the right hemisphere of the cerebellum. The mass effect on the fourth ventricle is not yet apparent.

Fig. 3.**30 a, b   Atypical hemorrhage: cavernoma.**
a Plain CT demonstrates a small hemorrhage in the left anterior white matter.

b The postcontrast scan shows marked enhancement.

Fig. 3.**31   Atypical hemorrhage: vascular malformation.** An arteriovenous malformation was confirmed as the cause of parenchymal hemorrhage in a 4-year-old child.

Fig. 3.**32   Atypical hemorrhage: cerebral infarction.** The location of the hemorrhage in the posterior circulation identifies it as a hemorrhagic infarct.

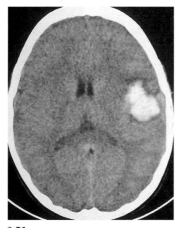

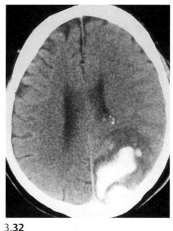

3.**31**

3.**32**

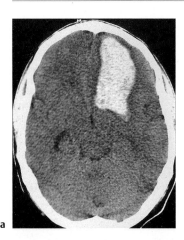

a

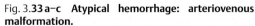

Fig. 3.**33 a–c** **Atypical hemorrhage: arteriovenous malformation.**
a The location in the frontal lobe characterizes the hemorrhage as atypical.
b, c Angiograms demonstrate that the cause is a small arteriovenous malformation.

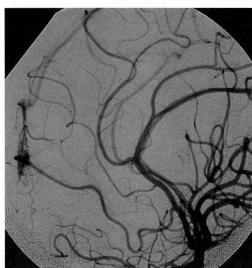

b

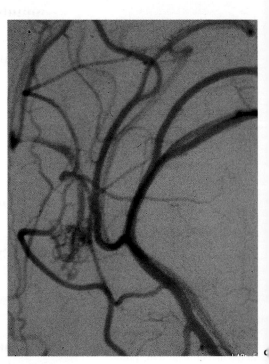

c

CT localization of the hemorrhage to the basal ganglia region in a hypertensive patient confirms a "typical" pathogenesis. Neither perifocal edema nor a faint peripheral ring of contrast enhancement (Fig. 3.**34**) would be inconsistent with hypertensive hemorrhage.

The differentiating criteria from tumor are demonstrated somewhat better on MRI, where very extensive perifocal edema (grade II or III) and marked signal enhancement should raise suspicion of a metastasis. With a bleeding arteriovenous malformation (AVM), postcontrast CT can often demonstrate the AVM vessels. It cannot detect small dural fistulae, however, which require angiography. Amyloid angiopathy (Fig. 3.**28 e**) typically presents as a subcortical hemorrhage in the posterior watershed area.

Fig. 3.**34 a, b Atypical hemorrhage with no demonstrable cause.** This hemorrhage is classified as atypical by its location outside the basal ganglia region and the absence of a prior history of hypertension.
a Plain CT shows a hematoma with perifocal edema in the superior parietal region.
b Postcontrast CT demonstrates a thin enhancing rim. Despite repeated angiography, the source of the bleeding could not be identified. *Caution:* rim enhancement is not pathognomonic for a tumor.

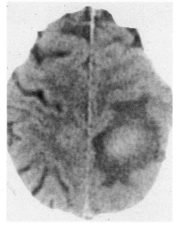
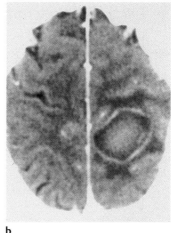

a   b

Fig. 3.**35 a–d Blood in the ventricles and subarachnoid spaces.**
a The comma-shaped hematoma in the left parietal area does not represent a parenchymal hemorrhage. Several other sulci also show slightly increased density, indicating the subarachnoid location of the hemorrhage. Blood in the cerebrospinal fluid spaces can have various causes. The morphology of intraventricular blood is largely independent of the cause.
b A ruptured basilar artery aneurysm has led to hydrocephalus, with a large blood clot in the left occipital horn.
c Following a subarachnoid hemorrhage, the fourth ventricle is enlarged and filled with blood. Blood is also visible in the prepontine cisterns. Hydrocephalus has already developed, as shown by the massive enlargement of the frontal horns.
d In addition to a large hemorrhage in the left occipital horn (**b**), this scan demonstrates a small fluid–blood level in the right occipital horn.

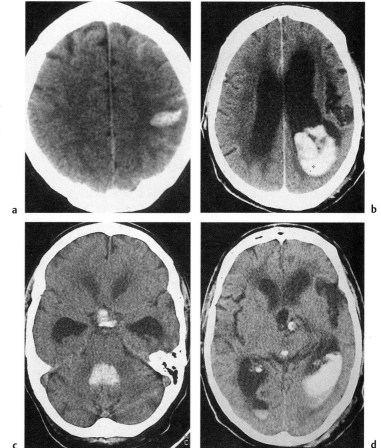

a   b

c   d

Arteriovenous Malformations

Frequency: according to some authors, approximately one AVM (or fewer) occurs for every ten subarachnoid hemorrhages from a basal cerebral artery aneurysm.

Suggestive morphologic findings: tubular structures on contrast-enhanced CT.

Procedure: angiography is indicated, as a prelude to interventional therapy if possible. CT angiography with bolus contrast injection and thin-slice spiral acquisition provides satisfactory visualization of the vascular malformation and also permits three-dimensional reconstructions.

Other studies: even extremely small AVMs can be defined by angiography.

Checklist for scan interpretation:
▶ Extent?
▶ Hemorrhage? Mass effect?
▶ Affected territories?
▶ Hydrocephalus?

■ Pathogenesis

Arteriovenous malformations (Fig. 3.**36**) represent an abnormal communication between intracerebral arteries and veins.

Congenital AVMs occur when arterial vessels connect to draining veins with no intervening capillaries. The feeding arteries often have paper-thin walls, while the draining veins are greatly enlarged due to the high arterial flow. This high flow into the vein of Galen, for example, can cause compression of the third ventricle, leading to hydrocephalus. The "nidus" of the AVM is the area of the actual arteriovenous shunts.

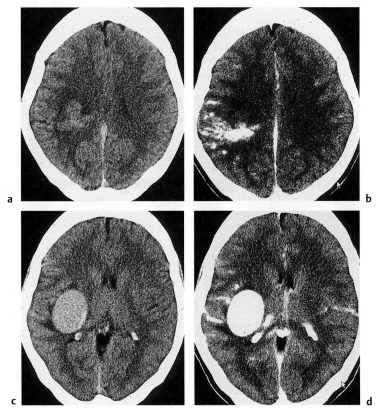

Fig. 3.36 a–h Structurally complex arteriovenous malformation (AVM): CT and angiography. The structure of AVMs is often complex and difficult to appreciate with CT alone, which generally does not document the time-varying enhancement characteristics of the lesion.

a, c Plain CT scans show a nonspecific hyperdensity in the superior parietal white matter (**a**) and a rounded hyperdensity with slight peripheral calcification in the basal ganglia region (**c**).

b, d The corresponding postcontrast scans show an enhancement pattern consisting of tortuous vascular channels at the parietal level (**b**). The intense enhancement of the rounded structure in the basal ganglia region (**d**) confirms its vascular nature.

Abb. 3.**36** e–h ▷

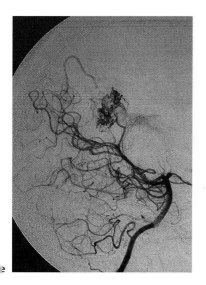

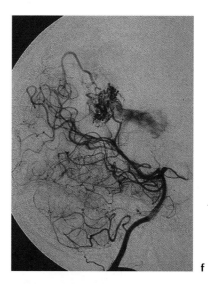

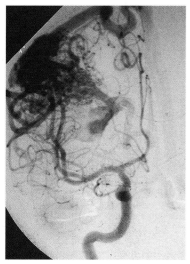

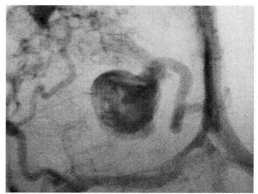

Fig. 3.**36 e–h** Angiograms demonstrate the nidus with its feeding arteries and draining veins, which encircle the AVM nodule.

■ Frequency

The prevalence of AVMs is probably higher than generally reported. It is approximately 0.14 % with a slight male predominance.

■ Clinical Manifestations

Nonbleeding intracerebral AVMs are often manifested by epileptic seizures and mild to severe headache. Bleeding lesions may also present with seizures or sudden onset of neurologic deficits.

■ CT Morphology

Plain CT findings in nonbleeding AVMs can be subtle (hypodensity, Fig. 3.**37;** very rarely, calcifications).

Bleeding may be so slight that local atrophy is the only result. Hemorrhage from an AVM appears hyperdense on plain CT (Fig. 3.**38**).

Characteristic changes are observed after intravenous contrast administration (Fig. 3.**39**). Enhancing tubular structures, often extending over a large area, can be seen along with hemorrhagic areas. It is common to find a wedge-shaped hyperdensity extending between the cerebral cortex and ventricle. The enlarged draining veins may reach considerable size.

■ Differential Diagnosis

Larger AVMs may appear as patchy hyperdensities on unenhanced scans, and can occasionally mimic other intrinsically hyperdense lesions (meningioma, lymphoma). Contrast administration, however, will generally demonstrate the tortuous vascular channels that are characteristic of AVMs. Of course, angiography is definitive for differential diagnosis when used to investigate an atypical hemorrhage. AVMs that have been embolized with hyperdense embolic material are easily identified when the surgical history is known. If the history is not known (unconscious patient, etc.), the finding may be misinterpreted and even mistaken for an oligodendroglioma or other lesion.

■ Follow-Up

Follow-ups are performed after embolization or surgical treatment of an AVM. The embolic material, usually in the form of microcoils introduced to thrombose the vessel, typically ap-

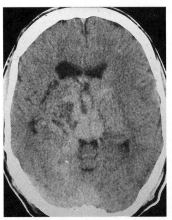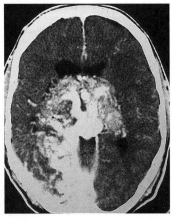

a
b

Fig. 3.**37 a, b   Arteriovenous malformations** (AVMs) may show mixed densities on unenhanced CT scans due to their complex structure.

- **a** This plain scan shows rounded and tubular hyperdensities around the basilar artery, chiefly on the rostral side, interrupted by hypodensities. The frontal horns of the lateral ventricles are displaced anteriorly.

- **b** The scan after intravenous contrast administration shows intense enhancement of the vascular loops. A large portion of the main mass of the AVM overlies the tentorium in the right hemisphere. The basal ganglia region shows intense bilateral enhancement.

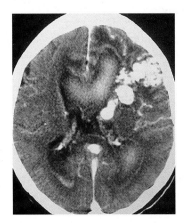

◁ Fig. 3.**38   Bleeding into the ventricles from an arteriovenous malformation.** Postcontrast CT shows a typical tangle of enhancing vessels, which here connect the basal ganglia region with the convexity.

Fig. 3.**39 a–d   Bleeding arteriovenous malformation** (AVM). Bleeding from an AVM appears on plain CT as an atypical hemorrhage (no history of hypertension, not localized to basal ganglia region).
a, b Plain scans show a hyperdense hemorrhage in the thalamic region of the left hemisphere.
c, d Contrast-enhanced scans show tortuous vascular channels at the periphery of the hemorrhage. This confirms the diagnosis and underscores the need for a detailed investigation of atypical hemorrhage.

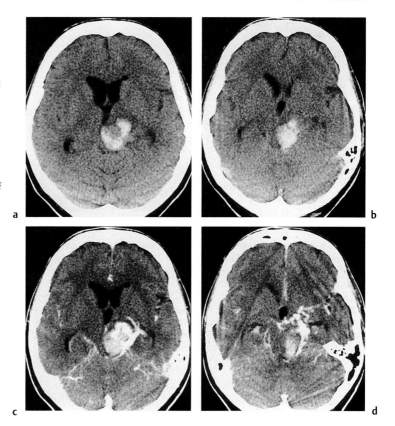

pears hyperdense on CT. The material may still define the course of the obliterated vessel. Intravenous contrast should be administered to detect persistent vessels.

Aneurysmal Subarachnoid Hemorrhage

Frequency: common CT finding in emergency examinations.

Suggestive morphologic findings: hyperdense basal cisterns.

Procedure: angiography, surgery (clipping), interventional therapy.

Other studies: angiography demonstrates aneurysms of the basal cerebral arteries as the underlying pathology.

Checklist for scan interpretation:
▶ Location of the hemorrhage?
▶ Involvement of fourth ventricle?
▶ Hydrocephalus?
▶ Detectable aneurysm?
▶ Left-sided or right-sided predominance?

Pathogenesis

The most frequent cause of subarachnoid hemorrhage is an aneurysm of the basal cerebral arteries (often at a bifurcation, Fig. 3.**48**).

If blood is detected on CT (Fig. 3.**40**) or lumbar puncture but angiography does not demonstrate an aneurysm, the less common etiologies justify an MRI examination, despite its very low yield.

The goal of diagnostic imaging in acute subarachnoid hemorrhage is to demonstrate the hemorrhage and ultimately detect its source along with any coexisting aneurysms. Follow-up attention should be given to the possible development of hydrocephalus (Fig. 3.**41**).

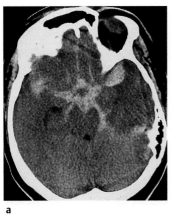 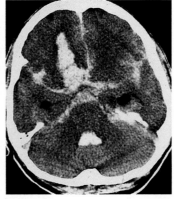 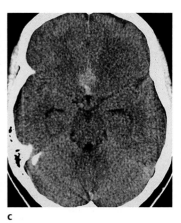

a   b   c

Fig. 3.40 a–c Contrast reversal of the basal cisterns in subarachnoid hemorrhage.

a Subarachnoid blood is responsible for the increased density that demarcates the brain stem in the occipital region. The pentagon-like figure outlines the periphery of the circle of Willis. The rounded hemorrhage near the right middle cerebral artery bifurcation should raise suspicion of a bifurcation aneurysm. A larger hematoma is also present at the left temporal pole.

b Copious intraparenchymal blood is present in the right frontal region and fourth ventricle. Blood in the fourth ventricle accounts for the possible development of hydrocephalus following a subarachnoid hemorrhage. The location of the aneurysm correlates (to a degree) with the location of the hemorrhage.

c Hemorrhage in the interhemispheric fissure due to an aneurysm of the pericallosal artery.

Rebleeding can be prevented by surgical clipping of the aneurysm.

■ Frequency

It is estimated that unruptured intracranial aneurysms are present in 2% of the population. The risk of aneurysm rupture increases with aging.

■ Clinical Manifestations

Subarachnoid hemorrhage may present with the following symptoms:

- Sudden headache of unprecedented severity
- Cranial nerve deficits (oculomotor dysfunction in cases of internal carotid artery aneurysms)
- Meningism

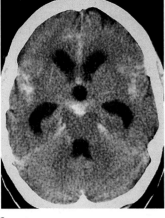 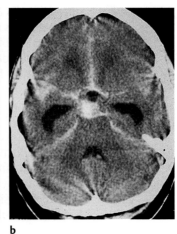

Fig. 3.41 a, b Hydrocephalus developing as a complication of subarachnoid hemorrhage. CT demonstrates subarachnoid blood in the extra-axial cerebrospinal fluid spaces, anterior interhemispheric fissure, and prepontine area, leading to hydrocephalus with expansion of the frontal horns, lateral ventricles, third ventricle, and temporal lobes.

a   b

- Impaired consciousness, ranging from lethargy to coma

The following diagnostic procedures are used:

- Unenhanced cerebral CT
- Lumbar puncture
- Angiographic visualization of the intradural arteries (four-vessel angiography)
- MRI

Subarachnoid hemorrhage can be graded using several different scales. The ones most commonly used are the Hunt and Hess scale (Table 3.**1**) and the World Federation of Neurosurgical Societies (WFNS) scale, which is largely based on the Glasgow Coma Score.

Table 3.**1** Hunt and Hess grading system for subarachnoid hemorrhage

Grade	Description
I	Asymptomatic or mild headache
II	Moderate to severe headache Nuchal rigidity No focal neurologic deficits
III	Lethargy Confusion Mild focal deficit
IV	Stupor Hemiparesis
V	Deep coma Decerebration

CT Morphology

Examination Technique

Localized blood can be detected using plain CT alone. Imaging with the usual slice thicknesses (8 mm supratentorial, 4 mm infratentorial) can be supplemented by acquiring thin slices at the level of the basal cerebral vessels. This should be considered if the standard CT examination does not detect blood, or gives equivocal findings. Intravenous contrast administration combined with spiral acquisition in the arterial phase can demonstrate larger aneurysms. This technique does not replace angiography. MRI is not useful for detecting acute subarachnoid hemorrhage.

Imaging Findings

The subarachnoid spaces are normally hypodense to the surrounding brain tissue. Blood in the subarachnoid spaces reverses this pattern, and the subarachnoid spaces become hyperdense to brain.

Blood is found in various portions of the subarachnoid space (Fig. 3.**42**). The distribution can often provide information on the location of the bleeding aneurysm (if present):

- Aneurysms of the internal carotid artery lead to blood in the suprasellar cisterns, often showing an asymmetric pattern when the sides are compared.

Fig. 3.**42 a, b** **Subtle CT presentation of subarachnoid hemorrhage. a** A small collection of blood is visible in the ambient cistern. **b** Subarachnoid blood collections overlie the brain stem and cerebellum.

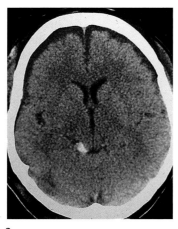
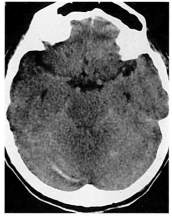

a   b

- Aneurysms of the middle cerebral artery lead to blood in the sylvian fissure.
- Aneurysms of the anterior communicating artery are manifested by blood in the basal portions of the frontal interhemispheric fissure.
- Aneurysms of the basilar artery present with blood in the posterior interhemispheric fissure, interpeduncular fossa, and sylvian fissure.
- "Perimesencephalic hemorrhages," characterized by blood in the interpeduncular fossa and ambient cistern, are not typical of aneurysms and are considered separately due to their benign course.

Hydrocephalus can develop as a complication of subarachnoid hemorrhage. It may go undetected until a repeat examination is performed.

Sensitivity

CT fails to detect blood in fewer than 2 % of patients with an acutely ruptured aneurysm (reports range from less than 2 % to less than 5 %). Once rupture has occurred, however, the high density rapidly declines. CT becomes

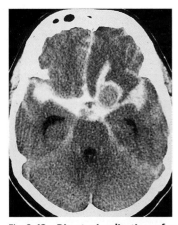

Fig. 3.**43 Direct visualization of an aneurysm.** An aneurysm of the left middle cerebral artery bifurcation appears on plain CT as a globular hypodensity within a large amount of blood in the pentagon region.

false-negative in 12 % of cases after 3 days, 50 % after 7 days, 80 % after 9 days, and in virtually all cases after 10 days.

Blood from a ruptured anterior inferior cerebellar artery aneurysm can be difficult to detect with CT. Posterior circle of Willis aneurysms also give rise to occasional false-negative scans. Blood in the prepontine cistern is frequently missed.

■ Differential Diagnosis

Other potential causes of increased subarachnoid density besides hemorrhage are intrathecal contrast administration (very high density affecting the entire subarachnoid space) and rare causes such as purulent leptomeningitis with exudation into the CSF. In the latter case, the finding is accentuated by concomitant hypodensity of the brain due to diffuse edema.

■ Additional Studies

Beyond the simple diagnosis of subarachnoid hemorrhage, CT can provide additional information on the location of the causative aneurysm. In some cases, an aneurysm is delineated as a round filling defect within a large subarachnoid hematoma (Fig. 3.**43**).

Thrombosed (Fig. 3.**44**) and naturally calcified aneurysms (Fig. 3.**45**) are also detectable on plain CT as structures of varying hyperdensity.

CT Angiography of the Circle of Willis

CT angiography using bolus contrast injection and spiral acquisition in the arterial phase can detect aneurysms larger than 5 mm (Fig. 3.**46**). This technique uses a slice thickness and table increment of 1 mm. Contrast administration should precede image acquisition by 8 seconds; the exact scan delay can be adjusted after estimating the circulation time. The image data set can be processed to reconstruct a three-dimensional image (Figs. 3.**47**, 3.**48**).

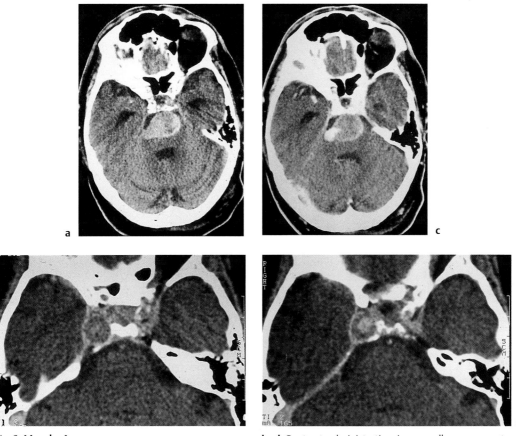

Fig. 3.**44 a–d   Aneurysm.**
a, c Plain CT suggests the diagnosis of a thrombosed aneurysm.

b, d Contrast administration is generally necessary to demonstrate the perfused portion of the aneurysm (basilar artery and internal carotid artery).

Fig. 3.**45 a, b   Heavily calcified aneurysm of the left internal carotid artery.**
a Plain CT shows only a circular pattern of wall calcification.
b Postcontrast CT demonstrates enhancement of the perfused residual lumen.

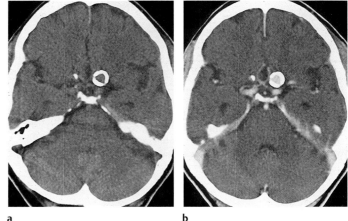

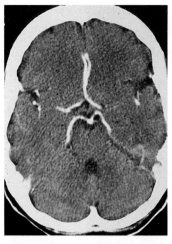

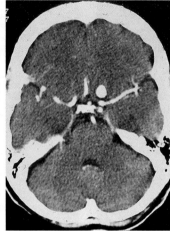

Fig. 3.**46 a, b Aneurysm visualized by spiral CT.** Thin-slice spiral CT images can demonstrate the circle of Willis (**a**) and can define small to medium-sized aneurysms (**b**), such as this aneurysm of the anterior communicating artery.

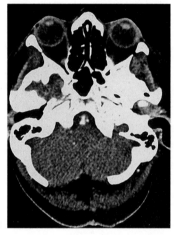

a

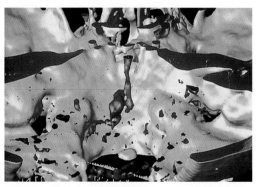

b

Fig. 3.**47 Three-dimensional reconstruction of a vascular segment with an aneurysm.** Today, spiral CT reconstructions can detect even very small aneurysms and define their relationship to the parent vessel.

a A very small aneurysm located near the union of the vertebral arteries.

b Three-dimensional reconstruction clearly shows the dilatation of the left vertebral artery.

MRI

Detection of a clinically suspected acute subarachnoid hemorrhage (day 1–3) is not an indication for MRI. The sensitivity of MRI at this stage is too low, regardless of the type of sequence used. But while CT becomes less sensitive for subacute (day 4–14) and chronic subarachnoid hemorrhage (after day 14) due to dilution effects, MRI becomes more sensitive, as an older hemorrhage generates higher signal intensities. Moderately T2-weighted images and proton-density sequences appear to be the most productive.

MRI is often used in patients with CT-confirmed subarachnoid hemorrhage in the absence of a demonstrable aneurysm. It is very rare, however, to identify a different cause of the hemorrhage or to detect an aneurysm that is angiographically occult due to thrombosis.

■ Follow-Up

Since endoluminal or surgical manipulations in the treatment of an aneurysm can lead to temporary or even permanent occlusion of cerebral supply arteries, and particularly because spastic vascular stenosis in response to hemorrhage can lead to regional ischemia or infarction, CT has an important follow-up role in detecting hypodense infarcted areas.

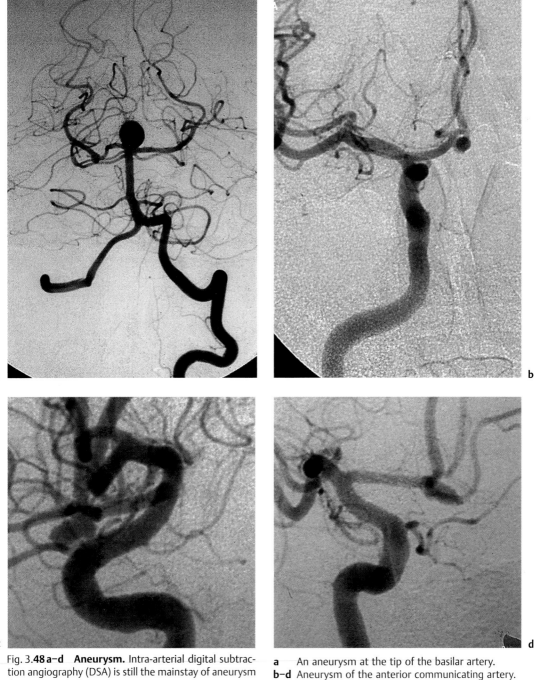

Fig. 3.**48 a–d   Aneurysm.** Intra-arterial digital subtraction angiography (DSA) is still the mainstay of aneurysm diagnosis.

a   An aneurysm at the tip of the basilar artery.
b–d Aneurysm of the anterior communicating artery.

Thromboses (Figs. 3.49–3.54)

Frequency: not a particularly rare CT finding, but easily missed.

Suggestive morphologic findings: bilateral, symmetrical, parasagittal lesions.

Procedure: MRI, angiography if required, conservative therapy.

Other studies: unenhanced MRI can demonstrate the thrombus.

Checklist for scan interpretation:
▶ Visible nonenhancing thrombus?
▶ Collaterals?
▶ Venous infarcts?
▶ Confirmation?

■ Pathogenesis

Thrombosis of the dural sinuses and deep and superficial cerebral veins is among the most commonly missed cerebral diseases. However, when the disease is included in the differential diagnosis, it is easy to make a presumptive diagnosis from the imaging findings.

Basically, all cerebral changes that show a bilateral distribution should raise a suspicion of dural sinus thrombosis, regardless of whether the lesions are hyperdense or hypodense. The bilateral distribution is based on the anatomy of

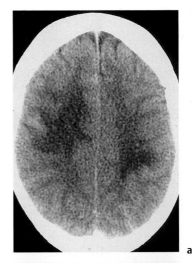

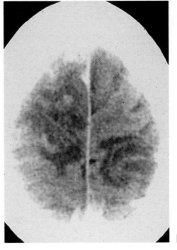

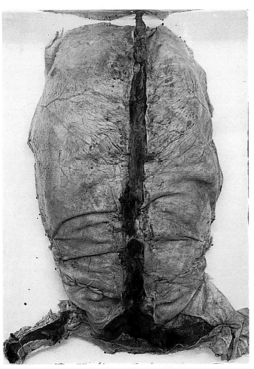

Fig. 3.**49 a–c Dural sinus thrombosis.**

a, b Plain CT shows nearly symmetrical bilateral lesions, suggestive of dural sinus thrombosis. The supraventricular axial scan shows patchy hypodensities with somewhat ill-defined margins in the white matter of both hemispheres. The bilateral, almost symmetrical distribution should raise suspicion of dural sinus thrombosis—specifically, of the superior sagittal sinus. Sinus thrombosis may appear on plain CT as a venous infarct.

c The gross pathologic specimen shows extensive thrombosis primarily of the superior sagittal sinus (from the pathology collection of the Charité Hospital, Berlin).

the venous drainage system, in which both hemispheres drain toward the midline. When this drainage is obstructed, the reflux effect leads to bilateral changes. The CT features of sinus thrombosis are reviewed in Table 3.**2**.

The mortality from undetected dural sinus thrombosis is very high. While the diagnosis of sinus thrombosis can be easily established today using noninvasive (MRI) and invasive studies (venous phase of cerebral angiography), a missed diagnosis will very likely have deleterious consequences. In most cases, however, CT is the initial imaging procedure.

Anatomy of the cerebral venous system. The dural sinuses are venous channels located between the periosteal and meningeal layers of the dura mater. The named sinuses are listed below:

- Superior sagittal sinus
- Inferior sagittal sinus
- Straight sinus
- Transverse sinus
- Sigmoid sinus
- Occipital sinus
- Cavernous sinus
- Sphenoparietal sinus
- Petrosal sinus

The sinuses drain into the internal jugular veins. There is also a system of superficial veins and a system of deep veins. The superficial veins drain into the sinuses, and the deep veins drain into the vein of Galen.

In the superficial venous system, the superior cerebral veins drain blood from the frontal and parietal brain into the superior sagittal sinus. The inferior cerebral veins drain the temporal lobes and portions of the occipital lobe into the transverse sinus and superior petrosal sinus. Anastomoses interconnect the superior and inferior veins and certain other veins (of Trolard, Roland, and Labbé).

One function of the deep veins is to drain portions of the hemispheric white matter and the diencephalon. The vein of Galen drains into the straight sinus, which in turn collects blood from thalamostriate branches, the basilar vein (of Rosenthal), and other veins.

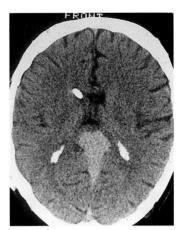

Fig. 3.**50 Hyperdense sinus.** Finding a hyperdense sinus on plain CT scans should raise suspicion of dural sinus thrombosis. Plain scan at the level of the lateral ventricles shows marked hyperdensity, probably of the great cerebral vein. Intraluminal thrombi remain hyperdense for 14 days.

Table 3.**2**   CT signs of venous sinus thrombosis

CT finding	Cause	Term
Plain CT		
• Hyperdense vein	Thrombus in the vein	
• (Bilateral) hypodensity	Venous infarcts	
• (Bilateral) hyperdensity	Intracerebral hemorrhage	
• Small ventricles	Increased intracranial pressure	
Postcontrast CT		
• Filling defect within sinus	Thrombus in the sinus, demarcated by collaterals and enhancing vessel wall	Empty triangle
• Cortical enhancement		
• Enhancement of tentorium	Opacified collaterals	Cord sign
	Dilated superficial veins	

The straight sinus, superior sagittal sinus, and paired transverse sinuses converge at the sinus confluence, which is located on the occipital aspect of the tentorium.

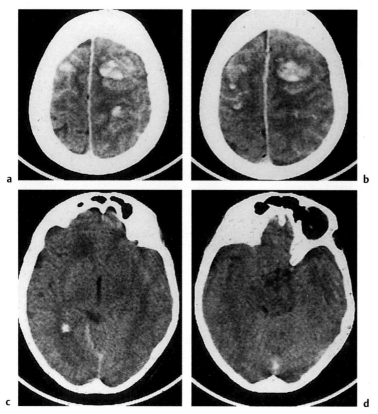

a

b

c

d

Fig. 3.**51 a–d Bilateral symmetrical hyperdensity.** Near-symmetrical bilateral hyperdensities suggest dural sinus thrombosis, regardless of their density. CT scans above and below the ventricular level show poorly marginated hyperdense areas of varying size that represent intracerebral hemorrhages. The patient presented clinically with thrombocytopenia, and the autopsy showed disseminated intravascular coagulation based on a hematologic disorder with initial thrombocytosis.

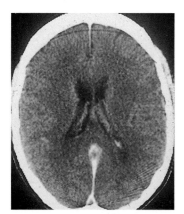

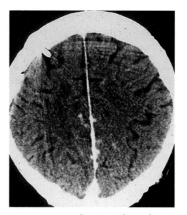

Fig. 3.**52 Dural sinus thrombosis: empty triangle sign.** Contrast-enhanced CT can demonstrate the empty triangle sign, which is characteristic of dural sinus thrombosis. Postcontrast scan at the ventricular level shows dense contrast material surrounding a nonenhancing triangular area (thrombus) in the sinus confluence. Because the sinuses are subject to numerous variations, the finding should be confirmed by magnetic resonance imaging or venography.

Fig. 3.**53 Dural sinus thrombosis: cord sign.** Contrast-enhanced CT shows massive expansion of the superior cerebral vein and incipient collaterals. Thrombosed veins were visible in this case even before contrast administration.

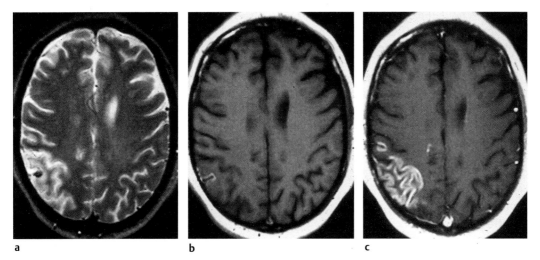

Fig. 3.54 a–c Gyral enhancement on magnetic resonance imaging.
a An infarct in the posterior middle cerebral artery territory is hyperintense on the T2-weighted image.

b Here, the infarct is slightly hemorrhagic.
c The infarct shows intense enhancement after contrast administration.

Emissary veins establish connections with the veins of the galea.

■ Frequency

Dural sinus thrombosis is not a rare condition, particularly in high-risk groups. A 1979 series indicated a postpartum incidence of one in 10,000 live births. Secondary sinus thrombosis has been found in up to 10% of head trauma patients, especially after penetrating injuries or fractures that cross a venous sinus.

■ Clinical Manifestations

Initial symptoms are headache, nausea, and vomiting. Focal and generalized seizures are common, followed by paralysis. Simple sinus thrombosis is often seen postoperatively, during the second half of pregnancy, and during the postpartum period. Purulent dural sinus thrombosis may be secondary to mastoiditis (transverse sinus) or inflammations in the facial region (cavernous sinus).

■ CT Morphology

A *fresh thrombus* leads to increased density of the thrombosed vessel, which appears as a hyperdense structure even on unenhanced scans (cord sign of superficial cerebral veins). After contrast administration, the intraluminal thrombus appears as a nonenhancing area within the opacified vessel (delta sign, empty triangle sign). With more extensive thrombosis, a normally enhancing sinus may not be seen, although one should consider the highly variable anatomy of the dural sinuses in individual patients. Protracted cases lead to *venous infarcts,* which appear as hypodensities or hyperdensities within the drained territory. If the thrombus occludes an unpaired vessel (superior sagittal sinus), the changes show a bilateral and almost symmetrical distribution as described above. *Older thrombi* become isodense on plain CT scans after about 14 days. Collateral signs are small ventricles, areas of cortical enhancement, and enhancement of the tentorium.

Although plain CT scans are crucial in the imaging evaluation of dural sinus thrombosis (clinical findings are often nonspecific), a tailored examination technique can assist in making the diagnosis. Thus, a liberal amount of contrast medium should be used for postcontrast scans: as much as 200 mL instead of the usual 100 mL, if this appears safe. If the material is injected with a pump, an adequate scan delay should be observed. Sagittal or coronal reconstructions are particularly useful for evaluating the deep veins and sigmoid sinus. Care should be taken that the range of coverage is sufficient to include the highest-level axial scan.

■ Differential Diagnosis

The differential diagnosis should include arterial infarcts, intratumoral hemorrhage, eclampsia, and meningitis/encephalitis.

■ References

Recommended for further study

Cerebral infarction
Egelhof T, Jansen O, Winter R, Sartor K. [CT angiography in dissections of the internal carotid artery: value of a new examination technique in comparison with DSA and Doppler ultrasound; in German]. Radiologe 1996; 36: 850–4.
- *Illustrates suggestive findings for various imaging procedures.*

Forsting M, Reith W, von Kummer R, Sartor K. [Radiology of stroke; in German]. Aktuelle Radiol 1993; 3: 209–16.
- *Contains all the information useful to the radiologist; good review of the literature.*

Kjos BO, Brant-Zawadzki M, Young RG. Early CT findings of global central nervous system hypoperfusion. AJNR Am J Neuroradiol 1983; 141: 1227–32.
- *Based on results in 10 patients, differentiates the CT findings of diffuse hypoperfusion from those of territorial and hemodynamic infarcts.*

von Kummer R, Meyding-Mamade U, Forsting M, et al. Sensitivity and prognostic value of early CT in occlusion of the middle cerebral artery trunk. AJNR Am J Neuroradiol 1994; 15: 9–15.
- *Investigates the prognostic value of early CT signs; includes pathophysiologic principles; emphasizes the role of CT vs. MRI in detecting early infarcts.*

Pfister HW, Borasio GD, Dirnagl U, Bauer M, Einhäupl KM. Cerebrovascular complications of bacterial meningitis in adults. Neurology 1992; 42: 1497–1504.
- *Describes complications that radiologists should consider.*

Tomsick TA. Sensitivity and prognostic value of early CT in occlusion of the middle cerebral artery trunk [commentary]. AJNR Am J Neuroradiol 1994; 15: 16–7.
- *A commentary on the preceding article.*

Hypertensive intracerebral hemorrhage
Haymann LA, Pagani JJ, Kirkpatrick JB, Hinck VC. Pathophysiology of acute intracerebral and subarachnoid hemorrhage: applications to MR imaging. Am J Neuroradiol 1989; 10: 457–61.
- *Very important and informative overview.*

Weisberg LA, Stazio A. Nontraumatic frontal lobe hemorrhages: clinical–computed tomographic correlations. Neuroradiology 1988; 30: 500–5.
- *Breakdown of etiologies in 25 patients, with open outcomes in nine.*

Aneurysmal subarachnoid hemorrhage
Mayberg MR, Batjer HH, Dacey R, et al. Guidelines for the management of aneurysmal subarachnoid hemorrhage: a statement for health-care professionals from a special writing group of the Stroke Council. American Heart Association. Stroke 1994; 25: 2315–28.
- *Basic principles for understanding the diagnostic imaging of subarachnoid hemorrhage.*

Vermeulen M. Subarachnoid hemorrhage: diagnosis and treatment. J Neurol 1996; 243: 496–501.
- *The best introduction the authors have found.*

Thrombosis
Kim KS, Walczak TS. Computed tomography of deep cerebral venous thrombosis. J Comput Assist Tomogr 1986; 10: 386–90.

Nagamoto Y, Yanaka K, Kamezaki T, Kobayashi E, Matsumura A, Nose T. Recovery from primary deep cerebral venous sinus thrombosis with recanalisation. Neuroradiology 1995; 37: 645–8.
- *Case report, interesting for its documentation of findings in recovery.*

Rao KCVG, Knipp HC, Wagner EJ. Computed tomographic findings in cerebral sinus and venous thrombosis. Radiology 1981; 140: 391–8.

Thron A, Wessel K, Linden D, Schroth G, Dichgans J. Superior sagittal sinus thrombosis: neuroradiological evaluation and clinical findings. J Neurol 1986; 233: 283–8.
- *Correlates CT and angiographic findings.*

Recent and basic works

Cerebral infarction
Bastianello S, Pierallini A, Colonnese C, et al. Hyperdense middle cerebral artery CT sign. Neuroradiology 1991; 33: 207–11.
- *Helps understand the hyperdense MCA sign.*

Bogousslavsky J, Regli F. Unilateral watershed cerebral infarcts. Neurology 1986; 36: 373–7.
- *Excellent diagrams on watershed infarction.*

Bozzao L, Bastianello S, Fantozzi LM, Angeloni U, Argentino C, Fieschi C. Correlation of angiographic and sequential CT findings in patients with evolving cerebral infarction. AJNR Am J Neuroradiol 1989; 10: 1215–22.
- *Reviews prognostic value of early CT signs of brain infarction.*

Brant-Zawadzki M. CT angiography in acute ischemic stroke: the right tool for the job? AJNR Am J Neuroradiol 1997; 18: 1021–3.
- *Commentary.*

Brown JJ, Hesselink JR, Rothrock JF. MR and CT of lacunar infarcts. AJNR Am J Neuroradiol 1988; 9: 477–82.
- *Describes the higher sensitivity of MRI; includes a concise discussion of lacunar infarcts.*

Duna GF, Calabrese LH. Limitations of invasive modalities in the diagnosis of primary angiitis of the central nervous system. J Rheumatol 1995; 22: 662–7.
- *Table of differential diagnoses for primary vasculitis.*

Fisher CM. Lacunar strokes and infarcts: a review. Neurology 1982; 32: 871–6.
- *Reviews lacunar syndromes from a neurologic perspective.*

Flacke S, Urbach H, Keller E, et al. Middle cerebral artery (MCA) susceptibility sign at susceptibility-based perfusion MR imaging: clinical importance and comparison with hyperdense MCA sign at CT. Radiology 2000; 215: 476–82.
- *Comparison of methods for the diagnosis of acute stroke.*

Knauth M, von Kummer R, Jansen O, Hähnel S, Dörfler A, Sartor K. Potential of CT angiography in acute ischemic stroke. Am J Neuroradiol 1997; 18: 1001–10.
- *Methodologic comparison of CT angiography and digital subtraction angiography (DSA); emphasizes relative importance of CT angiography.*

von Kummer R, Holle R, Grzyska U, et al. Interobserver agreement in assessing early CT signs of middle cerebral artery infarction. AJNR Am J Neuroradiol 1996; 17: 1743–8.
- *Methodologic evaluation of early CT signs of stroke.*

Lev MH, Farkas J, Gemmete JJ et al. Acute stroke: improved nonenhanced CT detection—benefits of soft-copy interpretation by using variable window width and center level settings. Radiology 1999; 213: 150–5.
- ■*This paper emphasizes the advantages of variations in window settings for the diagnosis of stroke.*

Mascalchi M, Bianchi MC, Mangiafico S, et al. MRI and MR angiography of vertebral artery dissection. Neuroradiology 1997; 39: 329–40.
- *Detailed discussion of the disease, with comprehensive bibliography.*

Moore P. Diagnosis and management of isolated angiitis of the central nervous system. Neurology 1989; 39: 167–73.
- *Reviews clinical criteria for the diagnosis of cerebral vasculitis.*

Mull M, Schwarz M, Thron A. Cerebral hemispheric low-flow infarcts in arterial occlusive disease: lesion patterns and angiomorphologic conditions. Stroke 1997; 28: 118–23.
- *Well-organized, easy-to-understand correlation correlation of subcortical infarcts with vascluar findings.*

Nabavi DG, Cenic A, Craen RA et al. CT assessment of cerebral perfusion: experimental validation and initial clinical experience. Radiology 1999; 213: 141–9.

Roberts JM, Redman CWG. Pre-eclampsia: more than pregnancy-induced hypertension. Lancet 1993; 341: 1447–51.
- *Pathophysiologic principles; covers all organ systems.*

Sanders TG, Clayman DA, Sanchez-Ramos L, Vines FS, Russo L. Brain in eclampsia: MR imaging with clinical correlation. Radiology 1991; 180: 475–8.
- *MRI findings in eight women with eclampsia and seizures.*

Schuknecht B, Ratzka M, Hofmann E. The "dense artery sign": major cerebral artery thromboembolism demonstrated by computed tomography. Neuroradiology 1990; 32: 98–103.

Wardlaw JM, Sellar R. A simple practical classification of cerebral infarcts on CT and its interobserver reliability. AJNR Am J Neuroradiol 1994; 15: 1933–9.
- *Includes an interesting literature review.*

Zeumer H, Schonsky B, Sturm KW. Predominant white matter involvement in subcortical arteriosclerotic encephalopathy (Binswanger disease). J Comput Assist Tomogr 1980; 4: 14–9.
- *Presents CT findings in Binswanger disease and correlates them with histology in one case; informative illustrations.*
- *Hypertensive intracerebral hemorrhage*

Pierce JN, Taber KH, Hayman LA. Acute intracranial hemorrhage secondary to thrombocytopenia: CT appearances unaffected by absence of clot retraction. AJNR Am J Neuroradiol 1994; 15: 213–5.
- *Important minor aspect.*

Arteriovenous malformation

Awad IA, Little JR, Akrawi WP, Ahl J. Intracranial dural arteriovenous malformations: factors predisposing to an aggressive neurological course. J Neurosurg 1990; 72: 839–50.
- *Seventeen original cases and meta-analysis of 360 patients.*

Rieger J, Hosten N, Neumann K, et al. Initial clinical experience with spiral CT and 3 D arterial reconstruction in intracranial aneurysms and arteriovenous malformations. Neuroradiology 1996; 38: 245–51.
- *Includes a detailed description of examination technique.*

Reul J, Thron A, Laborde G, Brückmann H. Dural arteriovenous malformations at the base of the anterior cranial fossa: report of nine cases. Neuroradiology 1993; 35: 388–93.
- *Correlates CT and angiographic findings in nine patients.*

Aneurysmal subarachnoid hemorrhage

Chakeres DW, Bryan RN. Acute subarachnoid hemorrhage: in vitro comparison of magnetic resonance and computed tomography. AJNR Am J Neuroradiol 1986; 7: 223–8.
- *Clear explanation of the phenomena underlying the contrasts between the two modalities.*

Chrysikopoulos H, Papanikolaou N, Pappas J, et al. Acute subarachnoid hemorrhage: detection with magnetic resonance imaging. Br J Radiol 1996; 69: 601–9.
- *Describes a promising approach to the MRI diagnosis of subarachnoid hemorrhage.*

Dillo W, Brassel F, Becker H. [Possibilities and limitations of CT angiography in comparison to DSA in intracranial aneurysm; in German]. RöFo Fortschr Geb Röntgenstr Neuen Bildgeb Verfahr 1996; 165: 227–31.
- *Somewhat pessimistic assessment of CT angiography—compare with more optimistic assessments: Casey SO et al., "Operator dependence of cerebral CT angiography in the detection of aneurysms," AJNR Am J Neuroradiol 1997; 18: 790–2; and Heinz ER, "Prospective evaluation of the circle of Willis with three-dimensional CT angiography in patients with suspected intracranial aneurysms," AJNR Am J Neuroradiol 1995; 16: 1579.*

Duong H, Melancon D, Tampieri D, Ethier E. The negative angiogram in subarachnoid hemorrhage. Neuroradiology 1996; 38: 15–9.
- *Also important for understanding the clinical presentation in sectional imaging studies.*

Durand ML, Calderwood SB, Weber DJ, et al. Acute bacterial meningitis in adults: a review of 493 episodes. N Engl J Med 1993; 328: 21–8.

Gosselin MV, Vieco PT. Active hemorrhage of intracranial aneurysms: diagnosis by CT angiography. J Comput Assist Tomogr 1997; 21: 22–4.
- *Provides a realistic assessment of the importance of CT angiography.*

Ida M, Kurisu Y, Yamashita M. MR angiography of ruptured aneurysms in acute subarachnoid hemorrhage. AJNR Am J Neuroradiol 1997; 18: 1025–32.
- *Update on state-of-the-art diagnosis.*

Korogi Y, Takahashi M, Katada K et al. Intracranial aneurysms: detection with three-dimensional CT angiography with volume rendering—comparison with conventional angiographic and surgical findings. Radiology 1999; 211: 497–506.
- *CT angiography in the diagnosis of intracranial aneurysms.*

Liu Y, Hopper KD, Mauger DT, Addis KA. CT angiographic measurement of the carotid artery: optimizing visualization by manipulating window and level settings and contrast material attenuation. Radiology 2000; 217: 494–500.

Liu Y, Hopper KD, Mauger DT et al. Can noninvasive imaging accurately depict intracranial aneurysms? A systematic review. Radiology 2000; 217: 361–70.
- *CT angiography in the diagnosis of intracranial aneurysms.*

Mendelsohn DB, Moss ML, Chason DP, Muphree S, Casey S. Acute purulent leptomeningitis mimicking subarachnoid hemorrhage on CT. J Comput Assist Tomogr 1994; 18: 126–8.
- *A rare differential diagnosis that should nevertheless not be missed.*

Noguchi K, Ogawa T, Fujita H, et al. Filling defect sign in CT diagnosis of ruptured aneurysm. Neuroradiology 1997; 39: 480–2.
- *Aid to locating aneurysms in CT.*

Rieger J, Hosten N, Lemke AJ, Langer R, Lanksch WR, Felix R. [Cerebral aneurysms: their 3-dimensional imaging with spiral CT; in German]. RöFo Fortschr Geb Röntgenstr Neuen Bildgeb Verfahr 1994; 160: 204–9.

Quagliarello V, Scheld WM. Bacterial meningitis: pathogenesis, pathophysiology, and progress. N Engl J Med 1992; 327: 864–72.

Sadato N, Numaguchi Y, Rigamonti D, Salcman M, Gellad FE, Kishikawa T. Bleeding patterns in ruptured posterior fossa aneurysms: a CT study. J Comput Assist Tomogr 1991; 15: 612–7.

van der Wee N, Rinkel GJE, Hasan D, van Gijn J. Detection of subarachnoid haemorrhage on early CT: is lumbar puncture still needed after a negative scan? J Neurol Neurosurg Psychiatry 1995; 58: 357–9.
- *Includes a description of false-negative CT findings.*

Yoshimoto Y, Ochiai C, Kawamata K, Endo M, Nagai M. Aqueductal blood clot as a cause of acute hydrocephalus in subarachnoid hemorrhage. AJNR Am J Neuroradiol 1996; 17: 1183–6.
- *Focuses on MRI but describes a CT pitfall.*

Thrombosis

Kesava PP. Recanalization of the falcine sinus after venous sinus thrombosis. Am J Neuroradiol 1996; 17: 1646–8.

Konno S, Numaguchi Y, Shrier DA, Qian J, Sinkin RA. Unusual manifestation of a vein of Galen malformation: value of CT angiography. AJNR Am J Neuroradiol 1996; 17: 1423–6.
- *Describes an effective application of spiral CT.*

Madan A, Sluzewski M, van Rooij WJJ, Tijssen CC, Teepen JJM. Thrombosis of the deep cerebral veins: CT and MRI findings with pathologic correlation. Neuroradiology 1997; 39: 777–80.
- *Case report, including illustration of autopsy findings.*

Numerow LM, Fong TC, Wallace CJ. Pseudodelta sign on computed tomography: an indication of bilateral interhemispheric hemorrhage. Can Assoc Radiol J 1994; 45: 23–7.

Oguz M, Aksungur EH, Soyupak SK, Yildirim AU. Vein of Galen and sinus thrombosis with bilateral thalamic infarcts in sickle cell anemia: CT follow-up and angiographic demonstration. Neuroradiology 1994; 36: 155–6.
- *Good image documentation and description of diagnostic signs.*

4 Inflammatory Diseases

Brain Abscess, Bacterial

Frequency: a common computed tomography (CT) diagnosis.

Suggestive morphologic findings: ring-enhancing lesion with smooth margins, often located near the frontal sinus or petrous temporal bone.

Procedure: antibiotic therapy, surgery if required.

Other studies: magnetic resonance imaging (MRI) can detect contrast enhancement with higher sensitivity. It is especially useful for detecting or excluding accompanying meningeal and ependymal reactions. Also better than CT for detection of complicating dural sinus thrombosis.

Checklist for scan interpretation:
▶ Number and location of enhancing lesions?
▶ Proximity to frontal sinus or petrous bone?
▶ Inflammatory changes in frontal sinus or petrous bone (bone window)?
▶ Meningeal enhancement?
▶ Mass effect (midline shift, ventricular compression, etc.)?

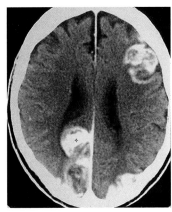

Fig. 4.**1 Otogenic brain abscess.** Postcontrast CT shows a digitate pattern of hypodensity in the left temporal lobe, representing perifocal edema. The abscess itself appears as a ring-enhancing structure bordering the calvarium above the petrous bone.

■ Pathogenesis

Bacterial brain abscesses can develop in a variety of clinical settings. Many brain abscesses result from an infection of the frontal sinus or petrous bone that has extended intracranially (Fig. 4.**1**). In both cases, the normally air-filled portions of these bones become filled with fluid, providing a clue to the etiology of the intraparenchymal changes.

Multiple brain abscesses may develop as a complication of sepsis (Fig. 4.**2**) or endocarditis (Fig. 4.**3**). In the latter case, infected thrombi are shed from the diseased valves and disseminate to the brain by the hematogenous route. The blood currents tend to carry the septic emboli through the internal carotid artery and

Fig. 4.**2 Septic brain embolism.** Postcontrast CT shows conspicuous enhancing lesions in the right occipital and left frontoparietal areas, and a less prominent lesion in the left occipital area. The gyral changes show the ring-enhancing pattern typical of brain abscess.

into the middle cerebral arteries. Once septic emboli have been seeded into the territory of the middle cerebral artery (MCA), a brain abscess begins to form. This occurs more or less independently of the specific etiology. The initial stage is a focal cerebritis, which soon develops central necrosis and is surrounded by perifocal edema. With time, the lesion forms a capsule and "ripens" into an established brain abscess.

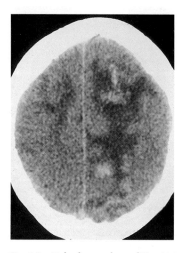

Fig. 4.**3** **Valvular endocarditis.** Noncontrast CT in a patient with clinically confirmed valvular endocarditis shows bilateral string-of-beads hypodensities with central hemorrhages, mainly on the right side. The hyperdense areas on the plain scan did not enhance after contrast administration.

The bacterial inflammatory process can have various central nervous system (CNS) manifestations. The brain abscess may be accompanied by localized or more extensive meningeal inflammation (Fig. 4.**4**), subdural empyema formation, ventriculitis (Fig. 4.**5**), or dural sinus thrombosis. Bacterial contamination from a penetrating head injury can also result in a brain abscess (Fig. 4.**6**).

■ Frequency

The incidence of brain abscess is increased in patients with pulmonary disease (especially pulmonary arteriovenous fistulae or bronchiectasis), patients with endocarditis, and immunosuppressed patients. Males predominate by about a 2:1 ratio.

■ Clinical Manifestations

While purulent forms of meningitis typically present with nuchal rigidity, headache, and hypersensitivity to light and sound, the clinical picture of brain abscess is dominated by focal neurologic symptoms. These may be accompanied by signs and symptoms of meningeal irritation.

■ CT Morphology

The typical CT appearance of brain abscess is that of a ring-enhancing lesion with central

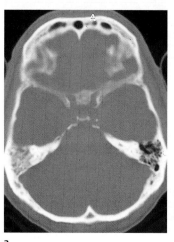

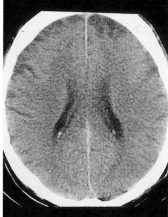

Fig. 4.**4 a, b** **Otogenic meningitis.**
a The bone-window scan shows opacification of the right mastoid due to inflammatory disease.
b Plain CT in a patient with clinically confirmed meningitis shows bilateral cortical hypodensities that represent secondary infarcts due to vasculitis. The meningitis itself is not demonstrable on CT scans.

a

b

Fig. 4.**5 a, b Brain abscess with ependymitis.**

a Noncontrast CT shows ventricular enlargement and bilateral occipital hypodensities, including a rounded hypodensity on the left side.

b A scan after intravenous contrast administration shows rim-enhancing lesions in the left and right occipital areas. The left occipital abscess appears to have ruptured into the ventricular system. Note the enhancing ventricular wall and the additional enhancing foci to the left of the ventricle.

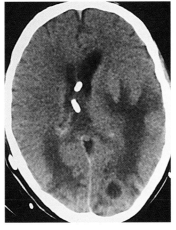 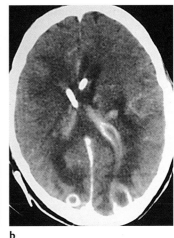

a   b

necrosis and perifocal edema (see Fig. 4.**1**). The ring is usually thin and uniform, without scalloping. As noted above, abscesses due to sinusitis are located either in the frontal lobe or in the middle or posterior cranial fossa in close proximity to the petrous bone. Brain abscesses secondary to endocarditis tend to be small, multiple, and located at the gray–white matter junction in the territory of the MCA.

The early cerebritis stage may not enhance after contrast administration. These patients require serial examinations at close intervals. If the initial examination is delayed, it can be difficult to distinguish brain abscess from other lesions that show a ring pattern of contrast enhancement. Metastases, glioblastoma, and other etiologies should be considered. CT may direct attention to complications that require surgical intervention, such as extensive mass effect. As stated earlier, it is important to recognize subdural fluid collections with accompanying meningeal enhancement that would signify a subdural empyema. Dural sinus thrombosis is not uncommon. A deep abscess may rupture into the ventricular system, giving rise to ventriculitis, with contrast enhancement of the ventricular wall (Fig. 4.**5**).

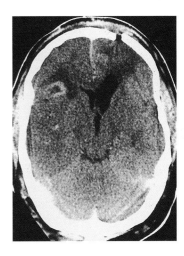

Fig. 4.**6 Abscess secondary to head trauma.** This scan demonstrates a gaping fracture site in the left frontal calvarium. To the right of the frontal horn there is a ring-enhancing lesion, representing an abscess.

■ Differential Diagnosis

Among the various diseases that can produce a ring-shaped enhancement pattern, the features of brain abscess are often the most characteristic. Apart from the typical location of sinugenic abscesses, the ring itself tends to have distinctive features: it is usually thin, circular, and of uniform diameter. By contrast, glioblastoma usually has a scalloped rim, while small tumors tend to have an enhancing rim of varying thickness.

Tuberculosis

Frequency: once very rare, but the incidence has been increasing in recent years.

Suggestive diagnostic findings: basal meningitis.

Procedure: cerebrospinal fluid (CSF) examination.

Other studies: MRI is much more sensitive than CT for detecting meningitis (the most common pattern of CNS involvement).

Checklist for scan interpretation:
▶ Hydrocephalus?
▶ Meningeal enhancement? Enhancement in the basal cisterns?
▶ Enhancement of the ventricular wall?
▶ Enhancing lesions in the brain parenchyma?
▶ Evidence of ischemic infarcts?

■ Pathogenesis

Cerebral or meningeal involvement by tuberculosis is almost always a result of hematogenous spread. The causative organism in nearly all cases is *Mycobacterium tuberculosis*.

Most cases start as a pulmonary infection that spreads swiftly to other organs by the hematogenous or lymphogenous route.

The most common CNS manifestation of the disease is meningitis (Fig. 4.**7**) or meningoencephalitis.

Other manifestations of intracranial infection are abscess formation and the development of multiple tuberculomas. Involvement of the cranium itself is extremely rare.

Involvement of the meninges, ependyma, and choroid plexus is characterized histologically by typical inflammatory reactions and, in severe cases, by caseating necrosis. Cranial nerve involvement is very common, and even the optic nerve may be affected. When meningitis develops, the associated vasculitis can result in areas of infarction. A frequent complication is hydrocephalus, with its associated clinical manifestations.

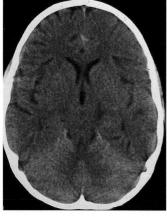 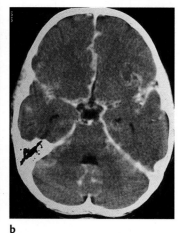

Fig. 4.7 a, b   Meningitis.
a Noncontrast CT scan in a 10-year-old child shows no significant abnormalities.
b Scan after contrast administration shows ubiquitous enhancement of the meninges, particularly in the tentorium and sylvian fissure on the left side and within the interhemispheric fissure. Changes over the hemispheres are less clearly defined due to the proximity of the calvarium.

a   b

■ Frequency

The incidence of tuberculosis has been rising, due in part to the increasing number of immunosuppressed patients. It is likely, therefore, that the incidence of CNS involvement by tuberculosis will also continue to increase.

■ Clinical Manifestations

Headache and nuchal rigidity are seen initially. Cranial nerve involvement is frequent, and is manifested by corresponding deficits. Consciousness changes range from confusion to neuropsychiatric disorders.

Focal neurologic deficits may result from vasculitis-induced infarction or intracerebral tuberculomas. Hydrocephalus is a frequent complication caused by involvement of the basal meninges and manifested by headache, nausea, vomiting, and impaired consciousness.

Children are commonly affected.

Untreated, the disease has a fatal outcome. If treatment is initiated in time, the patient may recover, although cranial nerve deficits and focal neurologic symptoms may persist. Even with adequate treatment, however, some patients may develop an organic brain syndrome or epileptic seizures.

CSF examination is diagnostic, showing a low glucose concentration, elevated protein, and a threefold to fourfold increase in cellularity. Lumbar spinal puncture should be withheld if obstructive hydrocephalus is present.

■ CT Morphology

Hydrocephalus is a frequent complication in many patients and must be described. If basal meningitis is present, it is often manifested on CT by contrast enhancement in the basal cisterns (Fig. 4.8).

Brain infarction due to vasculitis, seen also in other forms of meningitis, can have various CT manifestations. The infarcts may be unilateral or bilateral, symmetrical or asymmetrical, and may involve the cortex and white matter in various combinations. Perforating arteries may be affected by vasculitis.

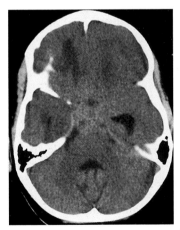 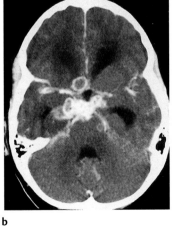 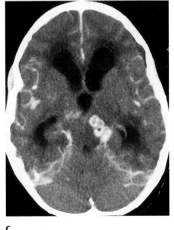

a   b   c

Fig. 4.8 a–c Tuberculous meningitis.
a Even plain CT in this 7-year-old child shows obliteration of the basal cisterns, with ill-defined hyperdensity.

b Scan after contrast administration shows the basal enhancement and ring-enhancing abscesses (mainly to the right of the midline) that are typical of tuberculous meningitis.
c Another abscess is compressing the brain stem from the left side. Hydrocephalus is also present.

Tuberculomas appear as intraparenchymal focal lesions, with a nodular or ring pattern of contrast enhancement. Tuberculous abscesses usually show a ring configuration, but are considerably larger than tuberculomas, which are distinguished by their small diameter. Meningeal involvement is marked by predominantly basal enhancement of the meninges, and ventricular involvement by enhancement of the ventricular wall. The choroid plexus shows marked contrast enhancement, even in the absence of disease.

Differential Diagnosis

Meningeal enhancement on postcontrast CT, even when basal and occurring in a pediatric patient, is seen in various types of meningitis and is not pathognomonic for the tuberculous form. The same is true of ventriculitis. When nodular or ring enhancement is seen with tuberculomas, it is necessary to consider the entire spectrum of differential diagnoses for ring-enhancing lesions. There is no morphologic characteristic that is specific for tuberculosis.

Brain infarcts due to vasculitis may be seen in all forms of meningitis. It is important to recognize the infarcts and relate them causally to meningitis, which is not always associated with meningeal enhancement.

Sarcoidosis

Frequency: cerebral involvement is rare.

Suggestive morphologic findings: enhancing tissue in the basal cisterns, optic chiasm, and pituitary stalk.

Procedure: watch for lesion regression in response to cortisone therapy.

Other studies: MRI is more accurate for the sagittal and coronal localization of lesions.

Checklist for scan interpretation:
▶ Involvement of the hypothalamus or pituitary?
▶ Hydrocephalus?

Pathogenesis

Sarcoidosis may have an infectious etiology, but this is unproved. Pulmonary involvement is most common. CNS involvement is rare, with an incidence rate in single figures.

Frequency

Approximately 3% of patients with sarcoidosis show isolated CNS involvement with no apparent involvement of other organ systems.

Clinical Manifestations

A great many patients with sarcoidosis also have diabetes insipidus. CNS involvement, including cervical cord disease, is very often misinterpreted as a tumor and is not correctly diagnosed until surgery. It is important to consider sarcoidosis in the differential diagnosis: the basal location of the lesions, together with involvement of the optic chiasm, should raise the possibility of sarcoidosis.

CT Morphology

CT after contrast administration shows enhancing, smoothly marginated tissue in the basal cisterns, which may extend into the brain parenchyma along small penetrating vessels. On the whole, the enhancing areas are clearly demarcated from the surrounding brain (noncaseating granulomas).

Unenhanced CT findings may be limited to nonvisualization of the basal CSF spaces.

Differential Diagnosis

The second major granulomatous disease, tuberculosis, may show features similar to those of sarcoidosis, but its clinical presentation is more dramatic. Low-grade primary brain tumors may also cause obstruction of the basal CSF spaces, in which case coronal MRI— e.g., using fluid-attenuated inversion recovery (FLAIR) sequences— can define the mass as originating in the brain parenchyma.

Herpes Simplex Encephalitis

Frequency: rare.

Suggestive morphologic findings: decreased density, followed in later stages by contrast enhancement and possible hemorrhagic imbibition in the mesial temporal lobe.

Procedure: immediate treatment.

Other studies: MRI is more sensitive than CT, especially for early detection, and is the imaging modality of choice. Single-photon emission computed tomography (SPECT) with ^{99m}Tc hexamethyl propyleneamine-oxime (HM-PAO) shows increased regional cerebral blood flow in the temporal region.

Checklist for scan interpretation:
▶ Decreased density in the sylvian fissure?
▶ Hemorrhages in that area?
▶ Give urgent recommendation for MRI.

Pathogenesis

Herpes simplex infections of the CNS are caused by two major types of organism: herpes simplex virus type 1 (HSV-1) and herpes simplex virus type 2 (HSV-2).

HSV-1, which persists in the gasserian ganglion and causes orofacial herpes, is responsible for encephalitis in adults.

HSV-2 causes genital herpes, and incites a diffuse encephalitis in neonates when transmitted from the infected maternal genitalia at birth. This diffuse encephalitis contrasts with the predominantly temporal-lobe encephalitis caused by HSV-1.

Frequency

Herpes encephalitis has an estimated annual incidence of one in 750 000 to one in 100 000. Males and females are affected equally.

Clinical Manifestations

The HSV-1 organism resides in the oropharynx of approximately 95 % of the adult population. HSV-1 encephalitis typically affects immunocompetent patients. HSV-2 encephalitis in newborns has an estimated incidence of one in 5000 to one in 10 000 births. HSV-2 neonatal encephalitis has a poor prognosis, both in terms of survival and in the persistence of serious sequelae. Impaired consciousness is the clinical hallmark of herpes encephalitis in the acute stage. Often this is preceded by a prodromal stage, with lethargy, fever, and sore neck. Epileptic seizures are not uncommon. While the disease is usually fatal when untreated, the mortality rate with virostatic therapy has fallen to less than one-third. Today the diffuse neonatal form of encephalitis is seen increasingly in patients with acquired immune deficiency syndrome (AIDS), and early trial administration of virostatic drugs is replacing the former practice of brain biopsy.

CT Morphology

MRI has become the imaging modality of choice for herpes simplex encephalitis owing to its higher sensitivity. CT is used only as an initial imaging procedure in cases that have not yet been definitively diagnosed.

Both plain and postcontrast CT scans generally show no abnormalities during the first two days after the infection is acquired. Starting on about the third day, CT shows increasing hypodensity in the temporal lobe region (Fig. 1.**19**). After intravenous contrast administration, the lesions may show a diffuse, striate, or gyral/meningeal pattern of enhancement. The region may show swelling, with a mass effect on the ventricular system. Increased density due to hemorrhage has also been described. If the patient survives the herpes encephalitis, the primarily affected brain areas generally show extensive atrophic changes due to volume loss.

■ Differential Diagnosis

The greatest aid to differential diagnosis is the typical location of the changes demonstrated by CT and MRI. Even atypical or normal-appearing findings on CT scans and even MRI do not exclude herpes simplex encephalitis in patients with equivocal clinical findings. Early treatment is crucial in all cases.

■ Follow-Up

In all cases in which the diagnosis of herpes encephalitis has been established or is merely suspected, MRI should be used for further investigation and follow-up.

Toxoplasmosis

Frequency: toxoplasmosis is the leading cause of radiologic brain abnormalities in AIDS patients.

Suggestive morphologic findings: ring-enhancing lesion that regresses in response to specific therapy.

Procedure: medical treatment for *Toxoplasma gondii*, follow-up.

Other studies: MRI is somewhat more sensitive, especially in detecting concomitant meningitic changes.

Checklist for scan interpretation:
▶ Calcifications?
▶ Contrast enhancement, including therapy-induced changes?

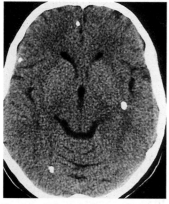

Fig. 4.**9 Congenital toxoplasmosis.** Noncontrast CT demonstrates multiple hyperdense lesions, which represent parenchymal calcifications due to congenital toxoplasmosis.

■ Pathogenesis

Cerebral toxoplasmosis is caused by the protozoan parasite *Toxoplasma gondii.* The course of the disease varies, depending on the patient's age and immune status.

An initial maternal infection can lead to congenital transmission by the transplacental route. The course depends on the age of the pregnancy, and can range from spontaneous abortion to an almost asymptomatic course characterized only by persistent intracerebral calcifications (Fig. 4.**9**).

Initial infection in adults is due to contact with infected cat feces or the ingestion of infected meat. Immunocompetent individuals become seropositive and may develop non-specific symptoms such as lymphadenitis. Cerebral manifestations are extremely rare.

Cerebral involvement is observed in immunosuppressed patients—those with congenital immune deficiency or acquired immune deficiency due to human immunodeficiency virus (HIV) infection, organ transplantation, etc.—and involves reactivation of a previous infection.

The disease is most prevalent in AIDS patients, in whom cerebral toxoplasmosis is perhaps the leading cause of focal neurologic symptoms.

■ Frequency

Toxoplasmosis is the most common opportunistic infection in immunosuppressed patients, and is particularly common in the HIV-infected population. In a series of 200 HIV patients with neurologic symptoms, an initial CT examination was negative in 40% of the patients, 5% of whom subsequently showed progression of symptoms and/or abnormalities on CT scans. Thirty-eight percent of the patients showed only cerebral atrophy, and 7% of those subsequently developed a detectable toxoplasmosis infection. The final 22% had at least one detectable lesion on initial CT examination.

■ Clinical Manifestations

Neonatal toxoplasmosis is characterized by a triad of signs:

- Chorioretinitis
- Hydrocephalus
- Intracranial calcifications

The very rare cerebral involvement in immunocompetent patients usually consists of a diffuse encephalitis, whereas focal changes tend to occur in immunosuppressed patients. The encephalitis in immunocompetent patients is manifested by headache, meningism, seizures, and mental disturbance.

Some 30–40% of AIDS patients develop cerebral toxoplasmosis during the course of their disease. The dominant clinical features are hemiparesis, sensory disturbances, and aphasia. Analgesic-resistant headache is also observed. Mental disturbance and epileptic seizures each occur in more than one-third of patients.

■ CT Morphology

Cerebral toxoplasmosis is of special importance in the imaging of AIDS, because positive serologic tests usually cannot be obtained in these immunoincompetent patients. As a rule, cases in which cerebral toxoplasmosis is suspected or focal brain lesions have already been detected by CT are managed by pharmacologic treatment with CT follow-up. Unenhanced CT frequently shows diffuse hypodensities in the white matter. Usually, the causative lesions in immunocompromised patients are toxoplasmosis foci, which enhance strongly after contrast administration (Fig. 4.**10**).

A typical feature on postcontrast scans is the "asymmetric target sign" (Fig. 4.**11**), which consists of an enhancing ring with a wall of irregular thickness.

The lesions are most commonly located in the basal ganglia region, at the subcortical gray–white matter junction, and in the thalamus. Since the CT findings are not

Fig. 4.**10 a, b** **Toxoplasmosis.** Postcontrast CT scans at two different levels through the ventricles show multiple intensely enhancing lesions. The outer margins of the lesions are ill-defined, and comparison with the hypodense, digitate edema shows that most of the lesions are located at the gray–white matter junction (differentiation from lymphoma).

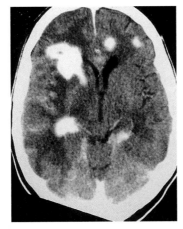

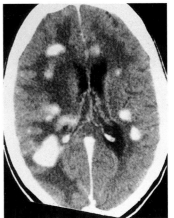

a   b

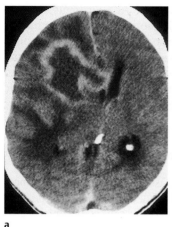 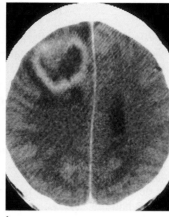

Fig. 4.**11 a, b Toxoplasmosis.** Both contrast-enhanced images (double-dose delay) demonstrate the asymmetric target sign that is characteristic of cerebral toxoplasmosis.

a   b

pathognomonic, stereotactic biopsy is of major importance in patients with therapy-resistant lesions. It is essential to exclude cerebral lymphoma, which is more common in immunosuppressed than immunocompetent patients and is highly responsive to radiotherapy.

Problems relating to the diagnosis of congenital toxoplasmosis and infections in the immune-competent population are of minor interest compared with the problems of CT neuroimaging in patients with AIDS.

Intrauterine infection leads to intracerebral calcifications that can be detected throughout the patient's lifetime. No detailed reports are available on the CT appearance of toxoplasmosis in immunocompetent individuals.

■ Differential Diagnosis

It should be borne in mind that even findings that are characteristic of toxoplasmosis may have other causes. Differential diagnosis in the AIDS population should include tuberculous lesions and cryptococcosis.

Differentiation from CNS lymphoma is of major clinical importance. A periventricular location is more characteristic of lymphoma, while lesions located at the gray–white junction are more typical of toxoplasmosis. These diseases cannot be differentiated with complete confidence, however, and enhancing cerebral lesions that are refractory to treatment should be evaluated by stereotactic biopsy to ensure that the opportunity for radiotherapy is not missed.

■ Follow-Up

CT has a particularly important role in evaluating the response to antitoxoplasmotic therapy. It is essential to distinguish the disease from CNS lymphoma, but often this is not accomplished at the initial diagnosis.

Cryptococcosis

Frequency: rare, but reported to be the second most common opportunistic CNS infection, after toxoplasmosis, in the HIV-infected population.

Suggestive morphologic findings: CT often shows multiple ring-enhancing lesions with accompanying edema. Basal meningitis or granuloma may be present.

Procedure: CSF examination.

Other studies: MRI is more sensitive.

Pathogenesis

Cryptococcosis is caused by the fungus *Cryptococcus neoformans.* The lung is almost always the primary site, and the infection then spreads hematogenously to other sites.

Frequency

Cryptococcosis is the second most common opportunistic CNS infection in HIV-infected patients after toxoplasmosis, accounting for approximately 13% of complications (including tumors and viral infections).

Clinical Manifestations

CNS manifestations range from granulomatous and gelatinous parenchymal involvement to meningitis. Cryptococcosis granulomas are very characteristic tumor-like lesions, and are known as *torulomas* or cryptococcomas.

The disease starts with nonspecific symptoms such as headache and nausea. The incidence is higher in AIDS patients (Fig. 4.**12**).

CT Morphology

As in other forms of meningitis, CT changes are visible only in pronounced cases. They include contrast enhancement in the basal cisterns, creating a pattern that is easily mistaken for tuberculous meningitis.

The torulomas of cryptococcosis resemble metastatic tumors on CT scans, appearing as focal lesions with a nodular or ring pattern of contrast enhancement.

Differential Diagnosis

As mentioned, the CT findings are nonspecific and may be confused with metastases, meningioma, and tuberculoma.

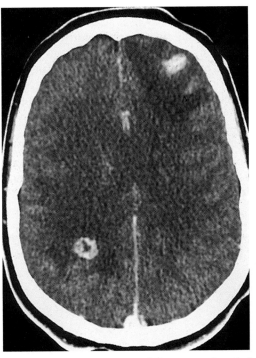

Fig. 4.**12** **Cryptococcosis.** CT defines two subcortical white-matter lesions: a ring-shaped lesion in the right parieto-occipital area and a more nodular lesion in the left frontal area. Both are associated with white-matter edema. These lesions are not specific for cryptococcosis. The patient also had thoracic involvement with spinal symptoms. Biopsy of the left frontal cerebral lesion established the diagnosis.

Neurocysticercosis

Frequency: rare, seen only after residence in an endemic area.

Suggestive morphologic findings: cystic lesion with an enhancing rim.

Procedure: diagnosis is based on history, serology, and imaging findings. Anthelmintic therapy is indicated.

Other studies: MRI is more sensitive for detecting subarachnoid dissemination.

Checklist for scan interpretation:
▶ Cellular or racemose form?
▶ Hydrocephalus?

■ Pathogenesis

Neurocysticercosis refers to invasion of the brain by larvae of the pork tapeworm *Taenia solium.* The infection is acquired in endemic areas, usually third-world countries. Ingested organisms invade the intestinal mucosa and spread hematogenously to various organs, very often including the brain, where larvae develop and may infest the cerebral parenchyma, subarachnoid space, ventricular system, and even the spinal canal.

Muscle is another very common site of involvement. Encysted larvae within muscle are especially prone to form calcifications. Larvae in human tissue incite an inflammatory reaction that is responsible for the clinical symptoms and imaging findings.

■ Frequency

The infection rate approaches 4% of the population in some infested regions. CNS involvement occurs in 60–92% of infected patients.

■ Clinical Manifestations

Neurocysticercosis may present clinically with seizures, hydrocephalus, or mental disturbance, depending on the pattern of CNS involvement.

Epileptic seizures are most common with parenchymal involvement. This may consist of multiple lesions, and can lead to focal neurologic symptoms.

The cysts (Fig. 4.**13**) can also occur within the ventricles or in the subarachnoid spaces.

Involvement of the basal cisterns is common, and leads to hydrocephalus with signs of increased intracranial pressure. The racemose form of cysticercus is an extreme variant that may occur at this location. Large racemose cysts in the basal cisterns have a doubtful prognosis.

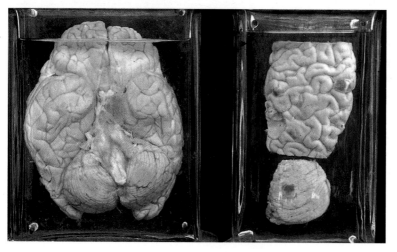

Fig. 4.**13 Neurocysticercosis.** Cystic lesions in the basal cisterns and on the surface of the brain are due to disseminated subarachnoid cysticercosis.

CT Morphology

CT imaging of the brain shows abnormalities in the majority of patients with neurocysticercosis. It is common to find cystic lesions of the brain parenchyma, which may produce a local or more extensive mass effect (sulcal effacement, ventricular compression). The cysts often show a circular or elliptical pattern of peripheral rim enhancement (Fig. 4.**14**). Evolution of the lesion is characterized by a fading of contrast enhancement (Fig. 4.**15**), followed by calcification of the cyst wall. MRI, with its higher contrast resolution, is better for evaluating contrast enhancement (Fig. 4.**16**).

In the frequent cases in which subarachnoid cysts cause hydrocephalus, CT can demonstrate the resulting ventricular enlargement.

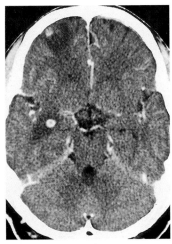

Fig. 4.**14** **Neurocysticercosis.** Typical CT appearance. CT shows a ring-enhancing lesion approximately 1 cm in diameter in the right temporal lobe, and another in the right frontal lobe. Each lesion is associated with a small area of perifocal edema.

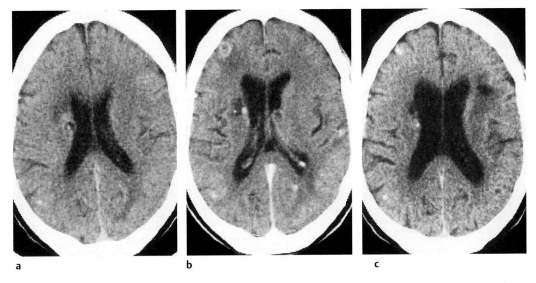

a b c

Fig. 4.**15 a–c** **Evolution of neurocysticercosis.**
a The initial CT examination demonstrates a cystic-solid lesion with mild perifocal edema and a faintly enhancing rim next to the right lateral ventricle.
b Scan 6 months later shows cystic transformation of this lesion, as well as a new ring-enhancing lesion in the right frontal lobe.

c Scan 18 months after the initial examination shows regression of the right periventricular cystic lesion, which no longer enhances. Contrast enhancement of the right frontal lesion has diminished, and there is less perifocal edema.

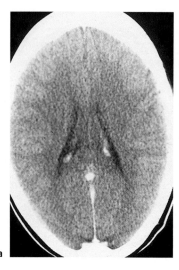

a

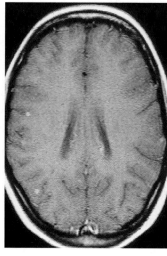

b

Fig. 4.**16 a, b Neurocysticerco-sis.** These images illustrate the superior sensitivity of magnetic resonance imaging (MRI) in neurocysticercosis.
a Contrast-enhanced CT shows no abnormalities.
b Contrast-enhanced MRI shows at least three small enhancing lesions in the right parietal area and equivocal lesions in the left parietal area.

■ **Differential Diagnosis**

The differential diagnosis in later stages should include other brain diseases that can lead to calcifications: infectious diseases, brain tumors such as oligodendroglioma, and tuberous sclerosis.

Nocardiosis

> **Frequency:** rare; occurs in immunosuppressed patients.
>
> **Suggestive morphologic findings:** multiple, more or less well-circumscribed nodules or cystic abscesses.
>
> **Procedure:** the diagnosis is established by isolating the organism in culture.
>
> **Other studies:** MRI is more sensitive for demonstrating contrast enhancement and defining the cystic nature of the lesion in T2-weighted images.
>
> **Checklist for scan interpretation:**
> ▶ Solitary lesion or multiple lesions?

■ **Pathogenesis**

Nocardia is a gram-positive aerobic bacterium that most commonly infects patients who are immunosuppressed. The infection may involve the lung, bone, CNS, and other organs. It may be acquired by dust inhalation or by direct inoculation through an opening in the skin (trauma, drug abuse, dialysis fistula, etc.).

Hematogenous dissemination to the CNS leads to formation of a brain abscess.

■ **Frequency**

Nocardiosis, like cryptococcosis, is rare in Europe, but is more common in the United States, where it is endemic in some areas.

■ **Clinical Manifestations**

Nocardial brain abscesses lead to various focal neurologic deficits, depending on their location.

■ **CT Morphology**

CT demonstrates brain abscesses with nonspecific morphologic features (Fig. 4.**17**).

Fig. 4.**17 a, b Nocardial brain abscess.**
a Postcontrast CT demonstrates a large lesion with central necrosis and a thin, enhancing abscess wall on the right side of the posterior fossa. The lesion on its anterior aspect is a smaller abscess.
b Multiloculated nocardial abscess (rarely described in the literature).

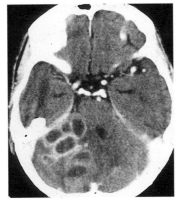 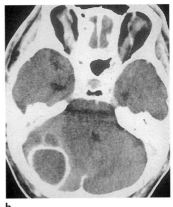

a   b

The lesions are usually large, with perifocal edema, and they tend to undergo central lique-faction, with the formation of granulation tissue or an abscess membrane that walls off the lesion. Like other abscesses, the lesion may rupture into the ventricular system and cause ventriculitis. It has been reported that subependymal nodules (microabscesses) are relatively frequent in nocardiosis.

■ **Differential Diagnosis**

Since the findings of nocardiosis are non-specific, the differential diagnosis should include all other potential causes of brain abscess. Biopsy material can be obtained from the lung, bone, or soft tissues. Involvement of the lung or bone should suggest the correct diagnosis, however.

Listeriosis

Frequency: rare.
Suggestive morphologic findings: encephalitis, rhombencephalitis; meningitis.
Procedure: the diagnosis is made by isolating the organism in culture.
Other studies: MRI is specific for encephalitis.

■ **Pathogenesis**

Listeriosis is caused by the bacterium *Listeria monocytogenes.* The CNS, particularly the brain stem (rhombencephalitis), is most commonly involved.

■ **Frequency**

Listeriosis is a rare disease, although instances of endemic occurrence have repeatedly been described. Most such cases affect members of special high-risk groups such as veterinarians or farmers, since the infection is often trans-

mitted from animals to humans. Infected or contaminated foods are another potential source of endemic outbreaks. A special form of listeriosis occurs as an intrauterine infection, leading to abortion or prematurity.

■ **Clinical Manifestations**

Encephalitis, especially of the brain stem, is by far the main determinant of clinical manifestations. Brain abscesses and even meningitis are much less common. Brain-stem encephalitis leads swiftly to respiratory failure.

■ **CT Morphology**

CT shows decreased density and slightly increased volume in the affected brain areas (rhombencephalon). Faint contrast enhancement may be evident. MRI is considerably more sensitive than CT in most respects, and it has become the preferred modality for evaluating listeriosis.

Lyme Disease

Frequency: fairly rare, but with a higher incidence in endemic areas.

Suggestive morphologic findings: multiple enhancing or nonenhancing white-matter lesions.

Procedure: the diagnosis is made serologically (titers). Erythema migrans is often present.

Other studies: MRI is more sensitive.

Checklist for scan interpretation:
▶ Presence of white-matter hypodensities?
▶ Contrast enhancement?
▶ Location?
▶ Meningeal enhancement?
▶ Spinal MRI necessary for a complete work-up?

■ Pathogenesis

Lyme disease is caused by a tick-borne spirochete, *Borrelia burgdorferi,* that resides in the saliva and bowel contents of the tick.

■ Frequency

Lyme disease has a low overall incidence, and CNS involvement by the disease (neuroborreliosis) is correspondingly rare. Usually it is diagnosed by the exclusion of other causes. There are endemic regions in which the tick vector is particularly common and the incidence of the disease is increased.

■ Clinical Manifestations

A considerable time may pass between the tick bite and the appearance of significant neurologic symptoms. Consequently, it is often difficult to establish a causal relationship.

The early symptoms following a tick bite are nonspecific:

■ Differential Diagnosis

CT cannot confirm listeriosis as the cause of meningitis or encephalitis. The diagnosis is established by serologic methods.

● Fatigue
● Fever
● Arthralgia, etc.

Erythema chronicum migrans is more characteristic, but is not always present. In the next clinical stage, lymphadenitis develops and is accompanied by signs of meningitis and CNS infection. CSF examination in the presence of meningitis shows lymphocytic pleocytosis, with elevated proteins and oligoclonal bands. Cranial nerve deficits, when present, most commonly involve the facial nerve, and bilateral facial palsy is typical. Fully developed Lyme disease usually takes several years to appear, and it can present a broad range of symptoms.

■ CT Morphology

CNS involvement by Lyme disease can resemble multiple sclerosis in both its clinical and imaging features. Unlike multiple sclerosis, however, the focal white-matter hypodensities on CT scans tend to be peripheral rather than periventricular. Contrast enhancement may or may not occur and is seen more clearly on magnetic resonance images. If meningitis is present, meningeal enhancement will be seen if the findings are sufficiently pronounced.

■ Differential Diagnosis

Differentiation is required from all diseases that can cause hypodense lesions in the brain parenchyma. The lesions tend to occur near the gray–white matter junction, but often this cannot reliably distinguish Lyme disease from other metastatic, inflammatory, or demyelinating diseases. Differentiation is mainly required from multiple sclerosis, which also has non-specific clinical features and often produces similar CSF changes.

Follow-Up

The focus in follow-up is on assessing the treatment response. MRI is generally preferred for this purpose.

Progressive Multifocal Leukoencephalopathy

Frequency: relatively common CT finding in AIDS patients.

Suggestive morphologic findings: asymmetric subcortical hypodensities with no mass effect; no contrast enhancement.

Procedure: in immunosuppressed patients, requires differentiation from treatable diseases such as lymphoma and toxoplasmosis.

Other studies: MRI is more sensitive than CT.

Checklist for scan interpretation:
▶ Progressive multifocal leukoencephalopathy (PML) has to be distinguished from progressive diffuse leukoencephalopathy (PDL) due to the difference in the prognosis.

Pathogenesis

Progressive multifocal leukoencephalopathy was first described in patients with systemic hematologic diseases. Today the disease is most commonly seen in patients with acquired immune deficiency. The risk is highest in AIDS patients and in immunosuppressed patients after organ transplantation. PML is caused by infection with a virus of the papovavirus group.

Frequency

PML is a relatively common finding in cerebral CT examinations in AIDS patients. Contrast-enhanced cerebral CT is performed in AIDS patients with focal neurologic symptoms, to exclude treatable diseases such as lymphoma and toxoplasmosis.

Clinical Manifestations

Various focal neurologic deficits are observed:

- Pyramidal tract signs
- Sensory deficits
- Seizures

CT Morphology

PML is characterized by multiple circumscribed, patchy hypodensities in the white matter (Fig. 4.**18**). There is no associated mass effect. Contrast enhancement is rarely observed, and the lack of enhancement can provide a differentiating criterion from lymphoma and toxoplasmosis. The location of the lesion is mainly supratentorial, sparing the cortex. Cerebellar involvement is less common.

Differential Diagnosis

PML in AIDS patients should not be confused with progressive diffuse leukoencephalopathy (PDL). PDL is distinguished by largely symmetrical hypodensities located predominantly in the frontal white matter. PDL is not caused by a papovavirus, but by the HIV virus itself (see Figs. 4.**19** and 4.**20** for other white-matter changes).

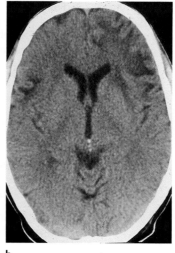

a b

Fig. 4.**18 a, b Progressive multifocal leukoencephalopathy** (PML). The typical CT appearance of PML in a patient with acquired immunodeficiency syndrome. Note the marked asymmetry of the white-matter hypodensity, which is most pronounced in the left frontal region and the area of the external capsule. Subtle lesions are also visible in the right parietal area.

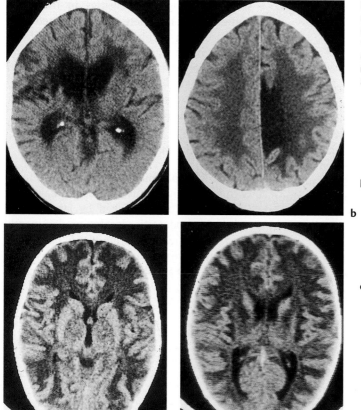

a b
c d

Fig. 4.**19 a–g Differential diagnosis of leukoencephalopathy** (1). White-matter hypodensities, which may be conspicuous and diffuse, are also found in cerebral microangiopathy.

a White-matter changes in microangiopathy are usually located adjacent to the frontal horns. Additional lacunar changes are seen in the right thalamus and elsewhere. Cerebral atrophy is pronounced.

b Radiotherapy to the skull causes a leukoencephalopathy that appears as symmetrical hypodense areas in the white matter. A postsurgical parenchymal defect is visible to the left of the midline.

c, d White-matter hypodensities in an 18-month-old child with Alexander's disease. The white-matter hypodensities are symmetrical, and show a predominantly frontal rather than occipital distribution.

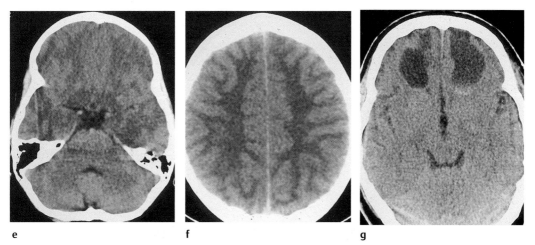

e   f   g

Abb. 4.**19 e–g**

e Hypoxic brain damage involves all of the white matter, exhibiting a somewhat irregular, patchy distribution.

f Here, the white-matter hypodensity is so uniform
that the net result is an increase in gray–white matter
contrast (a 7-year-old boy after diabetic coma).

g Postirradiation changes in the frontal lobes.

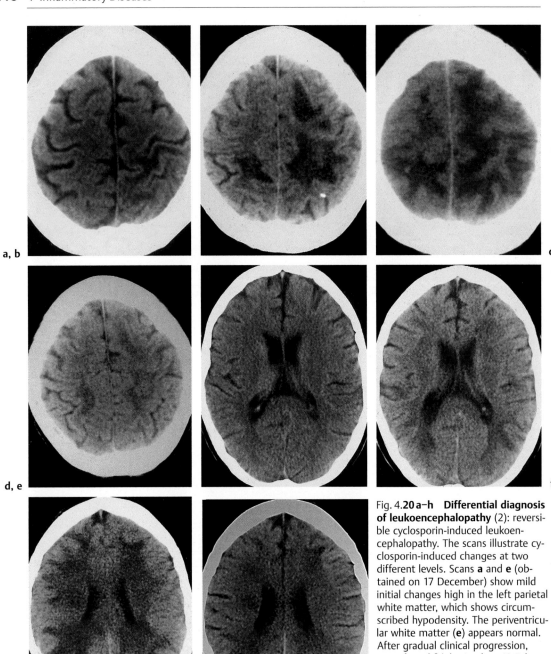

a, b

c

d, e

f

g

h

Fig. 4.20 a–h Differential diagnosis of leukoencephalopathy (2): reversible cyclosporin-induced leukoencephalopathy. The scans illustrate cyclosporin-induced changes at two different levels. Scans **a** and **e** (obtained on 17 December) show mild initial changes high in the left parietal white matter, which shows circumscribed hypodensity. The periventricular white matter (**e**) appears normal. After gradual clinical progression, scans **b** and **f** (obtained on 13 February) show a marked increase of changes both in the superior parietal region (**b**) and at the periventricular level (**f**). These changes progressed rapidly, and scans acquired the following day (**c, g**) show involvement of almost the entire white matter. When cyclosporin medication was discontinued, a gradual regression ensued. The changes were most persistent in the areas initially affected (scans **d** and **h**, acquired on 6 March).

Progressive Diffuse Leukoencephalopathy

Frequency: a relatively common CT finding in AIDS patients.

Suggestive morphologic findings: white-matter hypodensities, symmetrical, frontal.

Procedure: intravenous contrast administration is useful in differentiating from other causes of white-matter hypodensity.

Other studies: MRI is more sensitive.

Checklist for scan interpretation:
▶ Location in the white matter? Extent?
▶ Other changes such as atrophy or enhancing lesions?

■ Pathogenesis

PDL is thought to be caused by direct damage to oligodendrocytes by the HIV virus, leading to demyelination.

■ Frequency

PDL is found in a relatively high percentage of AIDS patients who undergo cerebral CT scanning to exclude lymphoma or toxoplasmosis. The changes are seen less frequently today than in the 1980's, however, owing to advances in therapeutic options.

■ Clinical Manifestations

The clinical manifestations are less specific than in PML, ranging from cognitive deficits to dementia-like symptoms.

■ CT Morphology

The white-matter hypodensities in PDL usually show a symmetrical or nearly symmetrical distribution on CT scans. The frontal white matter is affected initially, and with greater frequency. There is no mass effect, and the hypodensities do not enhance after contrast administration. The cortex is spared. Whereas the subcortical white matter is predominantly affected in PML, the changes in PDL mainly affect the centrum semiovale and periventricular white matter.

■ Differential Diagnosis

PML is most clearly distinguished from PDL by the asymmetric pattern of involvement in PDL. Contrast enhancement indicates the presence of toxoplasmosis, lymphoma, or another opportunistic infection.

■ References

Recommended for further study

Bacterial brain abscess
Hsu WC, Tang LM, Chen ST, Lyu RK. Multiple brain abscesses in chain and cluster: CT appearance. J Comput Assist Tomogr 1995; 19: 1004–6.
Kempf HG, Wiel J, Issing PR, Lenarz T. [Otogenic brain abscess; in German]. Laryngorhinootologie 1998; 77: 462–6.
● *Describes brain abscess as a potential complication of untreated cholesteatoma.*

Neurocysticercosis
Chang KH, Han MH. MRI of CNS parasitic diseases. J Magn Reson Imaging 1998; 8: 297–307.
● *Deals mainly with neurocysticercosis.*

Nocardiosis
LeBlang SD, Whiteman ML, Post MJ, Uttamchandani RB, Bell MD, Smirniotopoulos JG. CNS nocardia in AIDS patients: CT and MRI with pathologic correlation. J Comput Assist Tomogr 1995; 19: 15–22.
● *Presents nine cases with characteristic imaging findings and clinical features.*

Recent and basic works

Bacterial brain abscess
Benito Leon J, Munoz A, Leon PG, Rivas JJ, Ramos A. Actinomycotic brain abscess. Neurologia 1998; 13: 357–61.
Brightbill TC, Ihmeidan IH, Post MJ, Berger JR, Katz DA. Neurosyphilis in HIV-positive and HIV-negative patients: neuroimaging findings. AJNR Am J Neuroradiol 1995; 16: 703–11.
Caldemeyer KS, Mathews VP, Edwards-Brown MK, Smith RR. Central nervous system cryptococcosis: parenchymal calcification and large gelatinous pseudocysts. AJNR Am J Neuroradiol 1997; 18: 107–9.
Flinn IW, Ambinder RF. AIDS primary central nervous system lymphoma. Curr Opin Oncol 1996; 8: 373–6.
Miaux Y, Ribaud P, Williams M, et al. MRI of cerebral aspergillosis in patients who have had bone marrow transplantation. AJNR Am J Neuroradiol 1995; 16: 555–62.
● *Describes a case with an unusual cerebral manifestation.*
Piotin M, Cattin F, Kantelip B, Miralbes S, Godard J, Bonneville JF. Disseminated intracerebral alveolar echinococcosis: CT and MRI. Neuroradiology 1997; 39: 431–3.
Terk MR, Underwood DJ, Zee CS, Colletti PM. MR imaging in rhinocerebral and intracranial mucormycosis with

CT and pathologic correlation. Magn Reson Imaging 1992; 10: 81–7.

Thurnher MM, Thurnher SA, Schindler E. CNS involvement in AIDS: spectrum of CT and MR findings. Eur Radiol 1997; 7: 1091–7.
- *Overview illustrating the principal findings in CT and MRI.*

Tsuge I, Matsuoka H, Nakagawa A, et al. Necrotizing toxoplasmic encephalitis in a child with X-linked hyper-IgM syndrome. Eur J Pediatr 1998; 157: 735–7.

Yuh WT, Nguyen HD, Gao F, et al. Brain parenchymal infection in bone marrow transplantation patients: CT and MR findings. AJR Am J Roentgenol 1994; 162: 425–30.
- *Describes decreased contrast enhancement and edema following bone marrow transplantation.*

Tuberculosis

Berenguer J, Moreno S, Laguna F, et al. Tuberculous meningitis in patients infected with the human immunodeficiency virus. N Engl J Med 1992; 326: 668–72.

Lesprit P, Zagdanski AM, de La Blanchardiere A, et al. Cerebral tuberculosis in patients with acquired immunodeficiency syndrome (AIDS): report of six cases and review. Medicine (Baltimore) 1997; 76: 423–31.
- *Medical study that includes a review of imaging findings.*

Sarcoidosis

Stern BI, Krumholz A, Johns E, et al. Sarcoidosis and its neurological manifestations. Arch Neurol 1985; 42: 909–17.
- *Report on a very large series spanning a number of years.*
- *Herpes simplex encephalitis*

Neils EW, Lukin S, Tomsick TA. Magnetic resonance imaging and computerized tomography scanning of herpes simplex encephalitis. J Neurosurg 1987; 67: 592–4.

Schroth G, Gawehn J, Thron A. The early diagnosis of herpes simplex encephalitis by MRI. Neurology 1987; 37: 179–83.
- *Early study, includes correlation with CT.*

Toxoplasmosis

Laissy JP, Soyer P, Parlier C, et al. Persistent enhancement after treatment for cerebral toxoplasmosis in patients with AIDS: predictive value for subsequent recurrence. AJNR Am J Neuroradiol 1994; 15: 1773–8.
- *Describes 43 patients; addresses the key issue of recurrence.*

Raffi F, Aboulker JP, Michelet C, et al. A prospective study of criteria for the diagnosis of toxoplasmic encephalitis in 186 AIDS patients. The BIOTOXO Study Group. AIDS 1997; 11: 177–84.
- *Describes criteria useful in differentiating between toxoplasmosis and lymphoma.*

Ruiz A, Ganz WI, Post JJ, et al. Use of thallium-201 brain SPECT to differentiate cerebral lymphoma from toxoplasma encephalitis in AIDS patients. AJNR Am J Neuroradiol 1994; 15: 1885–94.
- *SPECT imaging in 37 AIDS patients correctly diagnosed 12 lymphomas.*

Cryptococcosis

Berkefeld J, Enzensberger W, Lanfermann H. Cryptococcus meningoencephalitis in AIDS: parenchymal and meningeal forms. Neuroradiology 1999; 41: 129–33
- *Describes one case of meningitis and one of multiple intraparenchymal abscesses.*

Schmidt S, Reiter-Owona I, Hotz M, Mewes J, Biniek R. An unusual case of central nervous system cryptococcosis. Clin Neurol Neurosurg 1995; 97: 23–7.
- *Case illustrating problems in the differential diagnosis of opportunistic CNS infection in the immunocompromised host.*

Neurocysticercosis

Palacio LG, Jimenez I, Garcia HH, et al. Neurocysticercosis in persons with epilepsy in Medellin, Colombia. The Neuroepidemiological Research Group of Antioquia. Epilepsia 1998; 39: 1334–9.
- *Series of several hundred patients; includes CT evaluation.*

Rahalkar MD, Shetty DD, Kelkar AB, Kinare AS, Ambardekar ST. The many faces of cysticercosis. Clin Radiol 2000; 55(9): 668–74.
- *Nocardiosis*

Mamelak AN, Obana WG, Flaherty JF, Rosenblum ML. Nocardial brain abscess: treatment strategies and factors influencing outcome. Neurosurgery 1994; 35: 622–31.
- *Report on 11 original cases and a review of 120 cases from the literature.*

Listeriosis

Aladro Y, Ponce P, Santullano V, Angel-Moreno A, Santana MA. Cerebritis due to *Listeria monocytogenes:* CT and MR findings. Eur Radiol 1996; 6: 188–91.
- *Describes CT and MR findings in three patients at diagnosis and during follow-up.*

Lyme disease

Demaerel P, Wilms G, Casteels K, Casaer P, Silberstein J, Baert AL. Childhood neuroborreliosis: clinicoradiological correlation. Neuroradiology 1995; 37: 578–81.
- *Describes CT and MRI findings in three children.*

Reik L Jr, Smith L, Khan A, Nelson W. Demyelinating encephalopathy in Lyme disease. Neurology 1985; 35: 267–9.
- *Case report describing an unusual CT manifestation.*
- *Progressive multifocal leukoencephalopathy*

Lanfermann H, Heindel W, Schröder R, Lackner K. [CT and MRI in progressive multifocal leukoencephalopathy (PML); in German]. RöFo Fortschr Geb Röntgenstr Neuen Bildgeb Verfahr 1994; 161: 38–43.
- *Describes radiologic findings and course in 14 patients.*

Progressive diffuse leukoencephalopathy

Berger JR, Pall L, Lanska D, Whiteman M. Progressive multifocal leukoencephalopathy in patients with HIV infection. J Neurovirol 1998; 4: 59–68.
- *Retrospective analysis of 250 AIDS patients, with cerebral CT evaluation.*

Bronster DJ, Lidov MW, Wolfe D, Schwartz ME, Miller CM. Progressive multifocal leukoencephalopathy after orthotopic liver transplantation. Liver Transpl Surg 1995; 1: 371–2.
- *Case report, confirmed by biopsy.*

Thurnher MM, Thurnher SA, Muhlbauer B, et al. Progressive multifocal leukoencephalopathy in AIDS: initial and follow-up CT and MRI. Neuroradiology 1997; 39: 611–8.
- *Retrospective analysis of initial CT and follow-up in 21 confirmed cases.*

Morriss MC, Rutstein RM, Rudy B, Desrocher C, Hunter JV, Zimmerman RA. Progressive multifocal leukoencephalopathy in an HIV-infected child. Neuroradiology 1997; 39: 142–4.
- *Case report.*

5 Intracranial Tumors

Among the many intra-axial and extra-axial brain tumors that are known, only a few types account for the majority of forms that are observed clinically. It should also be considered that the differential diagnosis of brain tumors in emergency situations is of less importance than detecting a potentially devastating mass effect involving a shift of the midline or a sub-falcial/transtentorial herniation. Magnetic resonance imaging (MRI) is generally superior to computed tomography (CT) for tumor differentiation and is the modality of choice for that application. The approximate prevalences of the various tumor types are reviewed in Table 5.1.

Table 5.1 Prevalence of brain tumors according to histologic subgroup. Metastases are disregarded*

Tumor	Prevalence (%)
Gliomas	50
Meningioma	10
Pituitary adenoma	7
Neuroma	7
Craniopharyngioma, dermoid, epidermoid, teratoma	4
Angioma	4
Sarcoma	4
Other	14
Total	100

* Cited after Adams RD, Victor M, *Principles of Neurology* (New York: McGraw-Hill, 3rd ed. 1985), based on a series of approximately 15 000 patients reviewed by Zülch, Cushing, and Olivecrona. The authors report the following figures for children: astrocytoma 48%, medulloblastoma 44%, ependymoma 8%.

Neuroepithelial Tumors

Gliomas (Figs. 5.1–5.18)

Frequency: gliomas account for approximately half of all intracranial tumors. Glioblastoma (grade IV glioma) predominates, accounting for about half of all gliomas. Low-grade astrocytomas account for 30%, and all others (oligodendroglioma, pilocytic astrocytoma) make up less than 10%.

Suggestive morphologic findings: white-matter hypodensity (low-grade forms) or mass with scalloped rim enhancement (higher-grade forms).

Procedure: biopsy confirmation and surgical treatment.

Other studies: MRI defines the tumor extent more accurately than CT. Positron-emission tomography (PET) is superior for detecting recurrence. CT is the method of choice for oligodendroglioma, due to frequent calcification.

Checklist for scan interpretation:
▶ Extent, edema, mass effect?
▶ Spread to contralateral hemisphere?
▶ Calcifications?

■ **Pathogenesis**

The "glial subgroup of neuroepithelial tumors," as gliomas are called in the World Health Organization (WHO) classification, consists of the following types:

Astrocytoma. Astrocytomas are gliomas derived from astrocytes. The subtypes in the WHO classification are indistinguishable by their imaging features.

Anaplastic astrocytoma. Anaplastic astrocytomas are grade III neoplasms characterized by rapid progression, transformation to glioblastoma, and enhancement on postcontrast CT.

Glioblastoma. Glioblastomas display a heterogeneous CT pattern of necrosis, hemorrhage, and contrast enhancement. They are classified according to their biologic behavior as grade IV gliomas. The histologic subtypes are indistinguishable by CT.

Pilocytic astrocytoma. Pilocytic astrocytomas are characterized by less infiltrative growth, a low propensity for malignant transformation, a protracted course, and a peak age incidence in adolescents. They are classified as grade I gliomas, which very rarely undergo malignant transformation to anaplastic pilocytic astrocytoma (grade III). CT can provide a presumptive diagnosis.

Pleomorphic xanthoastrocytoma. This tumor is a variant commonly found in patients with seizure disorder. With its relative lack of aggressiveness, it is classified as a grade II glioma. Malignant transformation is rare but can occur.

Subependymal giant-cell astrocytoma. This tumor occurs in tuberous sclerosis and has a characteristic CT appearance. Histologically, it is a grade I glioma.

Oligodendroglioma. Calcifications characterize both the histologic and CT appearance of oligodendrogliomas. These tumors often arise in the white matter or basal ganglia, and have a strong tendency to infiltrate the cortex and leptomeninges. Oligodendrogliomas are grade II neoplasms that have less malignant potential than astrocytomas.

Anaplastic oligodendroglioma. Anaplastic oligodendrogliomas are grade III gliomas. Malignant transformation to grade IV is usually indistinguishable from glioblastoma.

Grading of gliomas. The typical CT appearance of gliomas varies with the histologic grade of the neoplasm:

- *Grade I gliomas.* Grade I gliomas are characterized by their location (cerebellum, pons, optic tract), age of occurrence (mainly children and adolescents), and the CT appearance of a cyst and/or an enhancing tumor nodule (Figs. 5.**1**, 5.**2**). Subependymal giant-cell astrocytomas belong to this category.
- *Grade II gliomas.* These tumors usually appear as a hypodense area that exhibits little or no mass effect and no contrast enhancement. The absence of calcifications suggests astrocytoma, while the presence of calcifications is more consistent with oligodendroglioma (Figs. 5.**3**–5.**5**). Special forms include pleomorphic xanthoastrocytoma and gemistocytic astrocytoma.
- *Grade III gliomas.* Contrast enhancement occurs in portions of grade III gliomas (Figs. 5.**6**–5.**8**). Anaplastic astrocytomas and anaplastic oligodendrogliomas are observed.
- *Grade IV gliomas.* These tumors are characterized by a heterogeneous CT pattern with necrosis, hemorrhage, contrast enhancement, perifocal edema, and a scalloped or irregular enhancing rim. The histologic subtypes are glioblastoma, anaplastic astrocytoma, and anaplastic oligodendroglioma (Figs. 5.**9**, 5.**10**, 5.**15**).

In addition to these forms, there are also mixed gliomas in which two or more neoplastic glial cell types coexist in the same tumor, such as oligoastrocytoma and anaplastic oligoastrocytoma.

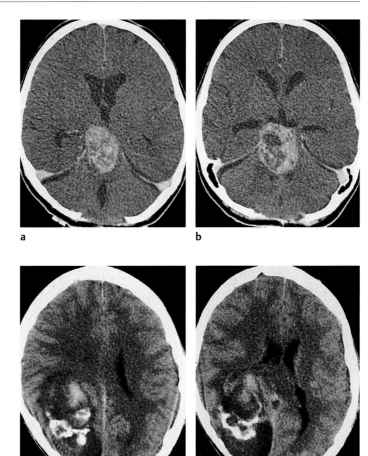

Fig. 5.**1 a, b   Pontine glioma.**
Pilocytic gliomas are classified as grade I tumors and include the pontine glioma shown here in a 9-year-old boy. Scans at two different levels demonstrate a large enhancing mass with central cystic lucencies.

a   b

Fig. 5.**2 a, b   Grade I glioma.**
The grade I gliomas found in children consistently enhance after contrast administration, but may also show extensive necrosis. In the case of this 14-year-old boy, contrast enhancement occurs in the rostral portions of the tumor. Calcifications are also visible within the hypodense glioma. There is a considerable mass effect, with anterior displacement of the right occipital horn.

a   b

■ Frequency

The incidence of supratentorial brain tumors correlates with their mortality rates, and considerable variation is seen in the geographic and histologic distribution of occurrence. For example, age-corrected incidence rates range from 1.5 per 100,000 (Singapore) to as much as 9.1–10 per 100,000 (Sweden and Israel). Incidence rates are generally higher in countries with a high socioeconomic status. A comparison of mortality rates in different countries shows a very broad range, from 1.1 per 100,000 in Mexico (1951–1958) to 10 per 100,000 in the Federal Republic of Germany (1967–1973). Rising mortality rates have been confirmed in a number of epidemiologic studies. The incidence of brain tumors in the United States is estimated at approximately 12,000 new cases per year.

The following statistical distribution has been calculated for the different grades of glioma:

Glioblastoma: anaplastic astrocytoma: low-grade astrocytoma = 5 : 3 : 2.

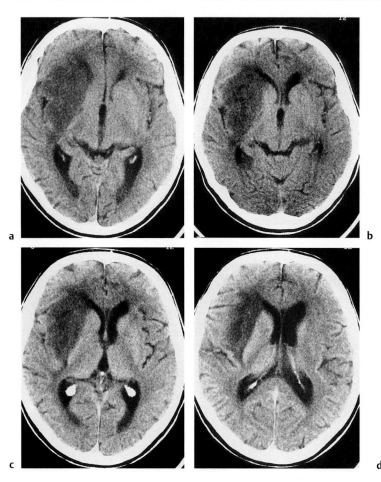

a

b

c

d

Fig. 5.**3 a–d Grade II oligoden-droglioma.** The prognostically favorable grade I gliomas found in children may show contrast enhancement, but grade II gliomas, unlike grade III and IV tumors, are nonenhancing. The scans illustrate a grade II oligodendroglioma of the right hemispheric white matter. The tumor appears as a hypodense area with an ill-defined peripheral margin on the cortical side, while the opposite margin is sharply demarcated from the basal ganglia. This pattern results from the initial sparing of non–white-matter structures at the center of the brain. This case shows that oligodendrogliomas do not necessarily contain calcifications. The absence of contrast enhancement characterizes the tumor as a grade II neoplasm.

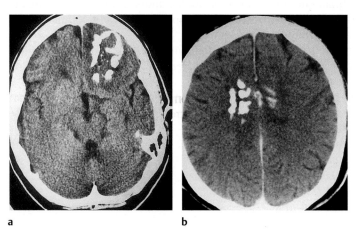

a

b

Fig. 5.**4 Oligodendroglioma.** Most oligodendrogliomas can be identified on CT by their calcifications. The two scans show typical coarse, irregular calcifications in the left frontal lobe and in the rostral portion of the corpus callosum. White-matter hypodensity is a far less important morphologic feature of oligodendroglioma than calcifications.
a Calcifications in the left frontal lobe.
b Calcifications in the corpus callosum.

Fig. 5.**5 a, b** **Oligodendroglioma involving the corpus callosum.** Postcontrast scans at two different levels show a calcified tumor with minimal contrast enhancement. Perifocal edema is pronounced, however.

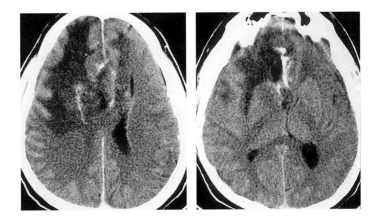

Fig. 5.**6** **Anaplastic astrocytoma.** Anaplastic astrocytomas are classified as grade III gliomas and show more or less intense contrast enhancement. Noncontrast CT shows a small lesion in the left parietal area, the attenuation of which is closer to that of the cerebral cortex than the white matter. Moderate enhancement occurs after contrast administration.
a Noncontrast scan.
b Postcontrast scan.

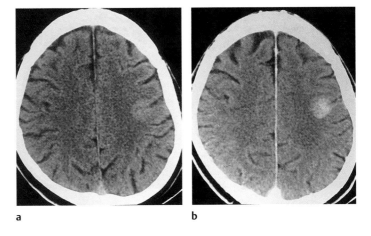

a b

Fig. 5.**7** **Grade III anaplastic astrocytoma.** CT shows a primary intraventricular brain tumor. This type of tumor can lead to ventricular expansion and pressure coning.

Fig. 5.**8** **Grade III glioma.** Grade III gliomas are indistinguishable from glioblastoma multiforme by their CT appearance. A tumor showing intense, scalloped rim enhancement is visible lateral to the left occipital horn.

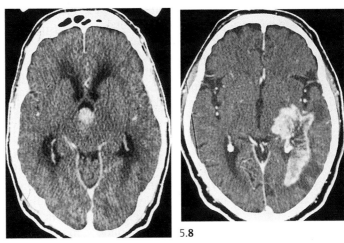

5.**8**

5.**7**

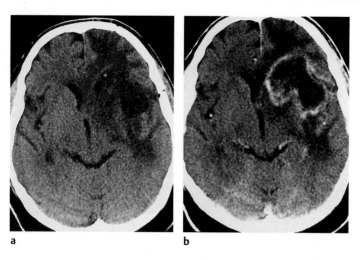

a   b

Fig. 5.**9** **Grade IV glioma (glioblastoma multiforme).** This glioma is characterized by mass effect, perifocal edema, and central necrosis on the unenhanced scan. Scalloped rim enhancement is characteristic after contrast administration.
a Noncontrast scan.
b Postcontrast scan.

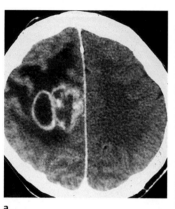
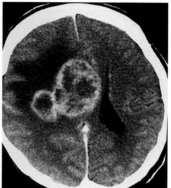

a   b

Fig. 5.**10 a, b** **Glioblastoma.** A scalloped or multi-ring pattern of contrast enhancement is characteristic of glioblastoma. These scans show extensive edema, involving almost all of the white matter in the right hemisphere.

■ Clinical Manifestations

Pilocytic astrocytomas occur predominantly in children and young adults. The peak age of occurrence is between 40 and 50 for astrocytomas and oligodendrogliomas, and somewhat later for glioblastomas. All higher-grade gliomas (III or IV) tend to occur at age 20 or older, and pilocytic astrocytomas may be diagnosed after age 20.

■ CT Morphology

Pilocytic astrocytoma. This tumor may occur in the cerebellum, brain stem, and less commonly at supratentorial sites. Infratentorial tumors can be distinguished from midline medulloblastoma by their eccentric location.

CT without intravenous contrast shows an ill-defined hypodense lesion with a mass effect or a corresponding cyst. Postcontrast CT often demonstrates nodular enhancement in the cyst wall.

Optic glioma. Most grade II–IV gliomas are supratentorial and appear as hypodense masses in the white matter. Only oligodendroglioma shows a predilection for the frontal or temporal lobe and infiltrates the cerebral cortex. The margins are ill-defined. Mass effects range from the effacement of individual sulci and subtle frontal-horn displacement to a shift of the midline and ventricular compression. The calcifications found in oligodendrogliomas are more common in lower-grade tumors than in the more malignant forms. The calcifications may be flocculent or stippled, and may follow the outline of the cerebral cortex. Contrast enhancement occurs in grade III and grade IV gliomas. The enhancement in grade III gliomas shows a patchy or bizarre pattern, while grade IV gliomas show a scalloped or irregular enhancing rim with central necrosis. Grade IV gliomas typically show a heterogeneous mix of enhancing and hypodense tumor tissue, necrosis or cysts, intratumoral hemorrhage, and mass effect.

Butterfly glioma. Butterfly glioma is a bihemispheric tumor that arises predominantly in the anterior or posterior commissure and infiltrates both hemispheres (Fig. 5.**11**).

Gliomatosis cerebri, or diffuse gliomatosis. Gliomatosis cerebri refers to a generalized malignant transformation that may involve all of the cerebral white matter. The course may span many years, and a mass effect may be ab-

sent or limited to mild compression of the frontal or occipital horns.

Multifocal gliomas. This is a pattern characterized by synchronous or metachronous development of multiple tumor foci (Fig. 5.**12**).

■ Differential Diagnosis

The imaging appearance of cerebral infarction most closely resembles that of gliomas (Fig. 5.**13**).

With cerebral infarction, however, the distribution of the hypodense area often conforms to a vascular territory or to a watershed area between two territories. Also, infarctions tend to involve the adjacent cortical gray matter more extensively, and they show predominantly cortical enhancement after contrast administration. Infarcts have an abrupt clinical onset that contrasts with the typically insidious onset of gliomas. Serial examinations after

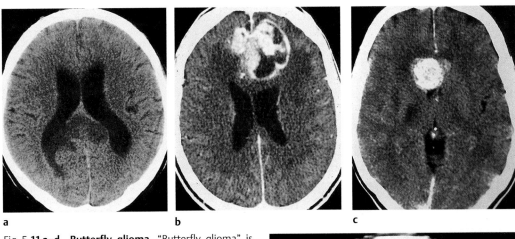

a   b   c

Fig. 5.**11 a–d** **Butterfly glioma.** "Butterfly glioma" is the term applied to primary brain tumors that extend across the anterior or posterior commissure or corpus callosum to involve both hemispheres.
- **a** The noncontrast scan shows a low-grade glioma of the posterior commissure.
- **b** This postcontrast scan in a different patient shows a glioblastoma with a scalloped, enhancing rim.
- **c** Corpus callosum glioma may also appear as a solid round mass.
- **d** The coronal reformatted image shows two ring-like masses located above the lateral ventricles.

d

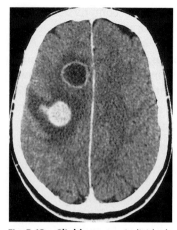

Fig. 5.**12** **Glioblastoma.** Individual glioblastomas can exhibit multiple tumor foci. This scan illustrates one ring-enhancing lesion and one nodular-enhancing lesion with perifocal edema. Similar patterns may be seen with metastases. However, it should be carefully checked whether there are bridging parts of the tumor connecting between lesions that appear to be solitary.

an infarction usually show a regression of changes with fading enhancement, whereas gliomas show either no significant change (low-grade forms) or marked progression (high-grade forms). As for inflammatory lesions, multiple sclerosis (Fig. 5.**14**) and granulomas (e.g., in tuberculosis) can sometimes mimic the neuroimaging features of higher-grade gliomas.

In the case of multiple sclerosis, examination of the cerebrospinal fluid (CSF) will help to narrow the differential diagnosis. It is rare, however, for multiple sclerosis to present with a large enhancing lesion, extensive perifocal edema, and an acute onset. In the case of metastases, multiplicity may not be a reliable differentiating criterion due to the potential multicentric occurrence of glioblastoma.

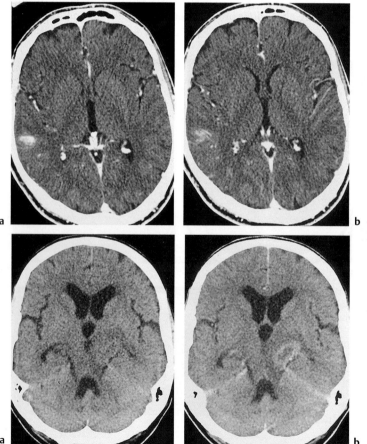

a

b

a

b

Fig. 5.**13 a, b** **Primary brain tumor mimicking cerebral infarction.** If the diagnosis is made promptly, there should be little danger of confusing primary brain tumors with infarction. These scans show a primary brain tumor that is manifested only by mild, ill-defined contrast enhancement in the right parietal area.

Fig. 5.**14 a, b** **Primary brain tumor mimicking a metastasis or demyelinating lesion.** The CT morphology of primary brain tumors can also mimic that of metastases. This tumor, located in the left cerebral peduncle, appears hypodense on plain CT and shows faint ring enhancement after contrast administration.
a Noncontrast scan.
b Postcontrast scan.

Fig. 5.**15 a, b   Grade IV glioma.**
Differential diagnosis is often difficult in cases of diffuse tumor involvement. These scans illustrate the postcontrast appearance of a very diffusely enhancing grade IV glioma. The tumor has spread across the anterior commissure to the left hemisphere.

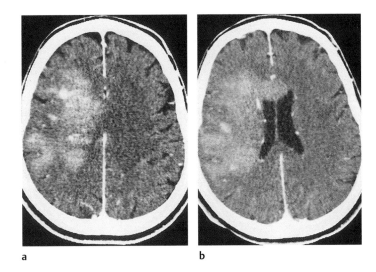

a

b

Fig. 5.**16 a, b   Parasagittal astrocytoma.** This parasagittal astrocytoma shows intense enhancement after contrast administration. It could be mistaken for a meningioma.

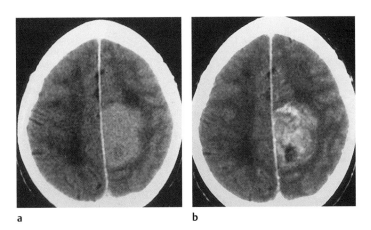

a

b

Fig. 5.**17   Glioblastoma.** The scalloped enhancing rim ▷ of glioblastoma can mimic other tumors in certain CT slices. Location aside, the enhancing rim, central necrosis, and enhancing nodular component of this glioblastoma could also suggest angioblastoma, although it is extremely rare for that type of tumor to occur at the supratentorial level.

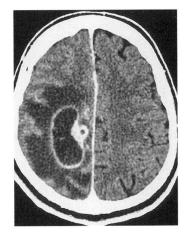

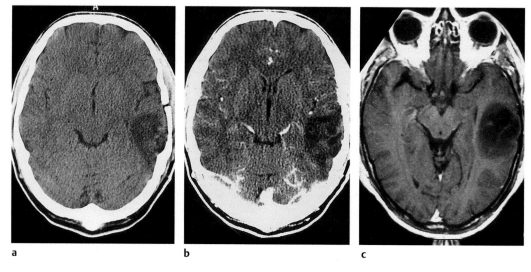

a b c

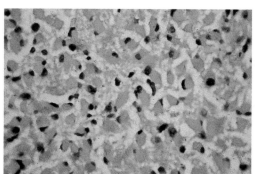

d

Fig. 5.**18 a–d Grade II gemistocytic astrocytoma**. The gemistocytic astrocytoma shown here is regarded as a special form of primary brain tumor, with a high malignant potential and a generally poor prognosis.

a, b Noncontrast CT (**a**) and postcontrast CT (**b**) show a relatively well-marginated, hypodense tumor in the left temporal lobe that does not enhance after contrast administration.

c   The postcontrast magnetic resonance image also shows no enhancement.

d   Typical histologic pattern, with plump eosinophilic cells and eccentric pleomorphic nuclei.

Even when all morphologic criteria have been evaluated, there will still be a certain percentage of cases in which only stereotactic biopsy can establish the diagnosis. The diverse imaging findings can lead to numerous misinterpretations, but these can be minimized by keeping in mind the frequency of glioblastoma.

■ Follow-Up

Two factors should be considered in the radiologic follow-up of brain tumor patients who have undergone surgical resection or radiotherapy:

- Both surgery and radiotherapy induce changes that can mimic a residual or recurrent tumor.

- Steroid therapy, by stabilizing defects in the blood–brain barrier, tends to reduce the size of perifocal edema and of enhancing tumor elements.

When a tumor has been surgically removed, the granulating resection margins will usually start to enhance on about the fifth postoperative day. This enhancement may persist for months. Thus, only an immediate postoperative examination can provide reliable information regarding residual tumor (assuming that the tumor enhanced prior to surgery).

Modern techniques of aggressive, selective radiotherapy can be very successful in inducing radiation necrosis at the tumor site. This necrotic area enhances after intravenous contrast administration and should not be mistaken for residual or recurrent tumor. The enhancement usually appears at about 4–8 months after the end of treatment and typically shows a ring pattern that is slightly larger than the original tumor.

It should be noted that perifocal edema and contrast enhancement may be decreased in volume and prominence by the initiation of steroid therapy, or by administering steroids at an excessive dosage. Consequently, these agents should be administered at a constant dosage for some time in order to allow accurate assessment of tumor regression or progression.

As for CT findings in patients who do not develop a recurrence, leukoencephalopathic changes and signs of cerebral atrophy begin to appear 6 months after surgery or radiotherapy. The CT hallmark of leukoencephalopathy is an accentuation of gray–white matter contrast due to a generalized decrease in white-matter density.

Pleomorphic Xanthoastrocytoma

Frequency: very rare.

Suggestive morphologic findings: hypodense mass located in the cortex or at the gray–white matter junction, often containing both cystic and solid components.

Procedure: treatment consists of surgical resection.

Other studies: as with all primary brain tumors, MRI is more sensitive than CT.

Checklist for scan interpretation:
▶ Location (precentral/postcentral)?
▶ Evidence of dural involvement?

■ Pathogenesis

Pleomorphic xanthoastrocytoma (Fig. 5.**19**) is a special form of astrocytoma that involves the cortex and leptomeninges. The prognosis is relatively good. Some cases of subarachnoid dissemination have been described in the literature.

■ Frequency

Pleomorphic xanthoastrocytoma is a very rare neoplasm (< 1 % of astrocytomas).

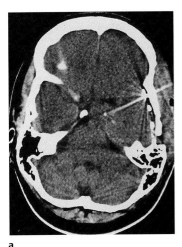
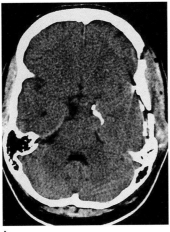
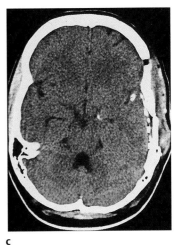

a   b   c

Fig. 5.**19 a–c Pleomorphic xanthoastrocytoma.** These CT scans were obtained after the placement of subdural electrodes.

a The scan at the basal level shows a mass lesion at the mesial left temporal pole.

b, c Scans at higher levels show linear calcification that is not specific for pleomorphic xanthoastrocytoma.

■ **Clinical Manifestations**

Children and young adults (< 30 years of age) are predominantly affected. Usually a long or short history of seizure is present. Headache is also a common symptom.

■ **CT Morphology**

Pleomorphic xanthoastrocytoma is character-ized mainly by its location. Arising from the cortex and leptomeninges, it shows a periph-eral location on CT scans. It appears on non-contrast scans as a hypodense mass with sharp or indistinct margins. Most of these tumors en-hance after contrast administration. Peripheral cysts are common, and calcifications are rare (Fig. 5.**19**). The tumors are always supraten-torial and usually occur in the temporal lobe. Perifocal edema is often present.

Despite the characteristic meningeal com-ponent, the detection of a dural tail on MRI is not typical of pleomorphic xanthoastrocytoma.

■ **Differential Diagnosis**

Differentiation is required from other tumors that abut the convexity and may infiltrate the dura. Pleomorphic xanthoastrocytoma is often misinterpreted as a glioblastoma or mening-ioma.

Subependymal Giant-Cell Astrocy-toma

Frequency: subependymal nodules are present in almost all tuberous sclerosis patients (98 % in some series), but subependymal giant-cell astrocytomas develop in only about 7–23 %.

Suggestive morphologic findings: subependy-mal enhancing mass located at the foramen of Monro.

Procedure: obtain delineation of subependymal nodules (contrast administration).

Other studies: MRI is superior for distinguishing subependymal tumors from heterotopic tissue (isointense to cortex in all sequences).

Checklist for scan interpretation:
▶ Number, location, size of tumors?
▶ Contrast enhancement?
▶ Signs of infiltrative growth?
▶ Other tumors or abnormalities?

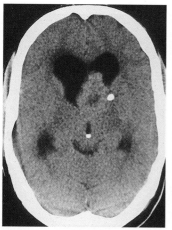
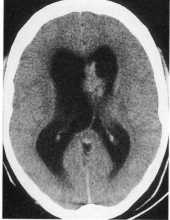
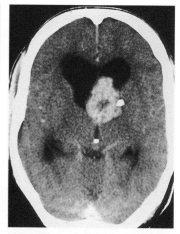

a b c

Fig. 5.**20 a–c Subependymal giant-cell astrocytoma.** CT demonstrates enlargement of the lateral ventricles due to obstruction of the foramen of Monro.
a, b Even without contrast administration, nodular

masses can be seen in the ventricular wall. A small calcification is visible on the left side.
c The mass enhances intensely after contrast admin-istration. Presumed infiltration of the basal ganglia was confirmed histologically.

■ Pathogenesis

Subependymal giant-cell astrocytomas (Fig. 5.**20**) are observed in tuberous sclerosis, one of the phakomatoses. They develop individually from subependymal tubers.

Subependymal giant-cell astrocytoma is an intermediate entity between heterotopia and neoplasia. Histologically, it does not exhibit mitoses or endothelial proliferation.

■ Frequency

Tuberous sclerosis has a reported annual incidence of approximately one per 178,000. Its prevalence is 10.6 per 100,000 population. Subependymal giant-cell astrocytomas develop in 7–23% of tuberous sclerosis patients, and in some cases may be the only detectable feature of the disease.

■ Clinical Manifestations

Subependymal giant-cell astrocytomas are usually benign and slow-growing. Clinical symptoms are caused chiefly by the mass effect on the foramen of Monro, leading to obstructive hydrocephalus.

■ CT Morphology

While subependymal nodules in patients with tuberous sclerosis do not show contrast enhancement, subependymal giant-cell astrocytomas enhance intensely after contrast administration. Serial observations published by one group of authors suggest that the onset of contrast enhancement signals the transformation of a subependymal tuber into a giant-cell astrocytoma. Both lesions may contain calcifications, and both may be hyperdense to the white matter.

■ Differential Diagnosis

The same diagnoses should be considered as with other subependymal masses:

- Ependymoma
- Subependymoma
- Heterotopic tissue

It is important to confirm or exclude tuberous sclerosis, which may present with the classic triad of adenoma sebaceum, seizures, and mental retardation.

■ Follow-Up

Subependymal giant-cell astrocytoma is rarely treated surgically, and there have been no reports on its propensity for recurrence.

Ependymal Tumors

Ependymoma

Frequency: makes up 2–8% of primary intracranial tumors, 15% of infratentorial posterior fossa tumors. In children, there appears to be a slight male predilection.

Suggestive morphologic findings: relation to ventricular ependyma, intense contrast enhancement, frequent calcification.

Procedure: only histologic examination can differentiate ependymoma from other tumors of ventricular origin. Seeding of CSF pathways may occur (spinal evaluation by MRI or myelography).

Other studies: the relation to the ventricle is often appreciated better on coronal or sagittal images (reformatted thin-slice CT or MRI).

Checklist for scan interpretation:
- ▶ Location?
- ▶ Hydrocephalus?
- ▶ Evidence of subarachnoid seeding?

Ependymomas arise from the ependyma lining the CSF spaces and may have a supratentorial, infratentorial, or spinal location. Infratentorial ependymoma (Figs. 5.**21**, 5.**22**) is common and mainly affects children under 4 years of age.

Supratentorial and spinal ependymomas are more common in young to middle-aged adults. The more benign forms grow by expansion and have well-defined margins on images; indistinct margins suggest a more malignant, infiltrative form. The potential for subarachnoid seeding to the spine necessitates adjunctive examinations of the spinal canal.

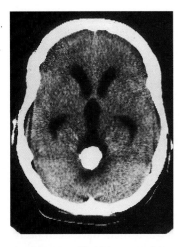

Fig. 5.**21** **Ependymoma.** CT demonstrates a heavily calcified mass in the fourth ventricle, causing hydrocephalus.

■ Pathogenesis

Ependymomas are classified as gliomas. The neuroepithelial forms arise from the ependymal lining of the CSF spaces. Mixed forms may occur. Intraparenchymal (ectopic) forms are usually supratentorial and arise from heterotopic ependymal cells.

The biologic behavior of ependymomas is variable, like that of other glial tumors. A highly malignant form is ependymoblastoma. The recurrence rate is relatively high, especially with infratentorial ependymomas that have invaded the cerebellopontine subarachnoid spaces. These tumors are difficult to resect completely because they tend to encase local blood vessels and cranial nerves (VII, IX, X). The potential for subarachnoid seeding also contributes to the generally poor prognosis.

■ Frequency

Ependymomas make up approximately 5–6% of intracranial gliomas, and 69% occur in children.

■ Clinical Manifestations

As with other posterior fossa tumors, the clinical hallmarks are nausea, vomiting, and gait disturbance.

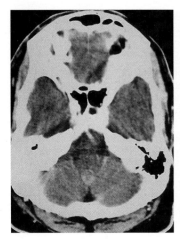

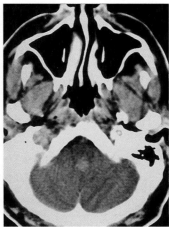

Fig. 5.**22 a, b** **Ependymoma.** Both postcontrast scans show a moderately enhancing infratentorial mass approximately 1 cm in diameter. The tumor is located in the fourth ventricle.

a   b

CT Morphology

In the small series that have been described to date, reports vary on the specific morphologic features of ependymomas, but the overall picture is as follows.

Supratentorial ependymomas may show intraventricular and extraventricular growth. Their density is highly variable on unenhanced scans, and the tumors may appear isodense, hypodense, or hyperdense to the white matter. They enhance after contrast administration (Fig. 5.**22**). Approximately half of the tumors contain calcifications, and many supratentorial ependymomas are partly or completely cystic. Supratentorial ventricular expansion may occur, depending on the tumor location. Tumors that are completely or predominantly extraventricular can lead to eventual hydrocephalus (Figs. 5.**21**, 5.**22**), by which time the tumor has often reached a considerable size (5–8 cm in diameter).

Infratentorial ependymomas generally arise from the floor of the fourth ventricle, the expanded walls of which form a hypodense halo. Hydrocephalus is invariably present at diagnosis. Authors consistently emphasize the "plasticity" of these tumors, or their tendency to squeeze through the foramina of the fourth ventricle and spread into the subarachnoid space of the posterior fossa. The tumors may extend through the foramen of Luschka into the cerebellopontine angle cisterns, or through the foramen of Magendie to the spinal subarachnoid space. Tumors located on the floor of the fourth ventricle tend to expand the superior portion of the ventricle. Like their supratentorial counterparts, approximately 50% of infratentorial ependymomas contain calcifications. This leaves a sizable number that show little or no density contrast to their surroundings on unenhanced scans, but ependymomas invariably show marked enhancement after contrast administration. Foci of intratumoral hemorrhage may be observed.

Differential Diagnosis

Infratentorial ependymoma in the pediatric age group requires differentiation from medulloblastoma (the most common posterior fossa tumor in children), from astrocytomas of the brain stem and cerebellum, and from rare tumors (ganglioglioma, hemangioblastoma, teratoma). Calcification is less common in medulloblastomas than in ependymomas. Medulloblastomas often show mixed density on plain CT scans due to intratumoral hemorrhage and necrosis. Ependymomas tend to show more conspicuous contrast enhancement.

The presence of cystic components helps to differentiate supratentorial ependymomas from other supratentorial tumors such as choroid plexus papilloma and meningioma. It is difficult to distinguish extraventricular ependymoma from other extraventricular tumors at a similar location, since any tumors in the glioma group may contain cysts and necrotic components.

Follow-Up

The standard criteria for the radiologic detection of recurrence are a reduction in the postoperative tissue defect, the appearance of new enhancing soft tissue, or progressive enlargement of enhancing tissue. Seeding into the subarachnoid space (including the spinal canal) may also be observed.

Subependymoma

Frequency: rare.

Suggestive morphologic findings: a solid mass in the ventricular wall, heterogeneous density, hyperdense with intratumoral hemorrhage, usually shows marked contrast enhancement. Calcification may be present.

Procedure: histologic evaluation is required, as subependymoma is not distinguishable from ependymoma by noninvasive methods.

Other studies: only MRI or myelography is suitable for spinal screening.

Checklist for scan interpretation:
▶ Location?
▶ Hydrocephalus?
▶ Evidence of subarachnoid seeding?

■ Pathogenesis

Like ependymomas, subependymomas are tumors that arise from the ventricular wall. Subependymomas originate from subependymal glial tissue and have much the same histology. Mixed forms, with elements of ependymoma and subependymoma, also occur, and a few subependymomas are relatively aggressive in their biologic behavior.

As a rule, subependymomas are benign tumors that rarely become symptomatic. They are detected incidentally in CT examinations performed for some other indication (or at autopsy). Invasive growth and subependymal spread are unusual.

■ Frequency

Subependymoma is a rare tumor that is usually asymptomatic and is mainly discovered at autopsy.

■ Clinical Manifestations

Supratentorial subependymomas generally do not cause clinical symptoms. It should be noted, however, that an absence of symptoms is mainly characteristic of supratentorial tumors. Infratentorial and spinal subependymomas lead to hydrocephalus or compression syndromes, even when biologically benign. Middle-aged and elderly adults are most commonly affected.

■ CT Morphology

Subependymomas form nodular masses of variable size in the ventricular wall. The tumor nodules are usually easy to distinguish from brain tissue and tend to have a small area of contact with it. Subependymomas may be hypodense or hyperdense. Extensive cystic change and extensive calcification appear to be unusual, although minute calcifications have been observed along with foci of intratumoral hemorrhage. Both changes may appear as hyperdense areas. Intense contrast enhancement does not rule out a diagnosis of subependymoma.

■ Differential Diagnosis

The differential diagnosis includes ependymoma, which is almost indistinguishable from subependymoma by its CT features. Subependymal giant-cell astrocytoma can be identified by noting the cerebral stigmata of tuberous sclerosis or other cerebral changes that occur in this phakomatosis. Nodular masses in the ventricular wall may also consist of heterotopic cortical tissue. Because this tissue represents periventricular gray matter located within the white matter, it is equivalent to gray matter in its unenhanced CT density, enhancement characteristics, and signal intensity on MRI.

Choroid Plexus Tumors

Choroid Plexus Papilloma and Carcinoma

> **Frequency:** generally rare, making up approximately 0.5% of intracranial tumors in adults. Accounts for 10% of intracranial tumors before 1 year of age, however, and 3–5% of intracranial tumors in children.
>
> **Suggestive morphologic findings:** "fern-like" pattern, intense enhancement.
>
> **Procedure:** coronal reformatted images can be helpful for differentiating choroid plexus tumor from secondary intraventricular tumor. Contrast administration is always indicated.
>
> **Other studies:** MRI is advantageous owing to arbitrary plane selection, and is useful for general screening of the neuraxis for CSF metastases.
>
> **Checklist for scan interpretation:**
> ▶ Location?
> ▶ Hydrocephalus?

Pathogenesis

Choroid plexus carcinoma is a highly malignant variant of choroid plexus papilloma. Infiltration of the white matter with extensive perifocal edema should raise suspicion of the malignant variant, which also causes seeding of CSF pathways. Choroid plexus papilloma is most common before 2 years of age but may also occur in adults.

Frequency

On the whole, choroid plexus tumors are rare. They make up approximately 0.4–1% of intracranial tumors, depending on the source. About 70% of patients are under 2 years of age.

Clinical Manifestations

A large percentage of choroid plexus papillomas are diagnosed in the first year of life, although the tumor may occur in later decades. The lateral ventricles are more commonly affected in children, and the fourth ventricle in adults. Males predominate. Severe hydro-

cephalus is almost always present and results from excessive CSF production by the tumor rather than obstruction.

CT Morphology

The tumors typically show an irregular, "fern-like" surface. Supratentorial tumors are often located in the trigone of the lateral ventricle, and infratentorial tumors are often found in the fourth ventricle (Fig. 5.**23**).

Choroid plexus tumors are isodense or slightly hyperdense to the white matter on noncontrast scans. Calcifications are frequent. Intense enhancement occurs after contrast administration. Papillomas are indistinguishable from carcinoma in the absence of infiltrative growth. Multiple tumors are occasionally observed.

Differential Diagnosis

Because of their intense contrast enhancement, at least on CT scans, vascular malformations of the choroid plexus are apt to be confused with choroid plexus papilloma. They can be differentiated by unenhanced MRI (vascular flow void) or by angiography. Cysts of the

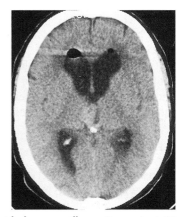

Fig. 5.**23 Choroid plexus papilloma.** Noncontrast CT demonstrates a hyperdense mass with smooth margins in the third ventricle, rostral to the calcified pineal gland.

choroid plexus are a more common finding. They are generally asymptomatic, but they may cause obstruction, and are occasionally mistaken for tumors. Cysts may be unilateral or bilateral. Older studies attributed them to cystic degeneration of the choroid plexus, but the same lesions have been described in children. Carcinoma can develop as a malignant variant of choroid plexus papilloma, and may show an infiltrative growth pattern on CT.

Neuroepithelial Tumors of Unknown Origin

Gliomatosis Cerebri

Frequency: rare.

Suggestive morphologic findings: increase in brain volume, hypodensities.

Procedure: no causal treatment, stereotactic biopsy.

Other studies: diagnosis requires demonstrating multiple-lobe involvement, so it is insufficient to biopsy a single site.

Checklist for scan interpretation:
▶ Enough evidence to make a presumptive diagnosis?

■ Pathogenesis

Gliomatosis cerebri is distinguished from primary brain tumors; this applies to unifocal gliomas, as well as multifocal and multicentric forms. Gliomatosis cerebri involves a diffuse infiltration of the brain by neoplastic astrocytes, often occurring along anatomic or functional structural units. White-matter tracts are predominantly affected. Brain anatomy is preserved.

Gliomatosis cerebri is slowly progressive, but published reports include cases with a peracute course as well as indolent cases that apparently develop over decades.

■ Frequency

Gliomatosis cerebri is a very rare disease. Accurate data have not been published regarding its incidence or prevalence.

■ Clinical Manifestations

Patients exhibit nonspecific personality changes.

■ CT Morphology

CT shows a substantial increase in brain volume accompanied by more or less diffuse hypodensity. The ventricles are correspondingly small, unless there has been outflow obstruction leading to localized expansion. There have been isolated reports of solitary or multiple hypodense foci that may show contrast enhancement.

■ Differential Diagnosis

A definitive diagnosis by brain biopsy is usually preceded by several misdiagnoses. An infiltrative glioma may be mistaken for gliomatosis cerebri, but generally a focal mass lesion can be identified somewhere in the brain. It is very difficult to distinguish gliomatosis cerebri from leukoencephalopathy, multifocal leukoencephalopathy, multiple sclerosis, and various ischemic changes. A helpful criterion is that leukoencephalopathy, unlike gliomatosis, never involves the gray matter.

Neuronal and Mixed Neuronal/Glial Tumors

Gangliocytoma

Frequency: very rare.

Suggestive morphologic findings: cystic and calcified tumor-like mass.

Procedure: MRI.

Other studies: MRI is more sensitive than CT (no beam-hardening artifact, Fig. 5.**24 b**).

Checklist for scan interpretation:
▶ Calcifications, cysts, enhancement characteristics?
▶ Compression of fourth ventricle? Hydrocephalus?

■ Pathogenesis

Gangliocytoma is a low-grade nerve cell tumor. A more malignant variant is ganglioglioma. Lhermitte–Duclos disease is a variant affecting the cerebellar hemispheres.

■ Frequency

Extremely rare.

■ Clinical Manifestations

Gangliocytoma is often located in the temporal lobe, where it typically produces seizures. Occurrence in the posterior fossa leads to cerebellar symptoms such as gait disturbance and vertigo. More extensive spread leads to cranial nerve deficits.

■ CT Morphology

Cystic and calcified structures are a typical finding. There is usually no contrast enhancement.

■ Differential Diagnosis

The main tumor to be considered in differential diagnosis is oligodendroglioma. Chondrosarcoma is a rare tumor that may present with similar features.

Ganglioglioma

Frequency: 0.3–0.9 % of brain tumors; more common in children and adolescents (up to 8 %).

Suggestive morphologic findings: hypodense (cystic) temporal mass, often with calcification or rim enhancement.

Procedure: temporal lobe CT projection.

Other studies: MRI can demonstrate temporal lobe tumors without artifacts.

Checklist for scan interpretation:
the diagnosis is rarely made prior to surgery. The key points are as follows:
▶ Location?
▶ Structure: cystic, solid, calcifications?
▶ Mass effect, edema?

Fig. 5.**24 a, b   Gangliocytoma.** The magnetic resonance imaging (MRI) sequence, chosen to optimize contrast between the white matter and the cortex, clearly demonstrates a rounded mass in the right mesial temporal lobe.
a CT clearly demonstrates the partially calcified mass. In addition, there is an arachnoid cyst adjacent to the temporal pole.
b MRI. The tumor is more clearly visualized.

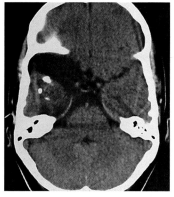
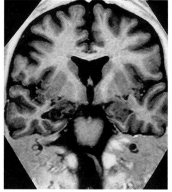

a   b

▪ Pathogenesis

Ganglioglioma is a low-grade, slow-growing neoplasm. Histologically, it consists of neural cells mixed with glial tissue.

▪ Frequency

Ganglioglioma, like gangliocytoma, is extremely rare. It mainly affects children and young adults. The peak incidence is at approximately age 11.

▪ Clinical Manifestations

Temporal lobe epilepsy is a common presenting feature in patients with ganglioglioma. Increasing frequency of seizures is an important clue to the underlying tumor. A long history of headaches is often present.

▪ CT Morphology

The CT appearance of gangliogliomas is somewhat variable. They are usually supratentorial, showing a preference for the temporal lobes. An infratentorial location is less characteristic.

One author, however, cites the floor of the third ventricle as a typical site of occurrence. The tumor is hypodense on noncontrast CT, and often contains one or more cysts, which appear as foci of water density. Calcifications are found in approximately one-third of gangliogliomas (Fig. 5.**25**).

Contrast enhancement of the solid portion of the tumor occurs in about half of the cases.

▪ Differential Diagnosis

Ganglioglioma may be omitted from the differential diagnosis because of its rarity, but should be considered in the differential diagnosis of infratentorial tumors, along with Lhermitte–Duclos disease, a hamartoma-like dysplasia.

▪ Follow-Up

The treatment of choice is surgical removal. Although the tumors appear to have well-defined margins, complete removal may not be possible, depending on the location. However, even an incomplete resection may be followed by good long-term survival, with clinical improvement and no significant tumor growth. Consequently, postoperative radiation and chemotherapy are usually withheld.

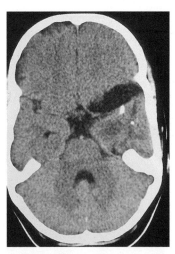

Fig. 5.**25** **Ganglioglioma.** Noncontrast CT in a 10-year-old girl shows expansion of the extra-axial cerebrospinal fluid spaces over the left temporal pole, accompanied by an intraparenchymal, hypodense mass approximately 2 cm in diameter, containing coarse calcifications.

Central Neurocytoma

Frequency: rare tumor, frequently mistaken for oligodendroglioma.

Suggestive morphologic findings: purely intraventricular mass with cysts and calcifications in young adults.

Procedure: a presumptive diagnosis can be made from CT findings.

Other studies: MRI is less rewarding, as it cannot confirm calcification. The angiographic findings are nonspecific.

Checklist for scan interpretation:
▸ Strictly intraventricular location?
▸ Calcifications?

Pathogenesis

The tumor cells closely resemble normal neurons; corresponding markers are used in neuropathologic analysis.

While neuroblastoma can be viewed as a more malignant type of neuroectodermal tumor, central neurocytoma is a benign but related variant of the latter type of lesion.

Frequency

Central neurocytoma has not been accepted as a separate entity for very long, and accurate data on its incidence and prevalence are therefore not yet available. On the whole, however, the tumor is rare.

Clinical Manifestations

Clinical symptoms are nonspecific. They include headache and symptoms caused by hydrocephalus.

CT Morphology

CT in typical cases demonstrates an intraventricular mass with moderately well-defined margins, mild to moderate contrast enhancement, and coarse calcifications. Multiple small cysts are also common. The tumor is isodense or slightly hypodense to the white matter on noncontrast scans. A frequent location is near the foramen of Monro, leading to expansion of the lateral ventricles. At least one case of noninvasive tumor extension through the third ventricle into the fourth ventricle has been described in the literature.

Differential Diagnosis

Among tumors that have a subependymal origin, ependymomas and subependymomas are typically located in the fourth ventricle. Ependymomas occur predominantly in children, while neurocytoma is a tumor of young adults. The differential diagnosis should include intraventricular gliomas, which are distinguished by edema of the peritumoral white matter. Choroid plexus papillomas enhance intensely after contrast administration, and occur mainly in children.

Follow-Up

With regard to the problem of residual or recurrent tumor, published studies indicate that even incomplete tumor removal leads to a regression of symptoms.

Esthesioneuroblastoma

Frequency: rare, but probably underdiagnosed.

Suggestive morphologic findings: mass below the cribriform plate.

Procedure: surgical removal.

Other studies: coronal MRI is useful for detecting intracranial extension.

Checklist for scan interpretation:
▶ Destruction of cribriform plate?
▶ Intracranial extension?
▶ What spaces are affected (paranasal sinuses, etc.)?
▶ Tumor stage according to Kadish et al. (1976) (see below).

Pathogenesis

Esthesioneuroblastoma arises from olfactory epithelial cells. Tumors such as neuroblastoma, pheochromocytoma, and the forms occurring in multiple endocrine neoplasia (MEN) syndromes have a related origin.

The following pretherapy staging system can be used:

● Stage A: tumor is limited to the nasal cavity.
● Stage B: tumor is localized to the nasal cavity and one or more paranasal sinuses.
● Stage C: tumor has infiltrated the orbits, skull base, or cervical lymph nodes, or there is other metastatic spread.

Therapeutic approaches vary. Given the relatively poor prognosis, surgical treatment is generally supplemented by radiotherapy, chemotherapy, or both.

■ Frequency

Esthesioneuroblastoma is an extremely rare tumor; only about 200 cases have been described in the literature.

■ Clinical Manifestations

Reports on affected age groups vary in different series. The case numbers are probably too small for reliable estimates. A slight male predominance has been noted in some series.

Symptoms result from the rich blood supply of the tumor (often supplied by the ophthalmic artery) and its location. Epistaxis and nasal airway obstruction are observed.

■ CT Morphology

Direct coronal CT scans (plain and postcontrast, soft-tissue window, bone window) are recommended (Fig. 5.**26**).

The typical site of occurrence is the upper nasal cavity, below the cribriform plate. The tumors display a very homogeneous density before and after contrast administration. Intratumoral hemorrhage and cysts are usually absent. Calcifications are common, but bone destruction is also common, making it difficult to distinguish tumoral calcification from displaced bone fragments. Erosive bone changes suggest extension into adjacent compartments (Fig. 5.**26**).

■ Differential Diagnosis

The radiologic differential diagnosis of esthesioneuroblastoma is difficult. The tumor should be considered in the evaluation of all midline masses that appear to be located in the anterior fossa. Differentiation is particularly required from frontobasal meningioma, which may show extracranial extension into the paranasal sinuses with a midline location. Bone-forming tumors, chondrosarcoma, and similar

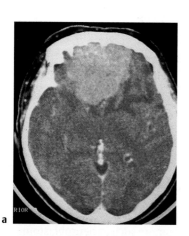

a

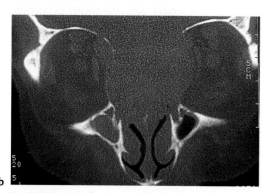

b

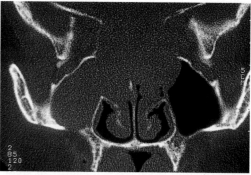

c

Fig. 5.**26 a–c** **Esthesioneuroblastoma.**
a An axial CT scan after contrast administration shows a very large mass with perifocal edema, abutting the anterior skull base.

b, c On direct coronal scans with a bone window, the very large extracerebral tumor component filling the ethmoid cells and sphenoid sinus and extending into the left frontal sinus helps to distinguish the tumor from meningioma.

entities are less homogeneous, consistently calcify, and show less contrast enhancement. Fibrous dysplasia also has a nonhomogeneous appearance. Squamous-cell carcinoma is the most common tumor that can mimic esthesioneuroblastoma in its imaging morphology.

Pineal Parenchymal Tumors

Pineocytoma, Pineoblastoma, Pineal Cyst

Frequency: rare; pineocytomas and pineoblastomas are considerably rarer than germinomas.

Suggestive morphologic findings: mass arising from the pineal region.

Procedure: MRI may be required. Contrast administration is essential.

Other studies: sagittal MRI contributes to accurate localization.

Checklist for scan interpretation:
▶ Hydrocephalus?
▶ Location in relation to third ventricle, vein of Galen, quadrigeminal plate?
▶ Calcifications, signs of infiltrative growth?

■ Pathogenesis

Pineocytoma is the more benign type of pineal parenchymal tumor. The more aggressive form is pineoblastoma.

■ Frequency

Pineal region tumors are relatively rare, making up approximately 3–8% of brain tumors in children and less than 1% in adults. Pineal cysts, by contrast, are a common incidental finding. In one large series, they were detected in about 4% of MRI examinations, and they are found in some 25–40% of autopsies. The frequency distribution of pineal region tumors in a series of 370 cases was as follows:

- Germinomas 27%
- Astrocytomas 26%
- Pineocytomas 12%
- Pineoblastomas 12%
- Ependymomas 4%
- Other tumors, including lymphomas and metastases, < 3%

■ Clinical Manifestations

Nearly all patients with pineal region tumors become symptomatic due to impairment of CSF circulation. The manifestations may be headache, vomiting, lethargy, or increased head circumference in children. Hormone-producing tumors can lead to precocious puberty and other endocrinopathies, depending on their specific substrates. A mass effect on the quadrigeminal plate may lead to Parinaud's syndrome.

■ CT Morphology

Published reports vary on the CT features of these rare tumors. They are usually described as appearing isodense or hyperdense to normal brain tissue and as showing moderate to marked contrast enhancement. Pineoblastomas show early infiltrative growth, while pineocytomas are more sharply marginated. Calcifications are found in pineocytoma, but less consistently than in germinoma. Calcifications apparently do not occur in pineoblastoma.

■ Differential Diagnosis

An aggressive pineoblastoma that infiltrates the cerebellar vermis may be mistaken for medulloblastoma.

Embryonal Tumors

Medulloepithelioma

> **Frequency:** very rare.
>
> **Suggestive morphologic findings:** smoothly marginated cystic/solid mass.
>
> **Procedure:** radical excision.
>
> **Other studies:** multiplanar MRI.
>
> **Checklist for scan interpretation:**
> ▶ Contrast enhancement (atypical)?
> ▶ Smooth margins (typical)?
> ▶ Intracranial or spinal metastases via CSF pathways?

■ **Pathogenesis**

Medulloepithelioma is included in the class of primitive neuroectodermal tumors (PNETs). It bears a close histologic resemblance to the primitive cells of the neural tube. Medulloepitheliomas are highly malignant, and survival is often less than one year. While cerebral medulloepithelioma has a poor prognosis, the ocular form of the tumor takes a much more favorable course. Children with ocular medulloepithelioma often remain disease-free after enucleation of the eye.

■ **Frequency**

Medulloepithelioma is extremely rare.

■ **Clinical Manifestations**

Medulloepithelioma is a tumor of early childhood. Most cases have been described during the first years of life, and occurrence after age 10 is very unusual.

■ **CT Morphology**

Medulloepitheliomas are usually located in the periventricular white matter. Occurrence in the brain stem has also been reported. Like other PNETs, they are sharply marginated. Generally they have both cystic and solid components. They are isodense or hypodense to surrounding tissues on noncontrast CT scans and usually do not enhance after contrast administration. Intratumoral hemorrhage is occasionally observed, but calcifications are absent.

■ **Differential Diagnosis**

Medulloepitheliomas located in the brain stem require differentiation from gliomas. This form is distinguished from pilocytic astrocytoma by its lack of enhancement after contrast administration and by its well-defined margins.

■ **Follow-Up**

Like other intracerebral tumors, medulloepitheliomas have a tendency to disseminate via CSF pathways. Consequently, the radiologist should look for intracranial and spinal metastases during the initial examination and in follow-ups.

Neuroblastoma

> **Frequency:** the primary intracerebral form is rare. Metastases are more common.
>
> **Suggestive morphologic findings:** supratentorial mass, frequently large, containing calcifications, hemorrhagic foci, and cysts.
>
> **Procedure:** seeding via CSF pathways, including the spinal canal, must be investigated.
>
> **Other studies:** MRI is superior for detecting CSF dissemination, particularly to the spine.
>
> **Checklist for scan interpretation:**
> ▶ Typical combination of intratumoral hemorrhage, calcifications, and cysts?
> ▶ Infiltration of dural sinuses (risk of distant metastasis with need to evaluate chest, etc.)?
> ▶ Relation to ventricles (CSF dissemination)?
> ▶ Hydrocephalus?
> ▶ Note necessity for MRI evaluation (for spinal metastases).

■ **Pathogenesis**

Neuroblastomas are highly malignant tumors, which frequently recur and are associated with a high incidence of CSF and non-CSF metastases. The precise histologic classification of neuroblastomas is controversial.

■ Frequency

Very rare.

■ Clinical Manifestations

Clinical symptoms vary with the site of occurrence. General signs of increased intracranial pressure are most commonly observed. Seizures and hemiparetic symptoms can also occur.

■ CT Morphology

The CT appearance of neuroblastoma (Fig. 5.**27**) is fairly characteristic.

The tumors are predominantly supratentorial and often show a relation to the ventricular system. Spontaneous intratumoral hemorrhage often leads to a patchy increase in density on unenhanced scans. Calcifications are common, as are cystic components of variable size. Marked enhancement occurs after contrast administration.

CSF dissemination is a frequent and specific feature of neuroblastoma. Nodular metastases may be found in the ventricles or extra-axial

CSF spaces, and there may be tumor encasement of the spinal cord.

■ Differential Diagnosis

A heterogeneous appearance is characteristic of various other tumors. Oligodendrogliomas, especially the more malignant forms, can have a variety of imaging features. This is also true of astrocytomas in children. Ependymomas and other PNETs should also be included in the differential diagnosis.

■ Follow-Up

Recurrences are common, and 5-year survival rates are often low even with comprehensive treatment.

Ependymoblastoma

This very rare tumor is included in the group of neuroblastomas, PNETs, and medulloblastomas in the WHO classification. It is a highly malignant, usually intraventricular tumor, with infiltrating margins and a poor prognosis. Ependymoblastoma cannot be reliably distinguished from other intraventricular tumors by CT.

Fig. 5.**27 a, b** **Metastatic neuroblastoma** in a 12-year-old child.
a Postcontrast CT shows an extensive mass involving the middle fossa and paranasal sinuses, with invasion of the left orbit.
   The bone-window scan reveals extensive bone destruction.

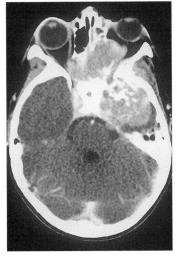
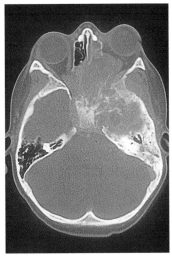

a   b

Primitive Neuroectodermal Tumor/ Medulloblastoma

Frequency: approximately every fifth or sixth brain tumor in children is a medulloblastoma, and it also accounts for one-third of posterior fossa tumors in the pediatric age group.

Suggestive morphologic findings: rounded midline mass, hyperdense on noncontrast CT, occurring in a child. Often located in the roof of the fourth ventricle (fastigium).

Procedure: spinal and cerebral MRI (to detect metastatic deposits).

Other studies: MRI is more sensitive than CT for detecting metastatic deposits and tumor recurrence (posterior fossa).

Checklist for scan interpretation:
▶ Location (midline/hemispheric, infratentorial)?
▶ Unenhanced density? Response to contrast administration?
▶ Calcifications, cysts, blood?
▶ Hydrocephalus?
▶ Tumor nodules located elsewhere in the brain or at the craniocervical junction?

■ Pathogenesis

Metastases from medulloblastoma are not uncommon and are seeded via CSF pathways. Accordingly, metastatic nodules may be found in the cisterns, spinal canal, and leptomeninges. Transpial spread can also occur via the Virchow–Robin perivascular spaces.

Medulloblastomas are classified as grade IV tumors and are among the most aggressive pediatric brain tumors.

■ Frequency

As a prototype PNET, medulloblastoma is the most common brain tumor in children. It accounts for approximately 20–25% of pediatric brain tumors, and has an incidence of 0.5 per 100 000 children. Some 70% of medulloblastomas are diagnosed in patients under 16 years of age, and 80% of affected adults are between age 21 and 40. The peak occurrence is at about 7 years of age. Approximately 65% of patients are male. Seventy-five percent of medulloblastomas arise from the cerebellar vermis.

■ Clinical Manifestations

Most patients are under 10 years of age, but a second peak occurs at the end of adolescence. Males predominate by a ratio of 4 : 1.

Symptoms result from hydrocephalus or vertigo and nausea. Cranial nerve deficits are most often caused by tumors that extend laterally to involve the cerebellopontine cistern.

■ CT Morphology

CT examination in most patients demonstrates a round or elliptical, infratentorial midline mass. The tumor arises from the cerebellar vermis and displaces the fourth ventricle rostrally. A striking feature is its mild hyperdensity on noncontrast CT scans (Fig. 5.**28**).

Medulloblastomas typically show moderate to intense contrast enhancement. Secondary hydrocephalus is almost always present. Calcifications are unusual. The tumors often appear remarkably well-demarcated on images (and at surgery), but this is often found to be misleading on histologic examination. Tumors in the lateral cerebellum are more likely to occur in young adults, and can be difficult to classify in the differential diagnosis.

Less typical cases are distinguished by their nonhomogeneity on noncontrast CT and by irregular or minimal contrast enhancement. Calcifications were found in 17% of tumors in one large series, but intratumoral hemorrhage is extremely rare.

With regard to invasiveness, some correlation has been noted between the sharp margins seen on CT scans and the good demarcation of the tumor found at surgery.

■ Differential Diagnosis

Astrocytomas are an important differential diagnosis. Unlike medulloblastomas, they usually appear hypodense on unenhanced scans. The presence of cysts does not exclude medulloblastoma, however. Similarly, calcifications do not favor a diagnosis of ependymoma over medulloblastoma, although it is important to note that medulloblastoma is a far more common tumor in children.

■ Follow-Up

Recurrent medulloblastoma resembles the primary tumor in that it also appears as a sharply marginated tumor nodule with homogeneous enhancement. Calcifications are more frequently described, however (56%). CSF dissemination may occur even without a recurrent tumor. The metastases may form a "sheet-like" growth, or discrete nodular deposits on enhancing sulci and cisterns.

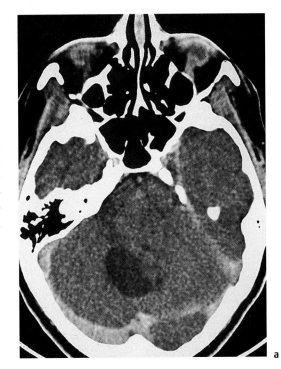

a

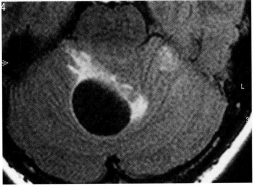

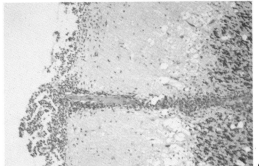

c

Fig. 5.**28 a–d Medulloblastoma** in a 30-year-old woman.
a Postcontrast CT demonstrates a large infratentorial tumor cyst. Nonenhancing soft tissue is visible to the left of the cyst.
b, c The tumor is defined most clearly by magnetic resonance imaging using a fluid-attenuated inversion recovery (FLAIR) sequence, with T2-weighted images in which the cerebrospinal fluid (CSF) appears hypointense. The sagittal image gives the best portrayal of tumor size.
d Histology. Leptomeningeal seeding with secondary infiltration of the cerebellum along the perivascular CSF spaces of the pial vessels.

d

Cranial Nerve Tumors

Schwannoma (Neurinoma)

Frequency: one of the most common intracranial tumors. The incidence is higher in neurofibromatosis.

Suggestive morphologic findings: cerebellopontine angle mass expanding the internal acoustic meatus (bone window). May appear as an enhancing intrameatal mass.

Procedure: CT imaging of the posterior fossa with a bone window and 2-mm slice thickness is performed to demonstrate the jugular bulb in relation to the tumor (a "high bulb" poses an obstacle to surgery).

Other studies: MRI demonstrates cerebellopontine angle tumors better than CT, owing to the lack of beam-hardening artifact. This applies to the differential diagnosis and the detection of spread.

Checklist for scan interpretation:
▶ Check for high position of the jugular bulb (Fig. 5.**29**).

■ Pathogenesis

Acoustic schwannomas may be unilateral or bilateral. Consistent with their clinical features, but contrary to their name, acoustic schwannomas arise from the vestibular nerve. The tumors are benign and require definitive surgical removal.

Some acoustic schwannomas occur in the setting of neurofibromatosis (Fig. 5.**30**). These tumors are often bilateral; they are diagnosed at an early age and coexist with meningiomas (bilateral acoustic schwannomas are pathognomonic for neurofibromatosis type 2).

Rarely, schwannomas occur within the brain parenchyma. With regard to the origin of these tumors, most authors agree that they arise from the Schwann cells of the perivascular neural plexus.

Another atypical site for schwannomas is the labyrinth. They can be detected on magnifi-

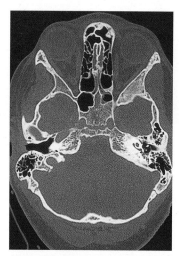

Fig. 5.**29 High position of the right jugular bulb.** The high jugular bulb appears as a rounded mass bounded by cortical bone in the posterior part of the petrous bone, contrasting with a normal appearance on the left side. The high bulb is situated within the surgical access route to the cerebellopontine angle. It should not be mistaken for an osteolytic lesion, associated with a glomus tumor, etc.

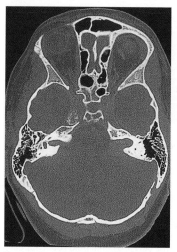

Fig. 5.**30 Expansion of the internal auditory canal.** Bilateral expansion of the internal acoustic meatus in bone-window CT is characteristic of acoustic neuromas in neurofibromatosis.

cation views of the petrous bone, appearing as soft-tissue masses located near the foramen rotundum. Differentiation is required from glomus tympanicum tumors. Except for the optic nerve, which is devoid of Schwann cells, schwannomas can arise from any of the cranial nerves. They are relatively easy to diagnose when they have an extra-axial location and have caused the expansion of bony canals.

Frequency

Acoustic schwannomas are among the most common intracranial tumors and make up about 5–10% of central nervous system (CNS) tumors in most series. The annual incidence is estimated at approximately 0.78–1.15 cases per 100000 population. The great majority of acoustic schwannomas (95%) are unilateral.

Clinical Manifestations

Acoustic schwannoma has an insidious clinical onset. Unilateral hearing loss is the initial symptom, followed later by ataxia and vertigo. Pressure on the brain stem from the tumor may lead to ischemic injury. Hypesthesia in the trigeminal nerve distribution and facial nerve paralysis are also observed. Late symptoms result from hydrocephalus. Cranial nerve deficits are the initial symptoms of cranial nerve schwannomas. Intraparenchymal schwannomas lead to focal neurologic deficits.

CT Morphology

On noncontrast scans of the posterior fossa using a 2-mm slice thickness, expansion of the bony porus acusticus may be the only evidence of an acoustic schwannoma, which is generally isodense to brain tissue. A nonisodense tumor of a relatively large size may appear as a semicircular cerebellopontine angle mass, the convexity of which points to the fourth ventricle (Fig. 5.**31**).

There is little or no evidence of perifocal edema. Larger tumors may displace or even compress the fourth ventricle, leading to hydrocephalus. The typical intrameatal extension

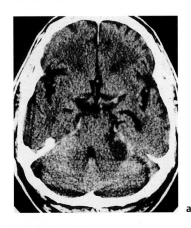

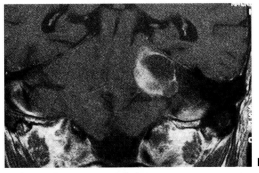

Fig. 5.**31 a, b   Acoustic schwannoma.**
a Noncontrast CT demonstrates a hypodense lesion in the left cerebellopontine angle. Its appearance would be consistent with an arachnoid cyst.
b A predominantly cystic acoustic schwannoma was detected by magnetic resonance imaging and intraoperatively.

of contrast enhancement can be seen only on thin CT slices (Fig. 5.**32**).

Differential Diagnosis

The main entities to be considered in the differential diagnosis of cerebellopontine angle masses are acoustic schwannoma and meningioma (Fig. 5.**33**).

Metastases and lymphomas are of secondary importance, and the latter are rare. Expansion of the bony porus acusticus is characteristic of acoustic schwannomas but generally does not occur with meningiomas. Other differentiating criteria are easier to evaluate

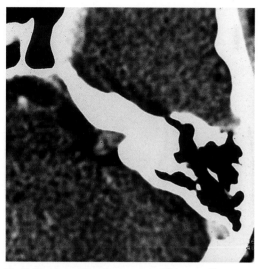

Fig. 5.**32** **Acoustic schwannoma.** This scan illustrates the typical CT appearance of an acoustic schwannoma: an enhancing cerebellopontine angle mass extending into the internal acoustic meatus.

with MRI. One such criterion is the intrameatal extension of contrast enhancement that occurs with schwannomas, compared with the meningeal enhancement that is seen with meningiomas. Although these signs are seen more clearly with MRI, they may cause confusion, since some schwannomas may show limited meningeal enhancement, while meningiomas often show a surprising degree of intrameatal extension. Meningioma should definitely be considered in cases in which hearing loss was not the initial presenting symptom. Other lesions to be considered are epidermoids, arachnoid cysts, and glomus jugulare tumors. These masses are almost always distinguishable by their prolonged T2 relaxation times on MRI.

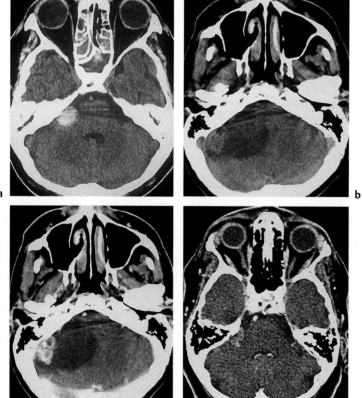

Fig. 5.**33 a–d** **Differential diagnosis of acoustic schwannoma.**
a   A hemorrhage in the cerebellopontine angle is markedly hyperdense on the noncontrast scan.
b, c Cystic metastases with mural nodules should not be mistaken for a cerebellopontine angle tumor with perifocal edema.
d   Meningiomas in this region are equally difficult to distinguish from acoustic schwannoma with CT and magnetic resonance imaging.

Neurofibroma

Frequency: generally rare, but more common in neurofibromatosis type 1.

Suggestive morphologic findings: periorbital soft-tissue masses, frequent sphenoid dysplasia.

Procedure: contrast-enhanced MRI of the head.

Other studies: MRI is generally superior to CT in the imaging of phakomatoses.

Checklist for scan interpretation:
▶ Other tumors (gliomas)?
▶ Sphenoid wing dysplasia?
▶ Size of globes in side-to-side comparison?
▶ Hamartia (MRI)?

■ Pathogenesis

Neurofibromas are composed of Schwann cells, fibroblasts, and perineural cells. They may occur as solitary lesions or in the setting of neurofibromatosis type 1 (classic Recklinghausen disease). They are benign tumors ("plexiform neurofibroma"), but a certain percentage undergo malignant transformation.

Sarcomatous degeneration occurs as a malignant variant. It is seen primarily in the setting of neurofibromatosis type 1.

■ Frequency

Neurofibromatosis type 1 is the most common phakomatosis, with an incidence of approximately one per 3000. Both sexes are affected equally.

■ Clinical Manifestations

Neurofibromatosis type 1 can have various manifestations, depending on the predominant tumor entity. Sphenoid wing dysplasia and retrobulbar masses can produce external signs. Optic gliomas can cause visual deterioration, depending on their location.

■ CT Morphology

Bone-window scans of the facial skeleton often show a size discrepancy between the sphenoid wings. A change in bone shape may also be observed. CT may also show disparate sizes of the ocular globes. Plexiform neurofibromas can vary greatly in size, ranging in appearance from plaque-like areas of increased density (Fig. 5.**34**) within the orbital fat to larger periorbital masses (e.g., within the bony orbit).

■ Differential Diagnosis

Neurofibromatosis type 2 is characterized by bilateral acoustic schwannomas. It may also be associated with multiple meningiomas and solitary neurofibromas.

Fig. 5.**34 a, b Multiple neurofibromas.** This patient presented with confluent tumors covering the entire right side of the face. CT shows marked deformation of the right sphenoid wing and extension of tumor nodules into the right orbit, which is communicating with the ethmoid cells in places. The tumors are hypodense without contrast medium, and enhance strongly after contrast administration.
a Noncontrast scan.
b Postcontrast scan.

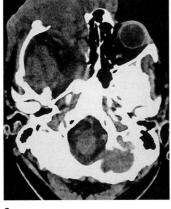

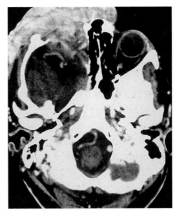

a   b

Meningeal Tumors

Meningioma

Frequency: 10–20% of intracranial tumors.

Suggestive morphologic findings: mass broadly based on the meninges, slightly hyperdense, enhances intensely after contrast administration.

Procedure: MRI on three planes is indicated prior to surgery. Angiography may be useful for detecting sinus infiltration, defining tumor blood supply, and for preoperative embolization.

Other studies: MRI is better for defining the relation to the meninges and showing peritumoral meningeal enhancement.

Checklist for scan interpretation:
▶ Bone infiltration?
▶ Ingrowth into foramina or optic canal?
▶ Multiple meningiomas or schwannomas suggesting neurofibromatosis?

■ Pathogenesis

Meningiomas arise from the dura mater, or more precisely from the arachnoid cells on its inner surface. Thus, meningiomas are classic extra-axial tumors. Not all meningiomas are in contact with the dura. Examples are tumors arising from the choroid plexus or tumors that have seeded from intraorbital meningioma. The incidence of meningiomas is highest in middle-aged women.

Since the great majority of meningiomas are benign, the prognosis is determined as much by location and resectability as by histologic type. Various histologic subtypes of meningioma have been described, including the common meningotheliomatous and fibrous subtypes. Hemangiopericytomas are a special type of vascular origin. Meningiosarcoma is a malignant form. Angiography can demonstrate a relationship between histologic subtype and vascularity. Endotheliomatous meningiomas, meningiosarcomas, and hemangiopericytomas have a rich blood supply, while the fibrous forms are less vascular.

In addition to these low-grade types of meningioma, there are more aggressive varieties characterized by infiltrative growth, necrosis, and metastasis. "Anaplastic" meningiomas are classified as grade III neoplasms.

The meninges can give rise to other tumors as well. The most notable of these are melanin-containing lesions (diffuse melanosis, melanocytoma, malignant melanoma, meningeal melanomatosis). Very little has been published on the CT appearance of these lesions, however.

■ Frequency

Meningiomas account for 14–19% of primary intracranial tumors, according to various series. The peak age incidence is 45 years, and females predominate by about 2 : 1. Only about 1.5% of meningiomas occur in children and adolescents, and many of these tumors result from neurofibromatosis.

■ Clinical Manifestations

A significant percentage of meningiomas are discovered incidentally. Because meningiomas can occur virtually anywhere in the cranial cavity (Fig. 5.**35**), a broad range of symptoms is observed.

Possible symptoms range from headache and focal seizures (convexity meningiomas), nausea and gait disturbance (tentorial meningiomas with secondary hydrocephalus) to visual disturbances and exophthalmos (sphenoid wing meningiomas). The spectrum of clinical features is too extensive to be covered here.

A large percentage of symptomatic meningiomas show perifocal edema when diagnosed. This phenomenon does not always correlate with tumor size: small meningiomas may be surrounded by extensive edema, while large meningiomas may show no edema. Malignant meningiomas are almost invariably associated with perifocal edema, however.

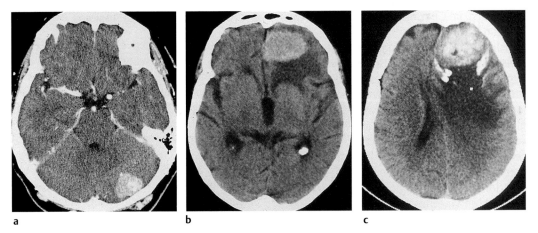

a   b   c

Fig. 5.**35 a–c** **Meningioma.** As extra-axial tumors, meningiomas are characterized by a broad dural base and sharp delineation from the brain tissue.

a This scan shows an intensely enhancing, smoothly marginated meningioma that extends inferiorly from the tentorium.

b It is not unusual to find marked peritumoral edema, which is here surrounding a meningioma arising from the anterior falx.

c The tumors often reach a large size before being diagnosed, and they may show a considerable mass effect in addition to perifocal edema.

■ CT Morphology

Aside from special forms such as meningioma en plaque, sphenoid wing meningioma, and intraventricular, intraorbital and ectopic forms (Figs. 5.**36**, 5.**37**), the appearance of mening-

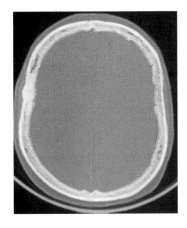

Fig. 5.**36** **Meningioma presenting only with bone** ▷ **changes.** This patient had normal-appearing soft-tissue scans (not shown), but the bone-window scan shows an osteoplastic reaction in the right parietal area. The inner and outer tables are thickened, the diploë is sclerotic, and spicules are visible on the inner calvarial surface.

Fig. 5.**37 a, b** **Sites of occurrence of meningioma.**

a In the slice shown, a lateral sphenoid-wing meningioma has the appearance of an intraaxial mass. A smaller, parasellar meningioma is also visible.

b A large petroclival meningioma with secondary hydrocephalus (enlargement of frontal and temporal horns) and pressure cones.

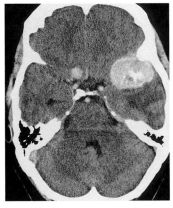 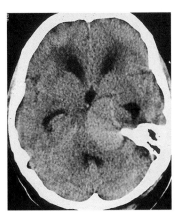

a   b

iomas on axial CT scans is determined by their location.

Almost all meningiomas are mildly hyperdense on noncontrast CT. Isodense or strongly hyperdense calcifications are found rarely. Intratumoral cysts are also uncommon. Meningiomas usually have smooth, well-defined margins, and the lesion typically appears as a convex, juxtadural mass projecting toward the center of the skull. Rapid, intense enhancement occurs after intravenous contrast administration. Since meningiomas are extra-axial, contrast enhancement in these lesions does not result from a defect in the blood–brain barrier (which is absent). As with extracranial tumors, the enhancement mechanism is based on tumor vascularity and contrast extravasation into the interstitium.

If the meningeal attachment lies in the plane of the axial scan, the meningioma can simulate a rounded intra-axial mass that is not obviously related to the dura (Fig. 5.**38**).

In addition to the characteristic soft-tissue mass described above, characteristic changes may be noted in the adjacent bone. Meningiomas lead to hyperostosis of the calvarium underlying the dural base. This hyperostosis may affect the inner table, outer table, and diploë separately or in varying combinations (Fig. 5.**36**). Many authors state that hyperostosis always signifies infiltration.

■ Growth Patterns of Meningioma

A particularly distinctive growth pattern is seen with sphenoid wing meningioma, which forms a plaque-like growth along the dura of the middle cranial fossa (meningioma en plaque). Often a substantial soft-tissue mass is visible only in the temporopolar area. A bone-window scan is necessary to detect the pronounced osseous component of the tumor (Fig. 5.**39**).

The bone-window scan demonstrates expansion of the sphenoid wing involving all three bony layers and frequently showing intraorbital extension (Figs. 5.**40**, 5.**41**).

Extension into the paranasal sinuses is also common, and is manifested by lucent areas within the diploë. These lucencies are found in proximity to meningioma cells and are useful for assessing maximum tumor extent. Often the involved anatomic structures will preclude a complete tumor resection. Brain-stem compression may occur in later stages.

Whenever a meningioma is growing in the vicinity of a dural sinus, there is a potential for dural sinus infiltration. Evidence of this can usually be found on standard contrast-enhanced scans. If the case cannot be investigated further by angiography, multiple CT scans acquired with a stationary table after bolus contrast injection can document the

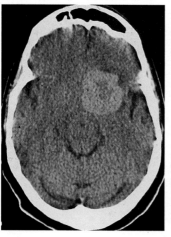
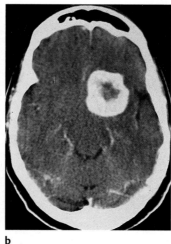

Fig. 5.**38 a, b Apparent intra-parenchymal meningioma.** If the dural attachment of a meningioma lies in the axial image plane, the tumor will mimic an intra-axial lesion in some slices. This medial sphenoid-wing meningioma is already markedly hyperdense on the noncontrast scan. The scan after contrast administration shows an intensely enhancing mass with a nonenhancing center. This pattern is not typical of meningioma, but it is not uncommon.
a Before contrast administration.
b After contrast administration.

a

b

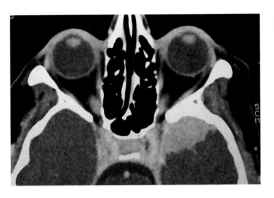

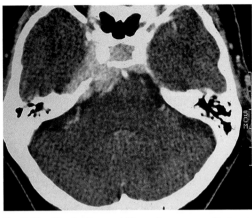

Fig. 5.**39 Sphenoid-wing meningioma.** Postcontrast CT shows an intensely enhancing mass broadly abutting on the dura of the left sphenoid wing. The medial aspect of the tumor is in broad contact with the cavernous sinus. There is evidence of slight reactive hyperostosis/osseous infiltration of the left sphenoid wing.

Fig. 5.**40 Meningioma at the petrous apex.** Postcontrast CT shows intense, somewhat inhomogeneous enhancement in the area of the left cavernous sinus. The enhancing tissue encompasses the petrous apex. The bone-window scan was normal.

filling defect within the affected sinus. Attention should also be given to venous collaterals, which can develop in response to occlusion of the sagittal sinus.

Multiple meningiomas are not uncommon; some authors state that 10% of meningiomas are multiple. When multiple meningiomas occur, of course, they are easily confused with meningeal metastases.

■ **Differential Diagnosis**

An intra-axial tumor located near the calvarium may be mistaken for the soft-tissue portion of a meningioma. Intracranial tumors that may show mild, homogeneous hyperdensity on plain scans include intracerebral lymphoma, gliomas, and medulloblastoma. Dural metastases may be indistinguishable from meningiomas. Extra-axial tumors can cause confusion, particularly when they are located in the cerebellopontine angle. Schwannomas are distinguished by their tendency to expand the porus acusticus. Aneurysms at the skull base (e.g., parasellar—Fig. 5.**42**) are also occasionally mistaken for meningiomas due to their intense contrast enhancement.

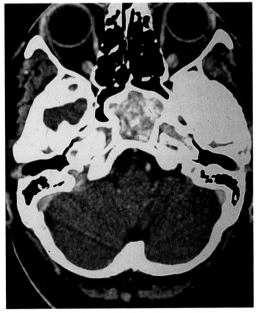

Fig. 5.**41 Infiltration of the sphenoid sinus by a meningioma.** Meningiomas in the anterior skull base region may be associated with bone changes and soft-tissue infiltration of the skull base. In the case shown, the sphenoid sinus is filled with material of soft-tissue attenuation.

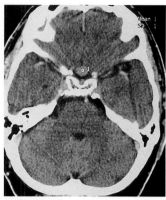
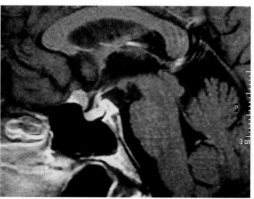

a

b

Fig. 5.**42 a, b Meningioma.** These images illustrate the superior sensitivity of magnetic resonance imaging for detecting small meningiomas. It is common for meningiomas in the cavernous sinus and sellar region to cause symptoms at an early stage. As a result, the tumors are often small at the time of the initial CT examination.

a The small tumor is very difficult to detect with CT.
b Magnetic resonance imaging plainly demonstrates a small meningioma on the roof of the sphenoid sinus.

The calvarial hyperostosis that accompanies meningioma can pose special problems of differential diagnosis. Similar changes are found in association with fibrous dysplasia and osteoma. In the absence of a soft-tissue mass, the following criteria can be applied. Fibrous dysplasia rarely involves the inner table and does not enhance after contrast administration. The bone changes tend to have smooth margins, contrasting with the more spiculated changes seen with meningioma. Involvement of the outer table is characteristic of osteoma (and of Paget disease). While meningioma can cross cranial suture lines because of its arachnoid origin, this is not characteristic of osteoma. Bone metastases arise from the diploë. The imaging appearance of meningiomas can mimic that of lymphomas and metastases (Fig. 5.**43**).

The differential diagnoses for various tumor locations are listed in Table 5.**2**.

CT can be an effective localizing study in meningioma patients. Three-dimensional re-

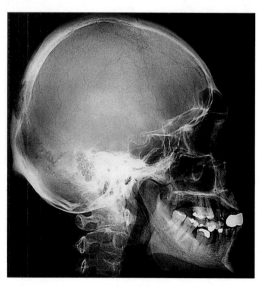

a

Fig. 5.**43 a–g Occipital meningioma with osteolysis.**
a The lateral skull film (obtained to investigate a palpable occipital nodule) demonstrates a lytic lesion.

Abb. 5.**43 b–g** ▷

Fig. 5.**43 b–g**

b, c CT shows a large occipital mass that is hyperdense on the noncontrast scan (**b**) and enhances strongly after contrast administration (**c**).

d The bone-window CT scan demonstrates the area of osteolysis.

e High-resolution magnetic resonance imaging shows a collar-button–shaped tumor extending through the lytic area into the subcutaneous tissue. The absence of dural sinus enhancement indicates sinus involvement.

f, g Angiography shows an intense tumor blush with a filling defect in the sinus.

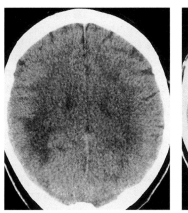

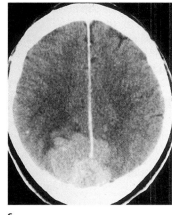

b

c

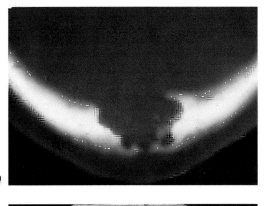

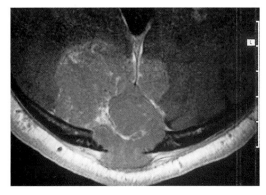

e

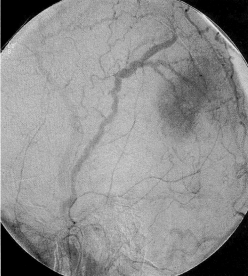

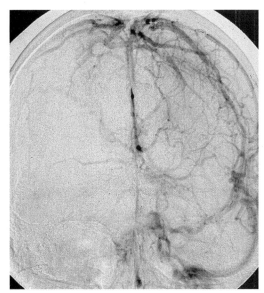

g

constructions can define the relationship of the tumor to the cranial sutures. Knowing this before opening the calvarium can help the surgeon select the best operative approach (Fig. 5.**44**).

Other forms of meningeal tumors, such as malignant melanoma, are rarely encountered.

Table 5.**2** Differential diagnosis of meningioma by tumor location

Location	Important differential diagnoses
Anterior skull base	Metastases Tumors of paranasal sinuses
Sella and parasellar region	Aneurysm Pituitary adenoma Craniopharyngioma Gliomas Tolosa–Hunt syndrome Metastases Chondroma
Convexity	Metastases Lymphoma
Sphenoid wing, middle cranial fossa	Trigeminal schwannoma Fibrous dysplasia
Tentorium, posterior cranial fossa	Medulloblastoma Hemangioblastoma Brain-stem glioma Schwannoma

■ Follow-Up

Meningioma can recur even after a complete resection, and a low tumor grade does not exclude recurrence. Nevertheless, it is still important to remove the tumor completely along with its dural attachment and the adjacent bone, because the recurrence rate is higher following a subtotal resection. Recurrence-free survival after a complete resection is approximately 90 % or more at 5 years, 80 % or more at 10 years, and 70 % or more at 15 years.

The CT detection of recurrent meningioma is relatively straightforward with regard to the soft-tissue portion of the tumor. Like the original tumor, it can be recognized as an intensely enhancing nodule. Dural and osseous recurrences are more difficult. CT can detect dural changes only to the extent that a definite soft-tissue mass is present. With a dural recurrence that consists only of slight dural thickening, MRI can demonstrate contrast enhancement of the recurrence, but it should be borne in mind that dural enhancement is frequently present as a normal postoperative finding. Osteoplastic changes, especially when involving the sphenoid bone due to sphenoid wing meningioma, signify invasion of the bone by tumor cells. Thin-slice CT scanning with a bone window is more rewarding in this situation than contrast-enhanced scanning with a soft-tissue window.

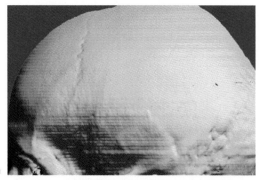

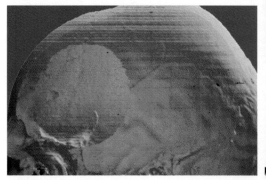

Fig. 5.**44 a, b Meningioma.** Three-dimensional views reconstructed from very thin CT slices (1 mm) can aid surgical planning by defining the relationship between the tumor and the cranial sutures.

a This surface-rendered view shows the coronal suture in a patient with frontobasal meningioma.

b Adjusting the window setting demonstrates a large underlying meningioma.

Expanding bony structures, spiculations, and lucent vesicles within the diploë are all indications of tumor recurrence.

Lipoma

> **Frequency:** very rare.
> **Suggestive morphologic findings:** mass containing both fat and calcifications, located between the frontal horns.
> **Procedure:** imaging findings have no therapeutic implications.
> **Other studies:** sagittal MRI for localization.
>
> **Checklist for scan interpretation:**
> ▶ Structure (fat, bone)?
> ▶ Location?
> ▶ Ventricular malformation?
> ▶ Other malformations?

■ Pathogenesis

The origin of intracranial lipomas is unclear. One theory holds that they are a congenital malformation caused by persistent rests of the primitive meninx. Lipomas may occur in isolation, or in conjunction with other anomalies. They are frequently associated with callosal dysgenesis.

■ Frequency

Intracranial lipomas are a rare incidental finding.

■ Clinical Manifestations

The clinical features of lipomas are location-dependent, ranging from hydrocephalus with its associated symptoms to focal neurologic symptoms.

■ CT Morphology

Lipoma typically appears on CT as a fat-density mass in the interhemispheric fissure. The size is highly variable, ranging from rounded basal cistern masses only a few millimeters in diameter (Fig. 5.**45**) or crescent-shaped fat-density masses abutting the corpus callosum to very large masses that occupy the place of a hypoplastic corpus callosum, extend far laterally from the midline, and contain plaque-like calcifications (Fig. 5.**46**).

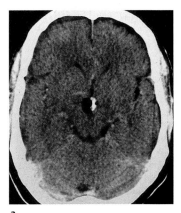 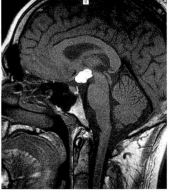 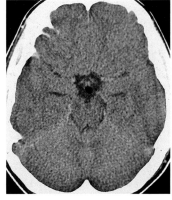

a   b   c

Fig. 5.**45 a–c** **Lipoma.**
a Noncontrast CT shows a calcium-containing mass of fat density at a typical location in the basal cisterns.
b Sagittal T1-weighted magnetic resonance imaging without contrast medium supports the diagnosis of lipoma by showing very high signal intensity, typical of fat.
c CT in a different patient shows a fatty, noncalcified mass at a typical location.

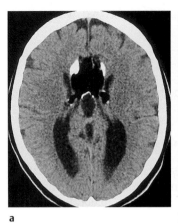
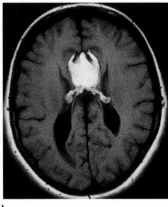

a   b

Fig. 5.**46 a, b Corpus callosum lipoma.** While lipomas of the basal cisterns are usually small, very extensive forms may occur in the corpus callosum.
a The steerhorn shape of the occipital horns of the lateral ventricles on noncontrast CT already suggests a malformation of the corpus callosum. A large fat-containing mass flanked by plaque-like calcifications is visible on the midline anterior to the third ventricle.
b T1-weighted magnetic resonance imaging in the same plane shows an identical pattern, except that the contrast between fat and calcification is reversed.

■ Differential Diagnosis

On cursory examination, small lipomas of the basal cisterns may be confused with aneurysms of the basal cerebral vessels. MRI can confirm the diagnosis of lipoma by demonstrating high fat signal intensity in the unenhanced T1-weighted image. Calcifications of the falx are more likely to be confused with lipomas on MRI than on CT scans. While CT shows falx calcifications as elongated calcium-dense structures in the interhemispheric fissure, the high signal intensity of the central fat marrow tends to dominate image contrast on MRI.

Fibrous Histiocytoma

Frequency: rare.

Suggestive morphologic findings: contact with bone and meninges (suggestive but not conclusive).

Procedure: thin-slice CT with a bone window.

Other studies: multiplanar imaging with MRI.

Checklist for scan interpretation:
▶ Fibrous histiocytoma can be included in the differential diagnosis of atypical meningiomas.

■ Pathogenesis

Malignant fibrous histiocytomas are soft-tissue sarcomas that are most commonly found at retroperitoneal and extremity sites in older patients. A CNS form, which always appears to abut the meninges, is extremely rare.

■ Frequency

Fibrous histiocytoma is an extremely rare tumor that is not seen in everyday clinical routine.

■ Clinical Manifestations

Focal neurologic deficits occur, depending on tumor location.

■ CT Morphology

Contact with the meninges appears to be an essential feature. Published cases have generally consisted of a cystic and solid component.

■ Differential Diagnosis

Malignant fibrous histiocytoma may be considered in the differential diagnosis of atypical-appearing meningiomas and other ring-shaped lesions that are in contact with the meninges. It does not have a characteristic appearance on CT or MRI.

Hemangiopericytoma

Frequency: < 1% of intracranial tumors.

Suggestive morphologic findings: the CT appearance is similar to that of meningioma, but without calcification or hyperostosis.

Procedure: the preoperative work-up includes angiography. Postoperative radiation and chemotherapy are indicated due to the high recurrence rate. Early postoperative MRI establishes a baseline for follow-ups.

Other studies: MRI and angiography are the modalities of choice.

Checklist for scan interpretation:
▶ Location?
▶ Osteolysis?
▶ Signs of invasion (sinus, falx, bone)?

■ Pathogenesis

Hemangiopericytomas arise from Zimmermann pericytes. Originally classified as "angioblastic meningioma," they are not meningiomas, despite their intracranial meningeal origin. They are considerably more aggressive than meningiomas, with a higher rate of invasion and recurrence and a significant rate of distant metastasis.

■ Frequency

Hemangiopericytoma is a very rare neoplasm.

■ Clinical Manifestations

Hemangiopericytomas generally present clinically with focal signs and possible development of hydrocephalus. The peak age incidence is at 30–50 years.

■ CT Morphology

The CT appearance resembles that of meningioma: an extra-axial mass with broad dural contact. Many hemangiopericytomas are located on the floor of one of the three cranial fossae. CT does not show the calcifications or bone reactions that are typical of meningiomas. Like meningiomas, however, the tumors are hyperdense on noncontrast scans and show intense but nonhomogeneous contrast enhancement. They may have lobulated margins.

■ Differential Diagnosis

Hemangiopericytomas cannot be consistently distinguished from meningiomas by their CT appearance. Aggressive features, osteolysis, and an absence of calcification and bone reaction with a presumed meningioma should raise the possibility of a hemangiopericytoma.

■ Follow-Up

Hemangiopericytomas have a strong tendency to recur, and MRI is usually better than CT for postoperative follow-up. Early examinations will provide an effective baseline for follow-ups.

Rhabdomyosarcoma (Fig. 5.47)

Frequency: more common in children than in adults (different manifestations in each group).

Suggestive morphologic findings: usually appears as a large mass of the paranasal sinuses or skull base with extensive bone destruction.

Procedure: MRI, surgery, chemotherapy.

Other studies: MRI directly demonstrates intracranial extension (early sign: meningeal enhancement).

Checklist for scan interpretation:
▶ Intracranial invasion (with common paranasal sinus tumors)?
▶ Bone destruction?
▶ Lymph-node involvement?
▶ Note the need for staging (distant metastases).

■ Pathogenesis

Several histologic types of rhabdomyosarcoma are known:

● Embryonal form (70–80%): the most prevalent type.
● Alveolar form (10–20%): second most prevalent type.
● Botryoid or pleomorphic form: less prevalent.

A botryoid or pleomorphic histology is most common in adults. The prognosis in children is better than in adults. Rhabdomyosarcoma is not limited to the head and neck but can occur anywhere in the body.

■ Frequency

Rhabdomyosarcoma is the second most common primary malignant orbital tumor in children, making up approximately 3–4% of orbital masses in that age group, but it is still generally rare. The peak occurrence is at about 7 years of age, with a male predominance.

■ Clinical Manifestations

Tumors of the head and neck most commonly affect the facial skeleton, including the skull base, paranasal sinuses, and orbits. Accordingly, local signs of a mass lesion are often the main presenting features (expansion, mucocele-like presentation).

■ CT Morphology

Coronal CT usually demonstrates the lesions most clearly.

Bone-window scans with a small slice thickness will often show destruction of the orbital roof (with orbital forms) or anterior skull base (with paranasal sinus tumors). Scans with a soft-tissue window often demonstrate large masses with moderate to marked contrast enhancement. If the tumor obstructs the sinus outlets, retained secretions can be found. Calcification and necrosis are generally absent.

■ Differential Diagnosis

Rhabdomyosarcoma is the most common tumor of this region in children. The differential diagnosis in all patients includes the following:

- Esthesioneuroblastoma
- Malignant lymphoma
- Meningioma
- Chondrosarcoma

An accurate delineation of tumor topography is generally more valuable than making an (often frustrated) attempt to narrow the differential diagnosis.

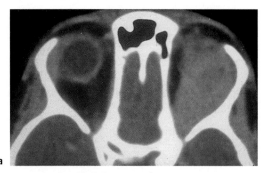

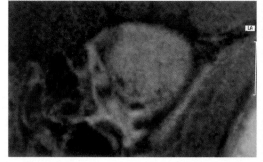

Fig. 5.**47 a, b Rhabdomyosarcoma.**
a Axial CT in a 7-year-old girl demonstrates a mass below the right orbital roof.
b Coronal magnetic resonance imaging resolves the key question of intracranial extension by demonstrating meningeal enhancement and a tumor nodule in the anterior cranial fossa.

Hemangioblastoma

Frequency: 10% of cerebellar tumors, 1.5% of brain tumors in general.

Suggestive morphologic findings: cerebellar cyst with an enhancing mural nodule. The solid form is difficult to recognize as angioblastoma.

Procedure: preoperative angiography, to exclude other sites of occurrence.

Other studies: angiography may demonstrate more tumor nodules than CT or MRI.

Checklist for scan interpretation:
▶ Characteristic imaging appearance?
▶ Compression of fourth ventricle?
▶ Hydrocephalus?

■ Pathogenesis

Hemangioblastomas are also found in Hippel–Lindau syndrome, a phakomatosis. In this setting, they are associated with retinal angiomatosis, as well as with tumors and cysts in the visceral organs.

Hemangioblastoma is essentially benign in its biologic behavior.

■ Frequency

Hemangioblastoma is the most common posterior fossa tumor in adults. Supratentorial occurrence is extremely rare, and fewer than 100 cases of supratentorial hemangioblastoma have been described in the literature. A familial incidence due to Hippel–Lindau syndrome is present in about 20% of cases. The average age of occurrence is 33 years. A slight male predilection exists for solitary hemangioblastoma, but a female predilection is noted in Hippel–Lindau syndrome (one in 36,000 live births).

■ Clinical Manifestations

Hemangioblastomas most commonly affect adults 30–50 years of age. The tumors have a high familial incidence, and multiple forms can occur. Cystic tumors of the posterior fossa are most likely to produce early clinical manifestations, due to compression of the fourth ventricle and hydrocephalus (gait disturbance, headache, personality change).

■ CT Morphology

Hemangioblastomas (Fig. 5.**48**) are usually found in the posterior fossa. Supratentorial forms are extremely rare.

In the series described to date, approximately three-quarters of hemangioblastomas are cystic, with one or more solid mural tumor nodules. The nodules are not visible on plain scans, but enhance intensely after contrast administration. The cyst wall is usually well-defined, and may or may not enhance. Perifocal edema is frequently present. Compression of the fourth ventricle leads to expansion of the supratentorial CSF spaces, with associated

Fig. 5.**48 a–c Angioblastoma.**
a Noncontrast CT demonstrates an infratentorial cystic mass on the left side. There is a large mural nodule with indistinct margins.
b The nodule shows moderate enhancement after contrast administration. A cyst wall is not defined.

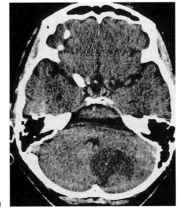
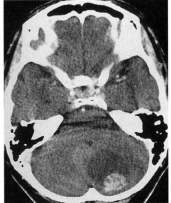

a   b

Abb. 5.**48 c** ▷

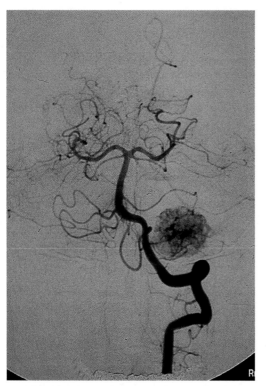

Fig. 5.**48 c** On angiography, the tumor nodule shows an intense blush in the arterial phase.

clinical signs. Solid angioblastomas are found in a quarter of the cases. Unlike cystic angioblastomas, this form cannot be confidently diagnosed by CT. Metastases and primary brain tumors are indistinguishable by their morphologic imaging features. The wall is often irregular, and intralesional hemorrhage is occasionally seen.

■ Differential Diagnosis

The differential diagnosis includes pilocytic and other astrocytomas. Unlike angioblastomas, these tumors sometimes calcify. The solid portion of cystic angioblastomas is located on the cerebellar surface, whereas astrocytomas tend to occur near the fourth ventricle. Cystic metastases are also found in the cerebellum but are usually distinguished by the absence of a tumor nodule.

■ Follow-Up

Angioblastomas have an average recurrence rate of 10%.

Lymphomas

Lymphoma

Frequency: 1–2% of brain tumors in immunocompetent patients; increasing in immunosuppressed populations.

Suggestive morphologic findings: location in basal ganglia, corpus callosum, or white matter; usually hyperdense on plain CT, enhance intensely after contrast administration.

Procedure: the primary treatment is radiotherapy (not surgery), and stereotactic biopsy is therefore necessary to establish the diagnosis.

Other studies: MRI demonstrates subependymal and subarachnoid spread. CT is not well suited for this purpose.

Checklist for scan interpretation:
▶ A presumptive diagnosis must be made.
▶ Periventricular location?
▶ Hyperdense on plain CT?

■ Pathogenesis

Two typical situations are encountered in patients with primary intracerebral lymphoma:

- Lymphoma is seldom included in the differential diagnosis of immunocompetent patients.
- In immunosuppressed patients, lymphoma can be difficult to distinguish from foci of cerebral toxoplasmosis.

If there is any doubt, and especially if the patient responds poorly to antitoxoplasmotic therapy, biopsy should be performed. A positive biopsy will then prompt the initiation of percutaneous radiotherapy. Secondary intracerebral lymphomas are not distinguishable by their imaging features.

Primary intracerebral lymphomas are almost always non-Hodgkin lesions of the B-cell type (Fig. 5.**49**).

Intracerebral tumors that arise from vascular elements infiltrate the surrounding brain tissue via the perivascular spaces. Contrast enhancement is not due to angiogenesis, with the formation of vessels lacking a blood–brain barrier, but is caused by perivascular invasion, with the destruction of vessel walls.

Intracerebral lymphomas generally respond well to percutaneous irradiation. It is

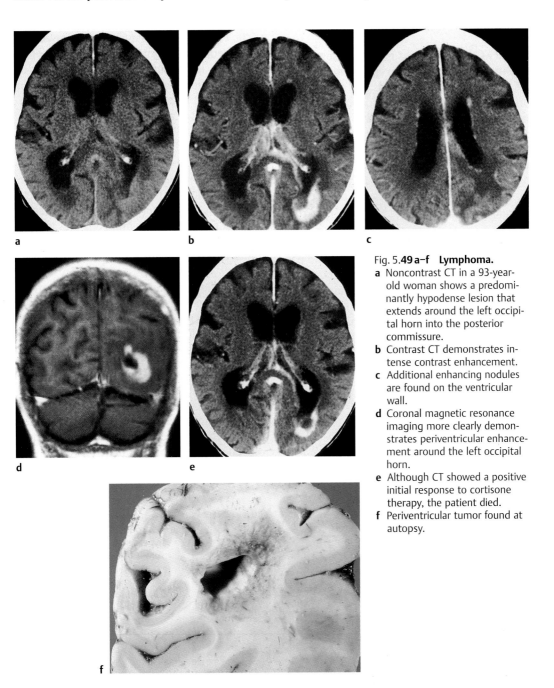

Fig. 5.**49 a–f   Lymphoma.**
a Noncontrast CT in a 93-year-old woman shows a predominantly hypodense lesion that extends around the left occipital horn into the posterior commissure.
b Contrast CT demonstrates intense contrast enhancement.
c Additional enhancing nodules are found on the ventricular wall.
d Coronal magnetic resonance imaging more clearly demonstrates periventricular enhancement around the left occipital horn.
e Although CT showed a positive initial response to cortisone therapy, the patient died.
f Periventricular tumor found at autopsy.

important, therefore, to establish the diagnosis by biopsy. Even so, the survival times are not encouraging. Unifocal lymphomas have a better prognosis than multifocal disease, but the average survival is only 1–2 years, even with prompt initiation of treatment.

■ Frequency

Primary CNS lymphomas have been somewhat rare in the past, making up approximately 0.2–2% of malignant lymphomas and 0.85–2% of primary CNS tumors. It is reasonable to expect, however, that their incidence will rise dramatically as the numbers of immunosuppressed patients increase. Moreover, the incidence of CNS lymphomas in the population as a whole has increased during the past 20 years.

■ Clinical Manifestations

The clinical features are nonspecific, and depend chiefly on the site of occurrence and pattern of involvement. They range from personality changes, signs of increased intracranial pressure, and focal or generalized seizures to sensorimotor deficits with hemiparetic symptoms. It is important to note that the symptoms of CNS lymphoma respond well to steroids, although this may cause confusion with inflammatory demyelinating disease.

■ CT Morphology

Lymphoma may present as a solitary focal lesion or as two or more lesions. Common sites of occurrence are the basal ganglia, corpus callosum, and the frontal and temporal lobes. Some authors state that the frequent approximation of lymphomas to the ependyma (ventricle, Fig. 5.**50**) or subarachnoid space results from seeding through CSF pathways.

Most lymphomas appear slightly or markedly hyperdense on noncontrast CT scans. Isodense and hypodense lesions are less common. Mass effects such as ventricular compression or gyral effacement can usually be demonstrated. Perifocal edema tends to be mild. Lymphomas show moderate or marked enhancement after contrast administration. Previous cortisone therapy may suppress contrast enhancement, but otherwise lack of enhancement is rare. While calcifications and hemorrhage are almost never observed, the tumors found in patients with acquired immune deficiency syndrome (AIDS) often show central necrosis. Nodular and scalloped configurations are common. Individual lesions are generally quite large. Other forms show a more diffuse pattern of infiltration. Additional patterns are listed below:

- Meningeal seeding
- Subependymal spread (with positive CSF examination)
- Ocular involvement, which is associated with the intracerebral form of lymphoma (subarachnoid spread), but may not be synchronous with intracerebral disease

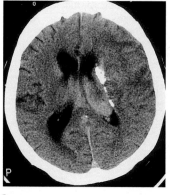 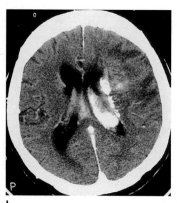

Fig. 5.**50 a, b Lymphoma.**
a Noncontrast CT demonstrates hyperdense intraventricular tumor tissue. The marked accompanying calcification is unusual for a lymphoma.
b The mass shows very intense contrast enhancement.

a   b

■ Differential Diagnosis

Lymphomas that broadly abut the meninges or show meningeal spread may be mistaken for meningiomas. MRI cannot significantly advance the differential diagnosis by detecting or excluding meningeal enhancement. Angiography contributes more by demonstrating the typical vascularization pattern of meningioma. Rarely, glioma-like patterns with irregular rim enhancement are seen. Cerebral metastases are generally associated with extensive perifocal edema, which distinguishes them from multiple lymphomas. As for inflammatory lesions, abscess-like patterns are occasionally seen with lymphoma. There is also reference in the literature to the ventricular changes caused by ependymitis, which may be mistaken for lymphoma in immunosuppressed patients. Contrast enhancement in ependymitis is confined to the ventricular wall, however, whereas with lymphoma it extends into the deep white matter or basal ganglia.

Plasmacytoma (Multiple Myeloma)

Frequency: rare.

Suggestive morphologic findings: punched-out lytic lesions in the skull, often visible in the lateral scout view.

Procedure: make a presumptive diagnosis and confirm prior to surgery and radiotherapy.

Other studies: MRI is sensitive for medullary involvement beyond immediate osteolysis.

Checklist for scan interpretation:
▶ Osteolysis?
▶ Soft-tissue mass?
▶ Extent of medullary involvement?
▶ Involvement of meninges, cerebrum?

■ Pathogenesis

Plasmacytoma is characterized by focal or disseminated proliferation of neoplastic plasma cells. The sites of occurrence correlate with sites of hematopoietic marrow. This accounts for the involvement of the skull, in which multiple punched-out lytic lesions are virtually pathognomonic for the disease. Extraosseous manifestations are less common. While plasmacytoma is generally considered a diffuse disease, there are solitary plasmacytomas with a single focus involving, say, the sphenoid wing. Overall, plasmacytoma is an uncommon disease that rarely affects the skull. Osteolytic lesions with a large soft-tissue component are occasionally found in the sphenoid wing. Meningeal and cerebral manifestations are very rare.

■ Frequency

Plasmacytoma is the most common generalized bone malignancy. The incidence in Europeans is approximately one to two per 100 000, and about twice that high in people of color. Males from 50 to 70 years of age are predominantly affected. Less than 2% of cases occur before age 40. The calvarium should be scrutinized along with the vertebral bodies as a site of predilection, as it contains abundant hematopoietic marrow.

■ Clinical Manifestations

Symptoms depend on the pattern of involvement. They are similar to those associated with a fast-growing meningioma, and indeed this tumor is a frequent clinical and radiologic differential diagnosis. Plasmacytoma located in the sphenoid wing may cause exophthalmos, oculomotor disturbances, and cranial nerve deficits.

■ CT Morphology

A consistent imaging feature of plasmacytoma is osteolysis (Fig. 5.**51**).

In some cases, the soft-tissue component may be so large that it mimics a meningioma. Soft-tissue tumors frequently extend onto the meninges. Plasmacytomas are slightly hyperdense to brain tissue on noncontrast CT scans, and enhance after contrast administration. Calcifications (bone fragments?) may be present. Extraosseous plasmacytoma can occur anywhere in the soft tissues of the skull base and

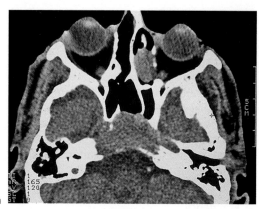

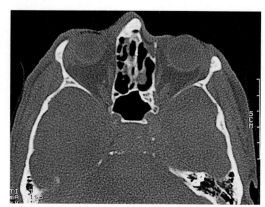

Fig. 5.**51 a, b** **Plasmacytoma.** The clivus and sphenoid wing are common sites for plasmacytoma. In the example shown, imaging was done to investigate oculomotor palsy.

a Bone-window CT without contrast medium demonstrates lytic splaying of the clivus. A second mass is located in the ethmoid cells on the left side.

b A bone-window scan at a slightly different gantry angle shows postoperative changes in the facial skeleton on the left side, additional masses in the ethmoid cells, and destruction of the dorsum sellae.

facial skeleton, appearing as a sharply marginated mass. With meningeal involvement, the pattern resembles that of leptomeningeal metastases.

■ Differential Diagnosis

Differential diagnosis should include the following tumors:

- Meningioma (sphenoid location and leptomeningeal soft-tissue masses)
- Metastases (from breast, renal-cell or bronchial carcinoma)
- Lymphomas
- Chondrosarcoma
- Hemangioma

Plasmacytoma should be considered even in the absence of conspicuous osteolysis. In cases in which the underlying disease has already been diagnosed, the intracranial foci should be easy to identify.

■ Follow-Up

Follow-up is of particular interest in patients with solitary plasmacytoma. An immediate postoperative contrast examination should be available to document the extent of soft-tissue proliferation.

Germ-Cell Tumors

Germinoma

Frequency: pineal tumors make up approximately 2 % of intracranial tumors (perhaps considerably more in Asia). Germinomas account for some 30–60 % of these lesions, depending on the source.

Suggestive morphologic findings: mass in the pineal region, hyperdense on plain scans, often with calcification.

Procedure: elevated tumor markers in serum and CSF (α-fetoprotein, human chorionic gonadotropin).

Other studies: sagittal MRI contributes to localization.

Checklist for scan interpretation:
▶ Hydrocephalus?
▶ Unenhanced density, calcification, contrast enhancement?
▶ Location in relation to third ventricle, vein of Galen, quadrigeminal plate?

Pathogenesis

The term "intracranial germ-cell tumors" is a collective one encompassing the following types:

- Germinoma
- Teratoma
- Teratocarcinoma
- Embryonal carcinoma
- Yolk-sac tumor (endodermal sinus tumor)
- Choriocarcinoma
- Mixed germ-cell tumors

Among pineal region masses, the tumors of pineal-cell origin described on pp. 143 f are also important: pineocytoma, pineoblastoma, and pineal cysts. Other common pineal region tumors are meningiomas and gliomas, but these are not masses typical of the pineal gland. The germ-cell tumors of the pineal region that have the greatest practical importance are germinomas.

Intracranial germinomas are classified as malignant tumors. They can spread intracranially by locally invasive growth, CSF metastasis, and (rarely) hematogenous metastasis.

The peak age incidence is from 20 to 40 years. Males are predominantly affected.

Frequency

Germinoma is the most common germ-cell tumor and also the most common pineal region tumor, accounting for approximately 2 % of intracranial tumors.

Clinical Manifestations

Germinomas of the pineal region cause aqueductal compression, leading to obstructive hydrocephalus and its manifestations. With dystopic germinomas, the clinical features are location-dependent. Suprasellar tumors may present with chiasmal symptoms.

CT Morphology

Germinomas are most commonly located in the pineal region. Dystopic forms occur at suprasellar and parasellar sites. Cases involving other structures, such as the basal ganglia, have also been described. Typical germinomas are markedly hyperdense to brain on noncontrast CT, have smooth margins, and show marked, homogeneous contrast enhancement. Many germinomas contains calcifications, depending on their location. Contrast enhancement in basal ganglia tumors has been described as irregular, however.

Differential Diagnosis

The location of the tumor in relation to the calcified pineal gland is useful for differentiating masses of the pineal region. If the tumor displaces the pineal gland anteriorly and superiorly, it is assumed to have an extrapineal origin. The differential diagnosis includes gliomas arising from the quadrigeminal plate and meningiomas arising from the falx or tela choroidea of the third ventricle. CT alone cannot differentiate between germinomas and pineal parenchymal tumors. One author claims that while this is true for males, a calcified pineal mass in a female is more likely to be a pineocytoma. The differential diagnosis of cystic lesions of the pineal region should include pineal cysts and epidermoids. This particularly applies to eccentric lesions.

Teratoma

Frequency: < 1 % of intracranial tumors.

Suggestive morphologic findings: mass of mixed density (with fat and calcifications), often located in the pineal gland; may enhance with contrast.

Procedure: surgical removal.

Other studies: sagittal MRI is better than CT for defining the topography of pineal masses.

Checklist for scan interpretation:
▶ Location, structure, size?
▶ Signs of rupture, hydrocephalus?
▶ Anatomic relationship to adjacent structures (vein of Galen, quadrigeminal plate, splenium, thalamus)?

■ Pathogenesis

Teratomas are classified as germ-cell tumors, along with germinomas, choriocarcinomas, and embryonal carcinomas.

■ Frequency

Like the other germ-cell tumors, teratomas are most commonly located in the pineal region. Within this group, which together make up about 2 % of brain tumors, teratomas are generally rare, accounting for less than 5 % in large reported series.

■ Clinical Manifestations

Clinical features are location-dependent. Tumors located in the pineal region cause hydrocephalus with signs of increased intracranial pressure.

■ CT Morphology

As noted, the pineal region is the most common site of occurrence. Teratomas have a heterogeneous composition that may include fat, calcifications, cystic areas, and solid elements. A fat-density mass in the pineal region should always raise a suspicion of teratoma. Intense contrast enhancement may be observed.

■ Differential Diagnosis

No method of noninvasive differential diagnosis between the various types of germ-cell tumor is available.

Cysts and Tumor-like Lesions

Rathke Cleft Cyst

> **Frequency:** a common autopsy finding; rarely symptomatic, detected incidentally.
> **Suggestive morphologic finding:** intrasellar cyst.
> **Procedure:** treatment is warranted only in symptomatic cases.
> **Other studies:** MRI far superior (sagittal).
>
> **Checklist for scan interpretation:**
> ▶ Size, density, location?
> ▶ Extension to optic chiasm?
> ▶ Displacement of pituitary or infundibulum?

■ Pathogenesis

Rathke cleft cysts arise from cellular rests of the craniopharyngeal duct. The lesions consist of epithelium-lined cysts with variable fluid contents. Rathke cleft cysts are related to craniopharyngioma.

■ Frequency

Because Rathke cleft cysts are usually asymptomatic and frequently small, they are seldom diagnosed by sectional imaging procedures. They are, however, detected incidentally in 13–23% of autopsies.

■ Clinical Manifestations

Rathke cleft cysts large enough to cause symptoms usually present with visual field defects, diabetes insipidus, or other endocrine disorders.

■ CT Morphology

CT demonstrates an intrasellar or parasellar cyst. The cyst wall may enhance after contrast administration, but there is no nodular component.

■ Differential Diagnosis

Differentiation from craniopharyngioma, which has a similar pathogenesis, can be very difficult. With craniopharyngioma, however, the cyst contents do not resemble CSF, especially on MRI.

Epidermoid

> **Frequency:** approximately 1% of intracranial tumors, but 7% of cerebellopontine angle masses.
> **Suggestive morphologic findings:** a CSF-dense mass, usually located in the cerebellopontine angle; suprasellar and parasellar occurrence is also seen.
> **Procedure:** surgical resection if symptoms are present (trigeminal neuralgia, etc.).
> **Other studies:** MRI can be used to avoid beam-hardening artifact near the skull base.
>
> **Checklist for scan interpretation:**
> ▶ Size and location of the tumor?
> ▶ Mass effect?
> ▶ Density, enhancement characteristics?
> ▶ Possible relationship to cranial nerves?

■ Pathogenesis

Epidermoids arise at the time of neural tube closure during embryonic development. Incomplete separation of the ectodermal elements that develop into skin and nerve tissue leads to inclusions ("right tissue in the wrong place"). Products formed by the skin (but not dermal appendages, as with dermoids) lead to secondary expansion of the cyst. Most intracranial epidermoids have an intradural location. Extradural lesions are located in the diploic space.

Epidermoids are characterized by their "mother-of-pearl" appearance at surgery.

■ Frequency

Epidermoid cysts are rare, accounting for less than 1% of intracranial masses. They have a strong predilection for the cerebellopontine angle and make up approximately 7% of cerebellopontine angle masses.

■ Clinical Manifestations

Clinical symptoms are location-dependent. Epidermoids located in Meckel's cave present with characteristic symptoms. (Meckel's cave is a dura-lined space located just rostral to the prepontine cistern at the medial aspect of the temporal lobe.) Possible complications are aseptic meningitis and vasospasm induced by epidermoid material.

■ CT Morphology

With its fluid contents, epidermoid appears as a CSF-density mass on CT. The cyst wall is usually thin and may enhance after contrast administration. Epidermoids have a characteristic location based on their pathogenesis. Most are located in the cerebellopontine cistern, or in parasellar or suprasellar cisterns. Less common sites are the CSF spaces around the pineal gland and the ventricles. Epidermoids are typically located off the midline (Figs. 5.**52**, 5.**53**), while dermoids tend to occur on the midline.

The mass effect is not pronounced, at least with small epidermoids.

■ Differential Diagnosis

Dermoids are clearly distinguished on CT by their fat density. Arachnoid cysts may occur at the same sites as epidermoids. Intralesional contrast enhancement reportedly suggests malignant degeneration or infection of an epidermoid cyst.

■ Follow-Up

If the tumor is not too large, there is generally no recurrence after a complete resection.

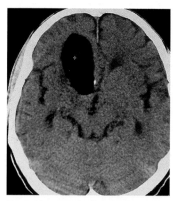

Fig. 5.**52** **Suprasellar epidermoid.** The typical appearance would be a mass with the density of cerebrospinal fluid, located in the cerebellopontine angle.

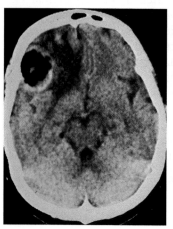
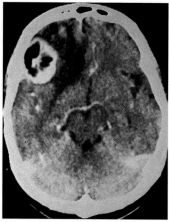

a   b

Fig. 5.**53 a, b** **Secretory meningioma simulating a dermoid/epidermoid.** The fat center is deceptive, but epidermoids do not enhance (**b**).

Dermoid

- **Frequency:** dermoids account for less than 1% of cerebral masses. Spinal lesions are more common.
  Suggestive morphologic findings: hypodense midline mass.
  Procedure: inspection of the skin (dermal sinus?), surgical resection.
  Other studies: MRI to document the cystic nature of the mass.
  Checklist for scan interpretation:
  ▶ Location, size?
  ▶ Sinus tract?
  ▶ Signs of rupture (disseminated subarachnoid fat)?
  ▶ Accompanying hydrocephalus?

■ Pathogenesis

Dermoids result from a developmental anomaly at the time of neural tube closure. Although they are histologically benign, dermoids can cause a chemical meningitis, due to rupture or gradual release of their contents. Hydrocephalus can develop as a late complication of postmeningitic adhesions.

■ Frequency

Dermoids are even less common than epidermoid cysts, making up only 0.3% of intracranial tumors.

■ Clinical Manifestations

Unlike epidermoids, dermoids are most often manifested in the pediatric age group. This is due to the somewhat more rapid enlargement of these tumors, which are present before birth. The possible coexistence of a dermal sinus is of diagnostic importance. The sinus may be visible externally as a hair-bearing or hairless "dimple" or pore on the skin. Often, a sinus tract is also visible on sagittal MRI.

Meningitis was mentioned above as a possible complication of dermoids. The lesion should be sought if corresponding symptoms are observed.

■ CT Morphology

Dermoid appears as a mass of very low density (negative Hounsfield units), due to its fatty contents. Dermoids are often located on the midline, distinguishing them from the off-midline location of epidermoids. Dermoid rupture is a significant complication. Dermoids may rupture spontaneously into the subarachnoid space or ventricular system. In this case, fat–CSF levels may be seen in the frontal horns of the lateral ventricles, for example, when the patient is supine.

■ Differential Diagnosis

Epidermoids are distinguished by their CSF density and off-midline location. Corpus callosum lipomas are not necessarily classified as dermoids, despite their midline location. They have a different pathogenic mechanism.

Colloid Cyst

- **Frequency:** 2% of gliomas, 0.5–1% of intracranial tumors.
  Suggestive morphologic findings: a CSF-density mass in the anterior part of the third ventricle.
  Procedure: endoscopic surgical removal in symptomatic cases (hydrocephalus).
  Other studies: MRI is better for demonstrating non-CSF signal intensity (multi-echo sequence, etc.).
  Checklist for scan interpretation:
  ▶ Hydrocephalus?
  ▶ Calcifications?

■ Pathogenesis

Colloid cysts are composed of an epithelialized wall enclosing colloid contents of variable composition. It was long believed that colloid cysts arise from the paraphysis, a rudimentary outpouching from the roof of the third ventricle. More recent studies support the theory that neuroepithelial cysts—an alternate term for colloid cysts—arise from the diencephalon (arcus postvelaris).

■ Frequency

Colloid cysts make up approximately 0.5–1 % of intracranial tumors. Most cases are diagnosed when the patients are between 20 and 50 years of age.

■ Clinical Manifestations

Obstruction of the foramen of Monro leads to paroxysmal headaches and finally to increased intracranial pressure.

■ CT Morphology

CT demonstrates a smoothly rounded cystic mass in the third ventricle. It may be detected incidentally or by a specific search in a patient with hydrocephalus. The density of the mass varies with its composition, and many colloid cysts are hyperdense. The cyst may completely obstruct the foramen of Monro, leading to hydrocephalus. This usually occurs in young adults. In other cases a ball-valve mechanism can cause intermittent obstruction, with intermittent elevation of intraventricular pressure. Contrast enhancement is usually absent, but rim enhancement may occur if a capsule is present. Whenever CT shows bilateral enlargement of the lateral ventricles with no apparent cause, thin-slice images should be obtained to exclude a small colloid cyst of the third ventricle.

■ Differential Diagnosis

The differential diagnosis is straightforward, owing to the typical location and appearance of the cyst.

Tumors of the Sellar Region

Pituitary Adenoma

Frequency: approximately 7 % of intracranial tumors are pituitary adenomas.

Suggestive morphologic findings: sellar mass.

Procedure: hormonal therapy if possible (prolactinoma), transsphenoidal and/or transcranial surgical resection if possible.

Other studies: today, MRI is used exclusively for tumor visualization. CT is used preoperatively to determine the surgical approach, as well as for postoperative follow-up.

Checklist for scan interpretationlz (preoperative coronal CT of paranasal sinuses):
▶ Inflammatory changes, ethmoid cells, sphenoid sinus?
▶ Changes in nasal skeleton (old fractures, etc.)?
▶ Sphenoid sinus topography (central position of septum, roof)?
▶ Position of the optic nerve (sphenoid sinus)?

■ Pathogenesis

Pituitary adenomas are histologically benign. Anterior lobe tumors may be classified as functioning (hormone-producing) or nonfunctioning. This term is not entirely accurate, however, since while "nonfunctioning" tumors do not produce hormones themselves, they can suppress physiologic hormone production by compressing the normal pituitary tissue. Functioning pituitary adenomas that produce growth hormone (GH) are distinguished from tumors that produce adrenocorticotropic hormone (ACTH) or prolactin. Prolactinomas are by far the most common. It is also useful to differentiate the tumors into microadenomas (< 10 mm in diameter) and macroadenomas. Pituitary carcinoma is a rare malignant variant.

■ Frequency

Pituitary tumors make up approximately 7–10 % of intracranial tumors, although a higher incidence is found at autopsy. Both sexes are affected equally. The incidence of pituitary adenomas is increased in multiple endocrine neoplasias (MEN I and II).

■ Clinical Manifestations

The main clinical manifestations of functioning adenomas depend on the hormone-mediated effects and may be seen long before local symptoms develop. Possible effects are as follows:

- GH: gigantism in children, acromegaly in adults; carpal tunnel syndrome and headache
- ACTH: Cushing disease
- Prolactinoma: galactorrhea in women, libido loss and impotence in men

Nonfunctioning adenomas lead to secondary hypogonadism.

Various mass effects can occur on adjacent tissues:

- Compression of the optic chiasm, with hemianopia, quadrantanopia, or scotoma
- Infiltration of the cavernous sinus
- Diplopia due to compression of the abducens or oculomotor nerve

Headaches, epileptic seizures due to temporal lobe compression, and hydrocephalus due to compression of the third ventricle are rare late manifestations of large tumors.

The classic triad of pituitary adenoma is as follows:

- Chiasmal visual field defect
- Endocrinopathy
- Sellar expansion on radiographs

■ CT Morphology

Pituitary adenomas (macroadenomas) appear as rounded midline masses on axial CT scans (Figs. 5.**54**, 5.**55**). They are isodense to brain tissue on noncontrast scans, and the extraaxial tumors show marked enhancement after contrast administration. Cysts and hemorrhage can be found in larger tumors.

The preoperative work-up for transsphenoidal surgery consists of coronal CT scans with a bone window and 2-mm slice thickness. Cicatricial changes following nasal fractures and inflammatory changes of the paranasal sinuses should be described. The configuration of the sphenoid sinus should also be noted. CT may show a centered septum, with bilateral symmetry of the sinus chambers or marked sinus asymmetry. In rare cases, the optic nerves may traverse the roof of the sphenoid sinus, with only a thin layer of bone separating them from the sinus lumen. With a larger adenoma, the sellar floor may be so depressed on one side that it almost occludes the sphenoid sinus lumen.

Pituitary adenomas have the same basic appearance on MRI and CT, but only MRI provides the contrast resolution necessary for a confident diagnosis. The tumors are best displayed

Fig. 5.**54 a, b Pituitary tumor.**
The typical CT appearance of a large pituitary tumor is that of a rounded mass projected over the basal cisterns.
a In the absence of intralesional cysts or hemorrhage, the mass appears isodense to brain parenchyma.
b The mass enhance intensely after contrast administration.

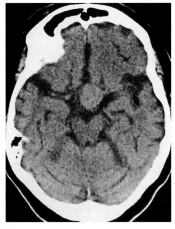

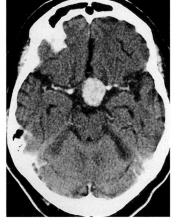

a
b

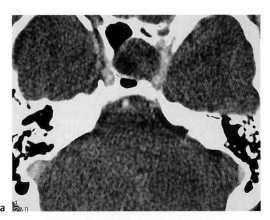

a

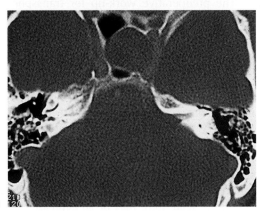

b

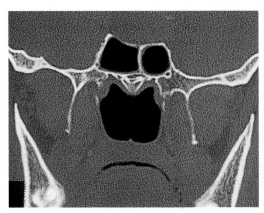

Fig. 5.**55 a–c** **Pituitary tumor.**
a This adenoma shows only minimal contrast enhancement. Its relatively low density clearly differentiates it from the adjacent, opacified cavernous sinus.
b, c Bone-window CT clearly demonstrates ballooning of the sella. The coronal scan (**c**) is an essential preoperative view, as the septum of the sphenoid sinus provides the surgeon with a landmark for tumor localization in the transsphenoidal approach. This is particularly important with small tumors.

on coronal images. The pituitary stalk is displayed away from the tumor, and the sellar floor is depressed on one or both sides. A concave superior border of the pituitary is not a tumor-related sign. Microadenomas can be seen only after contrast administration. Adenomas enhance less rapidly than normal pituitary tissue but retain their enhancement longer. As a result, they appear isodense to the pituitary on early dynamic images and hyperdense on delayed images. It is important to note and describe extension into the cavernous sinus, displacement or compression of the optic nerve, and tumor shape. A tumor that is hourglass-shaped on coronal images can be difficult to resect through the transsphenoidal approach. Infiltration of the cavernous sinus can be detected on postcontrast images acquired while the sinus is hyperdense but the tumor is still hypodense. MRI is better for this purpose.

▪ Differential Diagnosis

A brief rule of thumb for the differential diagnosis is outlined below:

- Chiasmal symptoms during the first two decades of life are caused by craniopharyngioma.
- The same symptoms from age 20 to 40 are caused by pituitary adenoma.
- After age 40, the most likely cause is meningioma.

Another clinical rule states that bitemporal hemianopia in a patient with an unenlarged sella (routine skull film, special sellar view) is probably caused by a circle of Willis aneurysm or a meningioma. Pituitary carcinomas are rare (Fig. 5.**56**).

■ Follow-Up

Residual tumor and hemorrhage are important postoperative concerns. In detecting a recurrence, it should be noted that recurrent tumors have nonhomogeneous margins, due to the absence of an intact capsule. Tumors that initially infiltrate the cavernous sinus or have a large suprasellar component may not be completely resectable.

Craniopharyngioma

Frequency: an important differential diagnosis of sellar masses in children.

Suggestive morphologic findings: cystic components and calcifications (CT).

Procedure: surgical removal.

Other studies: MRI is better for demonstrating extension to surrounding structures (coronal and sagittal images).

Checklist for scan interpretation:
▶ Calcifications? Large cysts, solid portions?
▶ Pituitary tissue?
▶ Relation to cavernous sinus, anterior cerebral artery, optic chiasm?
▶ Third ventricle compressed, hydrocephalus?

■ Pathogenesis

Craniopharyngioma (Fig. 5.**57**) is a benign congenital tumor that probably develops from rests of the craniopharyngeal duct.

■ Frequency

Craniopharyngiomas make up approximately 2.5–4% of brain tumors. About half of all cases are diagnosed in children. Peak occurrence is at 5–10 years of age.

■ Clinical Manifestations

Symptoms are determined by the relationship of the tumor to the pituitary, optic chiasm, and third ventricle. Tumors that compress the pituitary can cause precocious puberty, short stature, and diabetes insipidus. Suprasellar lesions can present with visual defects due to pressure on the chiasm. A very large tumor may compress the third ventricle or foramen of Monro, causing symptoms of obstructive hydrocephalus as well as lethargy (invasion of diencephalon).

■ CT Morphology

CT demonstrates a suprasellar or parasellar mass with coarse calcifications (Fig. 5.**57**).

Cystic components of CSF density are present along with solid tumor areas. The rela-

Fig. 5.**56 a, b** **Pituitary carcinoma.** The tumor, imaged here at two levels, has the same morphologic features as pituitary adenoma. Carcinoma was diagnosed histologically.

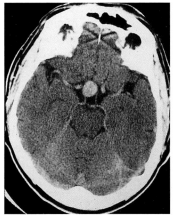

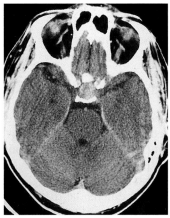

a   b

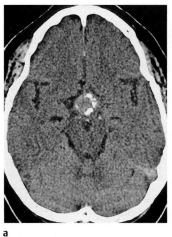
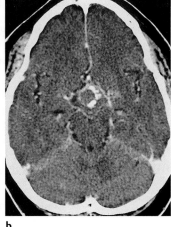

Fig. 5.**57 a–d Craniopharyngioma.** Craniopharyngioma is a suprasellar/parasellar mass characterized by calcifications and occasionally by intratumoral hemorrhage and cyst formation.
a, b The CT appearance of craniopharyngioma before (**a**) and after contrast administration (**b**). Smaller lesions are frequently missed on axial scans if the slice thickness is too large.

a b

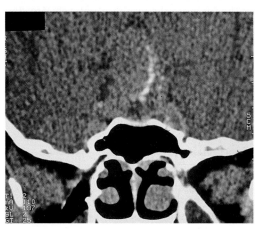
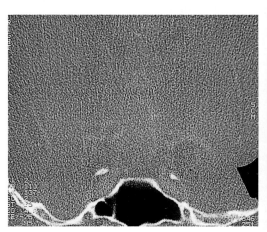

c

c, d The tumors are somewhat easier to detect on coronal scans. Soft-tissue window (**c**), bone window (**d**).

tionship of the various components is highly variable, but calcifications are almost always present.

Solid portions of the tumor show marked contrast enhancement.

■ Differential Diagnosis

The main differentiating criterion is the presence of calcifications. This gives CT an important role in the initial diagnosis. Both CT and MRI can demonstrate cystic components, which are also found in gliomas (Fig. 5.**58**).

The differential diagnosis includes germinoma, clivus chordoma, pituitary adenoma, and meningioma. Rathke cleft cyst should also be considered, as these lesions represent a minimal variant of craniopharyngioma, with an allied pathogenesis. Epidermoids are located off the midline.

■ Follow-Up

Given the complex anatomic environment and the many structures that must be preserved, a complete resection is difficult. Recurrences are common, therefore, and often display an even more heterogeneous structure (cystic, calcified, solid).

Fig. 5.**58 a, b Optic glioma in the differential diagnosis of sellar and parasellar masses.** Both precontrast and postcontrast CT demonstrate a rounded mass with central necrosis. The portion of an optic glioma located above the chiasm is particularly apt to cause morphologic confusion.
a Before contrast administration.
b After contrast administration.

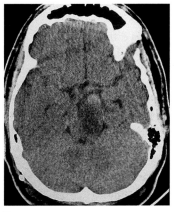
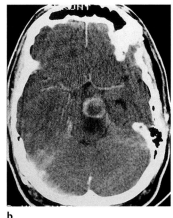

a　　　　　　　　b

Local Extension of Regional Tumors

Paraganglioma (Glomus Tumor)

Frequency: rare.

Suggestive morphologic findings: intensely enhancing mass in the skull base.

Procedure: angiography (for preoperative embolization).

Other studies: MRI more accurately defines tumor extent (no beam-hardening artifacts from bone).

Checklist for scan interpretation:
▶ Contrast enhancement (degree of vascularity)?
▶ Extent of bone destruction?
▶ Relationship to blood vessels?

■ Pathogenesis

Glomus tumors are neuroendocrine tumors that arise in the jugular fossa (cranial nerve IV or V) or inner ear (on cochlear promontory). They are accordingly designated as glomus jugulare or glomus tympanicum tumors. Glomus tumors are locally destructive growths that compress, rather than infiltrate, neighboring structures.

In addition to these typical locations, there are atypical forms, including solid tumors, that arise from the glomus pterygoideum and cause destruction of the anterior skull base.

■ Frequency

Glomus jugulare tumor, the prototypic paraganglioma, is generally rare and accounts for approximately 0.6% of head and neck tumors. It shows a marked female predilection, with about a 6: 1 ratio of females to males.

■ Clinical Manifestations

Clinical symptoms depend on the location of the tumor and the structures that it destroys (inner ear). Women are predominantly affected.

■ CT Morphology

These tumors enhance intensely because of their high vascularity. Calcifications are rare. The tumors are smoothly marginated, and foci of bone destruction, when present, appear as smooth-walled lytic defects.

■ Differential Diagnosis

Glomus jugulare tumor mainly requires differentiation from a high jugular bulb. The large jugular foramen associated with a high bulb (side-to-side comparison) should not be mistaken for local tumor-associated lysis. Glomus tumors have a characteristic "salt-and-pepper" appearance on MRI due to vascular flow voids, and this criterion is useful for differential diagnosis. Glomus tumors are very difficult to distinguish from hemangiopericytomas. Skull-base metastases from very vascular tumors (hypernephroma, etc.) are an important differential diagnosis. Radionuclide bone scanning may assist the differential diagnosis by demonstrating metastases in other body regions.

Chordoma

Frequency: rare.
Suggestive morphologic findings: midline mass with bone destruction (clivus).
Procedure: complete surgical removal is difficult.
Other studies: sagittal MRI is superior for defining the extent of the tumor.
Checklist for scan interpretation:
▶ Size, bone destruction, calcifications, enhancement pattern?
▶ Relationship to brain stem, pituitary, optic chiasm, third ventricle?
▶ Relationship to cavernous sinus (cranial nerves) in coronal image?

■ Pathogenesis

Chordomas arise in the region of the embryonic notochord. Fifty percent occur in the sacral/coccygeal region, one-third are intracranial, and the rest are mostly cervical. Although the term "clivus chordoma" is almost synonymous with chordoma, only 50% of intracranial chordomas are actually located on the midline and cause clivus destruction (Fig. 5.**59**).

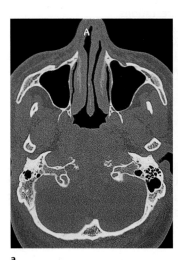

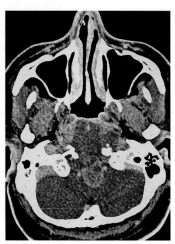

Fig. 5.**59 a, b   Clivus chordoma.**
a Clivus chordoma typically appears as an infrasellar mass with osteolytic destruction of the clivus.
b The scan with a soft-tissue window shows extensive involvement in front of and behind the clivus. The swallowing difficulties observed in this patient were due partly to a mechanical mass effect (anterior portion) and partly to compression of the brain stem and cranial nerve origins.

a   b

The rest are paramedian, with some lesions being parasellar and some occurring at the petrous apex. Chordomas are essentially benign, but they are difficult to resect completely, and this accounts for the high recurrence rate. The tumors are partly gelatinous at surgery, explaining their cystic appearance on CT and the prolonged T2 relaxation times in MRI. It should be noted that chordomas may be found in newborns.

■ Frequency

Chordomas are rare tumors. They usually produce clinical manifestations between 50 and 60 years of age.

■ Clinical Manifestations

Males are predominantly affected. Symptoms not caused by brain-stem compression or invasion of the nasopharynx may signify recurrent meningitis or recurrent mastoiditis.

■ CT Morphology

Characteristic CT features are areas of bone destruction, which are often extensive, calcifications, and cystic components. Destruction of the clivus accompanied by calcifications and cystic changes provides the clearest evidence of chordoma. When the extent is determined, attention should be given to possible intradural or nasopharyngeal extension. Metastatic seeding has also been observed.

■ Differential Diagnosis

Differentiation is mainly required from bone metastases and plasmacytoma. Differential diagnosis based on morphologic imaging features can be difficult in any given case. A lobulated mass with characteristic high signal intensity on MRI is suggestive of chordoma. The osteolytic lesions associated with plasmacytoma and bone metastases tend to arise from a single focus, whereas each lobule of a clivus chordoma can produce its own lytic focus, leaving residual bone between the lytic areas.

The homogeneous, dura-encompassing contrast enhancement of chordomas helps to differentiate them from meningioma. With pituitary adenoma, an intrasellar component can be demonstrated. Craniopharyngioma does not necessarily cause clivus bone destruction, and its characteristic calcifications are more pronounced.

■ Follow-Up

Most resections are subtotal, and adjuvant radiation is of little additional benefit. Recurrent tumor has the same imaging appearance as the original tumor. In patients who have received postoperative radiation, brain-stem symptoms may be radiation-induced, and do not necessarily signify recurrent tumor.

Chondroma, Chondrosarcoma

Frequency: rare.

Suggestive morphologic findings: a meningioma-like tumor, with flocculent calcifications.

Procedure: MRI, surgery.

Other studies: cartilage matrix shows high T2-weighted signal intensity on MRI.

Checklist for scan interpretation:
▶ Location, extent?
▶ Vascularity?

■ Pathogenesis

Intracranial chondromas usually arise from the synchondroses of the skull base. They may occur in isolation or in association with Ollier disease or Maffucci syndrome. The malignant variant is chondrosarcoma. A few cases arising from the falx have been described in the literature. Osseocartilaginous tumors include osteomas, which may also arise from the intracranial dura.

■ Frequency

Chondromas and chondrosarcomas of the CNS are extremely rare, but precise incidence data are not available.

■ Clinical Manifestations

Men and women are affected with about equal frequency. There is no apparent age predilection, but many tumors become clinically manifest in young adults. The actual symptoms depend on tumor location.

■ CT Morphology

Chondromas are usually hypodense on noncontrast CT scans. Moderate contrast enhancement and flocculent (popcorn-like) calcifications in a mass that otherwise resembles meningioma should suggest the diagnosis of chondroma.

Contrast enhancement is gradual, and delayed images may show quite a different enhancement pattern from that in early postcontrast scans.

Recurrent or locally invasive tumor should raise the possibility of chondrosarcoma (Figs. 5.**60**, 5.**61**).

■ Differential Diagnosis

As noted above, meningioma is among the tumors that can mimic the imaging features of chondroma. Meningioma is distinguished by a dural tail, and calcifications, when present in meningioma, are not characteristic of a cartilage-forming tumor.

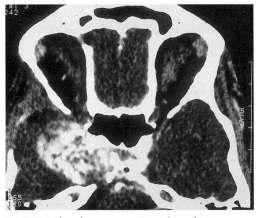

Fig. 5.**60 Chondrosarcoma.** Even the soft-tissue scan demonstrates flocculent calcifications in the parasellar mass.

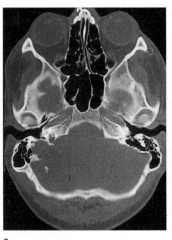
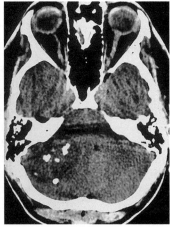
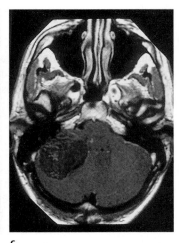

a
b
c

Fig. 5.**61 a–c Chondrosarcoma.**
a The mass, originally interpreted as a glomus tumor, has destroyed large portions of the right mastoid.
b The mild contrast enhancement is unusual for a glomus tumor.

c The tumor contains popcorn-like calcifications. Axial magnetic resonance imaging clearly demonstrates the extra-axial nature of the mass.

Carcinoma

> **Frequency:** intracranial extension is not uncommon in advanced stages.
>
> **Suggestive morphologic findings:** a soft-tissue mass, often arising from the paranasal sinuses or skull base.
>
> **Procedure:** MRI, surgery, chemotherapy, radiation.
>
> **Other studies:** intracranial extension (meningeal enhancement).
>
> **Checklist for scan interpretation:**
> ▶ Extent (secretion-filled cavities, soft tissue)?
> ▶ Bone destruction?
> ▶ Meninges, cavernous sinus, skull base foramina?

■ Pathogenesis

Epithelial tumors with very diverse origins may develop in the skull base region and paranasal sinuses. Squamous-cell carcinoma is by far the most common epithelial malignancy, but adenocarcinoma and anaplastic carcinoma are also found.

■ Clinical Manifestations

The symptoms are often nonspecific and suggest chronic sinusitis. Swallowing difficulties (Fig. 5.**62**) and local signs (swelling, etc.) are also observed.

■ CT Morphology

The main criterion for evaluating the intracranial extension is the integrity of the bony boundaries of the paranasal sinuses, orbital roof, etc. This is best evaluated on bone-window scans in axial and coronal planes. Contrast-enhanced images often improve the contrast between the intracranial portion of the tumor and brain tissue. In the paranasal sinuses themselves, secretion-filled cavities are easily distinguished from enhancing tumor tissue following contrast administration.

■ Differential Diagnosis

Generally, a differential diagnosis cannot be made without biopsy. Lymphomas are relatively common, while the various bone tumors and esthesioneuroblastoma are rarer. With large tumors, it may not be possible to determine the primary site of origin.

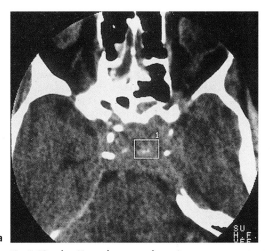

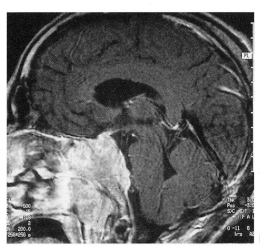

Fig. 5.**62 a, b Nasopharyngeal carcinoma.**
a Axial CT scan just below the sellar floor demonstrates an enhancing mass that has destroyed much of the clivus.

b Incipient brain-stem compression from the anterior side is seen more clearly with magnetic resonance imaging. The tumor shows intense contrast enhancement.

Metastases

Frequency: a common finding and a frequent indication for imaging.

Suggestive morphologic findings: multiple nodular or ring-like lesions.

Procedure: treatment by radiation or surgical resection.

Other studies: MRI is far more sensitive than CT.

Checklist for scan interpretation:
▶ Number of lesions?
▶ Presence and extent of perifocal edema and mass effect?
▶ Need for further investigation (MRI)?
▶ May note limitations of CT (meningeal metastases poorly visualized).

■ Pathogenesis

A variety of tumors can metastasize to the brain. The following principles should be noted when searching for a primary tumor:

The primary tumor cannot be identified based on the morphologic features of its intracranial metastases.

Tumors that frequently metastasize to the brain are not the only source of brain metastases. It is not unusual to discover that the source is a relatively common tumor that is not known for its tendency to spread to the brain.

The most common tumors that metastasize to the brain are bronchial and breast carcinoma. Intratumoral hemorrhage is relatively common in metastatic melanoma.

■ Frequency

Metastases are the second most common intracranial malignancies after higher-grade gliomas.

■ Clinical Manifestations

The clinical presentation is highly variable. It is common for patients with multiple brain metastases to have minimal clinical symptoms (Fig. 5.**63**). This is particularly characteristic of metastatic breast cancer. Large supratentorial metastases or smaller supratentorial metastases with mass effect and perifocal edema (Figs. 5.**64**, 5.**65**) may present with seizures.

With infratentorial metastases, the clinical presentation is often dominated by symptoms due to hydrocephalus.

■ CT Morphology

The key imaging criterion for brain metastases is their multiplicity. The following CT patterns are consistently encountered:

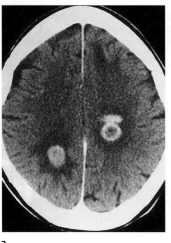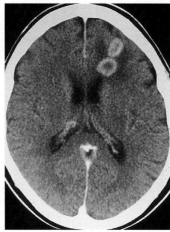

a   b

Fig. 5.**63 a, b   Multiple brain metastases.** CT scans at two different levels in a woman with intracranial metastases show multiple discrete supratentorial lesions. The rapid growth of the lesions outstrips their blood supply, creating a ring-like mass with a small necrotic center. Edema is often very pronounced, but may be suppressed by cortisone therapy. Supratentorial metastases, even when numerous, are often surprisingly asymptomatic.

- A relatively large solitary mass with circular or scalloped rim enhancement, resembling glioblastoma.
- Further investigation of a relatively large, presumably solitary cerebral mass reveals one or more additional lesions.
- Multiple small enhancing lesions with a large amount of surrounding edema.
- Multiple small, nodular-enhancing lesions with no significant mass effect and no significant edema.
- A single large infratentorial mass that compresses the fourth ventricle (Fig. 5.**66**) and has led to hydrocephalus.

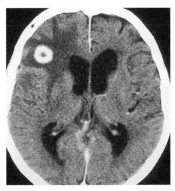

Fig. 5.**64 Metastasis.** The CT scan through a right frontal cerebral metastasis shows a typical digitate pattern of white matter edema. A significant mass effect is not yet apparent.

Even small metastases may be associated with a disproportionate amount of perifocal edema. Generally, the white matter is more susceptible to edema than the gray matter. As a result, small metastatic deposits in the cerebral cortex may be missed on unenhanced CT scans, and contrast administration is essential for excluding metastases when plain scans are negative.

Cystic metastases (Fig. 5.**67**) occur with bronchial carcinoma, but in principle may be seen with any underlying tumor.

The findings associated with brain metastases may be very pronounced. Some patients have extensive destruction of the cerebral hemispheres, which acquire a spongy appearance. Intralesional hemorrhage is not uncommon and shows increased density in the unenhanced scan. It should be noted that even isodense metastases may appear hyperdense,

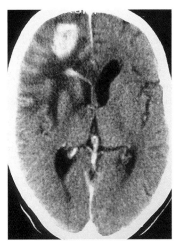

Fig. 5.**65 Metastasis.** This metastasis is associated with perifocal edema, disruption of the blood–brain barrier, and a mass effect, with displacement of the right frontal horn.

Fig. 5.**66 a, b Metastasis.**
a Noncontrast CT shows displacement of the fourth ventricle and very inhomogeneous density in the infratentorial brain tissue.
b Postcontrast CT reveals multiple metastases, showing a combination of scalloped and ring-shaped rim enhancement (bronchial carcinoma).

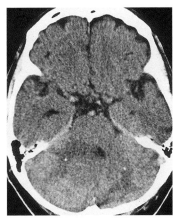

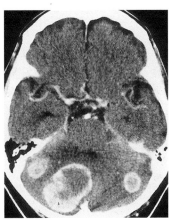

a

b

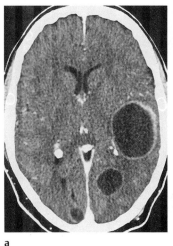
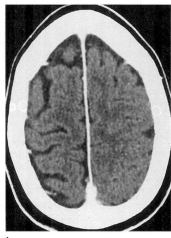

Fig. 5.**67 a, b   Metastasis.**
a These metastases have a cystic appearance—IE, large central necrosis with a very thin enhancing rim (breast carcinoma).
b The mass effect of the large lesions consists of sulcal effacement, seen more clearly at a higher level.

a   b

due to the low density of the surrounding white matter edema (Fig. 5.**68**).

Calcifications are found in metastases from ovarian carcinoma (Fig. 5.**69**). Rarely, calcified brain metastases are also seen with osteosarcoma.

Brain metastases most commonly appear as nodular or ring-enhancing lesions, but plane-of-section effects can mimic virtually any tumor morphology (Fig. 5.**70**).

MRI is markedly superior to CT for the detection of meningeal metastases, but even MRI is inferior to other tests such as CSF cytology (Fig. 5.**71**).

■ **Differential Diagnosis**

Different entities should be considered, depending on whether solitary or multiple lesions are found.

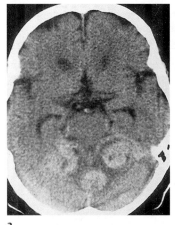
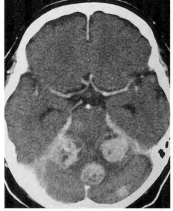

a   b   c

Fig. 5.**68 a–c   Metastasis.**
a Metastases may appear hyperdense on noncontrast CT because of the surrounding low-density edema.

b, c Postcontrast CT scans show intense enhancement of multiple metastases in the posterior fossa.

Solitary lesions. With a solitary lesion, differentiation is mainly required from glioblastoma. Generally, this will require stereotactic biopsy, since both entities may show a circular or scalloped pattern of rim enhancement (Fig. 5.**72**).

Often, it is easier to differentiate brain abscesses. Abscesses arising from mastoiditis or sinusitis are typically located in the middle fossa or in the rostral part of the frontal lobe. Thin-walled ring enhancement is observed. Metastases and glioblastoma are often diagnosed erroneously in patients with disseminated encephalomyelitis. Rarely, this disease presents with one or more enhancing rings on CT scans, but the patient's age and sex should help suggest the correct diagnosis.

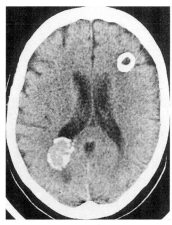

Fig. 5.**69 Metastasis.** Calcification occurs in metastases from ovarian carcinoma (shown here) and various other tumors. Differentiation is required from toxoplasmosis and other calcifying masses.

Fig. 5.**70 a, b Metastasis.** This type of metastasis is not always distinguishable from angioblastoma. The precontrast and postcontrast scans show a cystic mass with liquid contents and a thin, enhancing rim. Angiography can differentiate the lesion from hemangioblastoma. Metastases lack an enhancing nidus in the cyst wall.

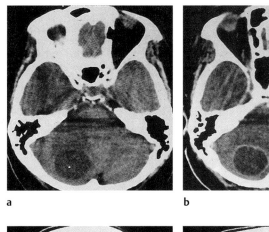

a   b

Fig. 5.**71 a, b Metastasis.** Solidappearing masses are rarely found accompanying meningeal carcinomatosis. These scans from a woman with metastatic breast carcinoma show extensive enhancement of the brain surface, with several nodular lesions.

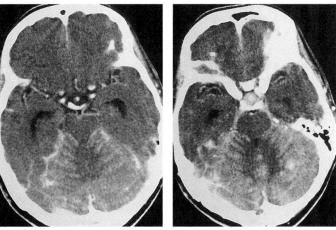

a   b

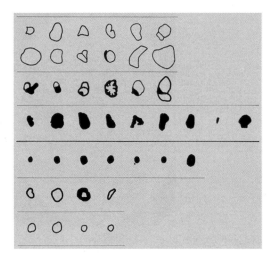

Fig. 5.72 Enhancement patterns found in metastases. The figure shows the outlines of 43 histologically confirmed intracranial metastases. The center line separates the lesions into two groups, with nodular-enhancing and ring-enhancing forms at the bottom and more irregular forms at the top. The lesions are also grouped according to size. It is clear that, starting at a certain size, all metastases exhibit central necrosis. Note also the diversity of the morphologic forms, which in some cases are indistinguishable from glioblastoma and other lesions, including brain abscess.

Multiple lesions. Glioblastoma should be considered when multiple clustered lesions are found within one hemisphere. Even if CT shows a dozen nodular and ring-enhancing lesions, glioblastoma should be at the forefront of differential diagnosis if the lesions are clustered. CSF findings are an important consideration, as they are suggestive in all inflammatory CNS diseases. Multiple dural-based lesions generally represent multiple metastases rather than small meningiomas. The differentiation of cavernomas from metastases is a recurring problem. Both lesions may be mildly or moderate hyperdense on noncontrast CT scans. If angiography is not used, very short-term serial examinations will sometimes show the progression that is characteristic of metastases.

■ Follow-Up

The follow-up of metastases is an important basic issue following the surgical resection of a solitary metastasis or after stereotactic or whole-brain irradiation. In many cases, however, the role of CT is limited to the initial detection of brain metastases and to immediate postoperative evaluation. Particular attention should be given to making an accurate description of any brain edema that is present. The question of hemorrhage or mass effect is of primary interest following surgery. MRI is better for resolving the question of residual or recurrent tumor, and PET is better for detecting radiation necrosis.

■ References

Recommended for further study
Gliomas
Albert FK, Zenner D, Forsting M. Radiologic monitoring after the extirpation of glioblastoma. Klin Neuroradiol 1994; 4: 203–19.
Burger PC, Heinz R, Shibata T, Kleihues P. Topographic anatomy and CT correlations in the untreated glioblastoma multiforme. J Neurosurg 1988; 68: 698–704.
● *Introduction to the basic problem of determining tumor extent by sectional imaging.*
Byrne TN. Imaging of gliomas. Semin Oncol 1994; 21: 162–71.
● *A review surveying all methods.*
Cairncross JG, Macdonald DR, Pexan JHW, Ives FJ. Steroid-induced CT changes in patients with recurrent malignant glioma. Neurology 1988; 38: 724–6.
● *Fundamental work on understanding imaging findings.*
Onda K, Tanaka R, Takahashi H, Takeda N, Ikuta F. Symptomatic cerebrospinal fluid dissemination of cerebral glioblastoma. Neuroradiology 1990; 32: 146–50.
● *Includes histologic correlations.*
Spetzger U, Thron A, Gilsbach JM. Immediate postoperative CT contrast enhancement following surgery of cerebral tumoral lesions. J Comput Assist Tomogr 1998; 22: 120–5.
● *CT findings in the initial hours after surgery.*
Steinhoff H, Lanksch W, Kazner E, et al. Computed tomography in the diagnosis and differential diagnosis of glioblastomas. Neuroradiology 1977; 14: 193–200.
● *Classic work on diagnosis and differential diagnosis.*
Tolly TL, Bruckman JE, Czarnecki DJ, et al. Early CT findings after interstitial radiation therapy for primary malignant brain tumors. AJNR Am J Neuroradiol 1988; 9: 1177–80.
● *Basic description of the problem.*

Pleomorphic xanthoastrocytoma
Blom RJ. Pleomorphic xanthoastrocytoma: CT appearance. J Comput Assist Tomogr 1988; 12: 351–4.
● *Case report with review of previously published cases.*
Levy RA, Allen R, McKeever P. Pleomorphic xanthoastrocytoma presenting with massive intracranial hemorrhage. AJNR Am J Neuroradiol 1996; 17: 154–6.
● *Case report with a clear description of the entity.*

Lipper MH, Eberhard DA, Phillips CD, Vezina LG, Cail WS. Pleomorphic xanthoastrocytoma, a distinctive astroglial tumor: neuroradiologic and pathologic features. AJNR Am J Neuroradiol 1993; 14: 1397–404.
- *CT and MRI findings in seven patients, with histologic confirmation.*

Subependymal giant-cell astrocytoma
McConachie NS, Worthington BS, Cornford EJ, Balsitis N, Kerslake RW, Jaspan T. Review article: computed tomography and magnetic resonance in the diagnosis of intraventricular cerebral masses. Br J Radiol 1994; 67: 223–43.
- *Overview based on 60 cases.*

Ependymoma and subependymoma
Furie DM, Provenzale JM. Supratentorial ependymomas and subependymomas: CT and MR appearance. J Comput Assist Tomogr 1995; 19: 518–26.

Plexus papilloma, carcinoma of choroid plexus
Buetwo PC, Smirniotopoulos JG, Done S. Congenital brain tumors: a review of 45 cases. AJNR Am J Neuroradiol 1990; 11: 793–9.
- *Review of this manifestation.*

Nakase H, Morimoto T, Sakaki T, et al. Bilateral choroid plexus cysts in the lateral ventricles. AJNR Am J Neuroradiol 1991; 12: 1204–5.
- *Describes cystic lesions that are occasionally mistaken for tumors.*

Numaguchi Y, Foster RW, Gum GK. Noncolloid neuroepithelial cysts in the lateral ventricle: CT and MR features. Neuroradiology 1989; 31: 98–101.
- *See Nakase et al. above.*

Gliomatosis cerebri
Pyhtinen J, Paakko E. A difficult diagnosis of gliomatosis cerebri. Neuroradiology 1996; 38: 444–8.

Ganglioglioma
Dorne HL, O'Gorman AM. Computed tomography of intracranial gangliogliomas. AJNR Am J Neuroradiol 1986; 7: 281–5.
- *Standard review of 13 original cases and review of 35 other published cases.*

Neurocytoma
Wichmann W, Schubiger O, von Deimling A, Schenker C, Valavanis A. Neuroradiology of central neurocytoma. Neuroradiology 1991; 33: 143–8.
- *■151, wingdings 2■ Reviews characteristics that may allow preoperative diagnosis.*

Esthesioneuroblastoma
Hurst RW, Erickson S, Cail WS, et al. Computed tomographic features of esthesioneuroblastoma. Neuroradiology 1989; 31: 253–7.
- *Good CT illustrations.*

Kadish S, Goodman M, Wang C. Olfactory esthesioneuroblastoma: a clinical analysis of 17 cases. Cancer 1976; 37: 1571–6.
- *Staging and prognosis.*

Pineocytoma, pineoblastoma, pineal cyst
Ganti SR, Hill SK, Stein BM, Silver AJ, Mawad M, Sane P. CT of pineal region tumors. AJNR Am J Neuroradiol 1986; 146: 451–8.
- *Review based on 60 histologically confirmed examinations.*

Medulloepithelioma
Molloy PT, Yachnis AT, Rorke LB, et al. Central nervous system medulloepithelioma: a series of eight cases including two arising in the pons. J Neurosurg 1996; 84: 430–6.
- *Comprehensive review; good magnetic resonance images, but no CT illustrations.*

Neuroblastoma
Davis PC, Wichman RD, Takei Y, Hoffman JC. Primary cerebral neuroblastoma: CT and MR findings in 12 cases. AJNR Am J Neuroradiol 1990; 11: 115–20.
- *Review of 12 cases with characteristic images.*

PNET/medulloblastoma
Bourgouin PM, Tampieri D, Grahovac SZ, Leger C, Del Carpio R, Melancon D. CT and MR imaging findings in adults with cerebellar medulloblastoma: comparison with findings in children. AJR Am J Roentgenol 1992; 159: 609–12.
- *Important review of adult manifestations.*

Lee YY, Glass JP, van Eys J, Wallace S. Medulloblastoma in infants and children: computed tomographic follow-up after treatment. Radiology 1985; 154: 677–82.
- *Methodological study and description of recurrent tumors in a large clinical population.*

Nelson M, Diebler C, Forbes WS. Paediatric medulloblastoma: atypical CT features at presentation in the SIOP II trial. Neuroradiology 1991; 33: 140–2.
- *Supplements the study by Lee et al., above.*

Sandhu A, Kendall B. Computed tomography in the management of medulloblastomas. Neuroradiology 1987; 29: 444–52.
- *Analysis of imaging features based on examinations in 116 patients; the image quality is dated.*

Schwannoma (neurinoma)
Curtin H. CT of acoustic neuroma and other tumors of the ear. Radiol Clin North Am 1984; 22: 77–105.
- *Comprehensive article for further study.*

DiBiasi C, Trasimeni G, Iannilli M, Polettini E, Gualdi G. Intracerebral schwannoma: CT and MR findings. AJNR Am J Neuroradiol 1994; 15: 1956–8.
- *Very rare manifestation.*

Mafee MF, Lachenauer CS, Kumar A, Arnold PM, Buckingham RA, Valvassori GE. CT and MRI of intralabyrinthine schwannoma: report of two cases and review of the literature. Radiology 1990; 174: 395–400.
- *A very rare manifestation.*

Wu EH, YS Tang, Zhang YT, Bai RJ. CT in the diagnosis of acoustic neuromas. AJNR Am J Neuroradiol 1986; 7: 645–50.
- *Still a remarkably up-to-date CT study, based on an analysis of 75 patients.*

Neurofibroma
Gardeur D, Palmieri A, Mashaly R. Cranial computed tomography in the phakomatoses. Neuroradiology 183; 25: 293–304.
- *Complete spectrum of findings in a series of 77 patients.*

Meningioma
Bradac GB, Ferszt R, Kendall BE. Cranial meningiomas: diagnosis, biology, therapy. Berlin: Springer, 1990.

Lipoma
Truwit CL, Barkovich AJ. Pathogenesis of intracranial lipoma: an MR study in 42 patients. AJNR Am J Neuroradiol 1990; 11: 665–74.

- *Illustrates a number of MRI cases; advances original theory.*

Rhabdomyosarcoma

Heiss E, Albert F. [Computed tomographic findings in cerebellar angioblastoma; in German.] RöFo Fortschr Geb Röntgenstr Nuklearmed 1982; 136: 151–6.
- *Clear and concise review of 16 cases evaluated by CT and angiography; the imaging material is still acceptable today.*

Lymphoma

Hartmann M, Sartor K. [Primary malignant lymphoma of the brain; in German]. Radiologe 1997; 37: 42–50.
- *Useful for further study.*

Plasmacytoma

Mäntylä R, Kinnunen J, Böhling T. Intracranial plasmacytoma: a case report. Neuroradiology 1996; 38: 646–9.
- *Describes a rare plasmacytoma infiltrating the meninges and temporal lobe; also reviews various intracranial manifestations.*

Germinoma

Chang T, Teng MMH, Guo WY, Sheng WC. CT of pineal tumors and intracranial germ-cell tumors. AJNR Am J Neuroradiol 1989; 10: 1039–44.
- *CT features of 59 pineal tumors; good CT documentation of all entities.*

Teratoma

Neuhold A, Fezoulidis I, Frühwald F, Wicke K, Stiskal M. [Space-occupying lesions of the pineal region in magnetic resonance tomography; in German]. RöFo Fortschr Geb Röntgenstr Neuen Bildgeb Verfahr 1989; 151: 210–5.
- *Compares preoperative CT and MRI findings in patients with pineal region masses, illustrates the relative importance of MRI.*

Rathke cleft cyst

Kucharczyk W, Peck WW, Kelly WM, Norman D, Newton TH. Rathke cleft cyst: CT, MR imaging and pathologic features. Radiology 1987; 165: 491–5
- *Presents typical imaging findings.*

Epidermoid

Hagen T, Kujat C, Donauer E, Piepgras U. [Neuroradiologic diagnosis of intracranial epidermoid tumors; in German]. Radiologe 1994; 34: 639–47.
- *CT images, including unusual cases; detailed coverage of basic principles.*
Sitoh YY, Tien RD. Neuroimaging in epilepsy. J Magn Reson Imaging 1998; 138: 277–88.
- *Detailed review of newer methods that can supplement CT.*
Uchino A, Hasuo K, Matsumoto S, et al. Intracranial epidermoid carcinoma: CT and MRI. Neuroradiology 1995; 37: 155–8.
- *Describes CT and MRI findings of this rare variant and summarizes 11 cases described in the literature.*

Dermoid

Gormley WB, Tomecek FJ, Qureshi N, Malik GM. Craniocerebral epidermoid and dermoid tumors: a review of 32 cases. Acta Neurochir 1994; 128: 115–21.
- *Review of clinical features, CT and intraoperative findings.*
Rubin G, Scienza R, Pasqualin A, Rosta L, Da-Pian R. Craniocerebral epidermoids and dermoids: a review of 44 cases. Acta Neurochir 1989; 97: 1–16.

- *Detailed review that includes orbital and diploic forms.*

Colloid cyst

Ciric I, Zivin I. Neuroepithelial (colloid) cysts of the septum pellucidum. J Neurosurg 1975; 43: 69–73.
- *Includes embryology.*
Kondziolka D, Lunsford LD. Stereotactic management of colloid cysts: factors predicting success. J Neurosurg 1991; 75: 45–51.
- *CT-guided biopsy of colloid cysts in two patients.*

Pituitary adenoma

Bonneville JF, Cattin F, Gorczyca W, Hardy J. Pituitary microadenomas: early enhancement with dynamic CT—implications of arterial blood supply and potential importance. Radiology 1993; 187: 857–61.
- *Interpretation of CT findings in 260 microadenoma patients.*
Sartor K, Karnaze MG, Winthrop JD, Gado M, Hodges FJ. MR imaging in infra-, para- and retrosellar mass lesions. Neuroradiology 1987; 29: 19–29.
- *Retrospective comparison of CT and MRI.*

Craniopharyngioma

Tsuda M, Takahashi S, Higano S, Kurihara N, Ikeda H, Sakamoto K. CT and MR imaging of craniopharyngioma. Eur Radiol 1997; 7: 464–9.
- *Twenty cases of craniopharyngioma.*

Paraganglioma

Mafee MF, Valvassori GE, Shugar MA, et al. High-resolution and dynamic sequential computed tomography: use in the evaluation of glomus complex tumors. Arch Otolaryngol 1983; 109: 691–6.
- *Describes an essential dynamic examination technique for glomus tumors.*

Chordoma

Sze G, Uichanco LS, Brant-Zawadzki MN, et al. Chordomas: MR imaging. Radiology 1988; 166: 187–91.
- *Very clear and informative work, also covers CT.*
Weber AL, Liebsch NJ, Sanchez R, Sweriduk ST. Chordomas of the skull base. Neuroimaging Clin N Am 1994; 4: 515–27.
- *Very informative article for further study.*

Chondroma, chondrosarcoma

Yang PY, Seeger JF, Carmody RF, Fleischer AS. Chondroma of falx: CT findings. J Comput Assist Tomogr 1986; 10: 1075–6.
- *Describes one case; adequate citations of literature and review of basics.*

Carcinoma

Hoe JW. Computed tomography of nasopharyngeal carcinoma: a review of CT appearances in 56 patients. Eur J Radiol 1989; 9: 83–90.
- *Investigates CT capabilities for TNM staging.*

Metastases

Pechova-Peterova V, Kalvach P. CT findings in cerebral metastases. Neuroradiology 1986; 28: 254–8.
- *A rare and relatively recent review work.*
Schumacher M, Orszagh M. Imaging techniques in neoplastic meningosis. J Neurooncol 1998; 38: 111–20.
- *Very informative review of this problem area in neuroimaging.*

Recent and basic works

Gliomas

Afra D, Osztie E. Histologically confirmed changes on CT of reoperated low-grade astrocytomas. Neuroradiology 1997; 39: 804–10.
- *Analysis of postoperative courses.*

Arita N, Taneda M, Hayakawa T. Leptomeningeal dissemination of malignant gliomas: incidence, diagnosis and outcome. Acta Neurochir 1994; 126: 84–92
- *Clinical study with CT illustrations.*

Bognar L, Turjman F, Villanyl E, et al. Tectal plate gliomas, 2: CT scans and MR imaging of tectal gliomas. Acta Neurochir 1994; 127: 48–54.
- *Part of comprehensive description; deals with imaging features.*

Geremia GK, Wollman R, Foust R. Computed tomography of gliomatosis cerebri. J Comput Assist Tomogr 1988; 12: 698–701.
- *One of numerous case reports on this entity.*

Ildan F, Gürsoy F, Gul B, Boyar B, Kilic C. Intracranial tuberculous abscess mimicking malignant glioma. Neurosurg Rev 1994; 17: 317–20.
- *Rare manifestation of tuberculosis; CT features well documented.*

Kendall BE, Jakubowski J, Pullicino P, Symon L. Difficulties in diagnosis of supratentorial gliomas by CAT scan. J Neurol Neurosurg Psychiatry 1979; 42: 485–92.
- *Much of this information is still of current interest.*

Lilja A, Lundqvist H, Olsson Y, et al. Positron emission tomography and computed tomography differential diagnosis between recurrent or residual glioma and treatment-induced brain lesions. Acta Radiol 1989; 30: 121–8.
- *Important because this is a major indication for cerebral positron-emission tomography (PET).*

McGahan JP, Ellis WG, Budenz RW, et al. Brain gliomas: sonographic characterization. Radiology 1986; 159: 485–92.
- *Case report.*

Stylopoulos LA, George AE, de Leon MJ, et al. Longitudinal CT study of parenchymal brain changes in glioma survivors. AJNR Am J Neuroradiol 1988; 9: 517–22.
- *Basic work dealing with the interpretation of imaging features.*

Tonami H, Kamehiro M, Oguchi M et al. Chordoid glioma of the third ventricle: CT and MR findings. J Comput Assist Tomogr 2000; 24(2): 336–8.

Vonofakos D, Marcu H, Hacker H. Oligodendrogliomas: CT patterns with emphasis on features indicating malignancy. J Comput Assist Tomogr 1979; 3: 783–8.
- *One of the few studies on oligodendroglioma.*

Wood JR, Green SB, Shapiro WR. The prognostic importance of tumor size in malignant gliomas: a computed tomographic study by the brain tumor cooperative group. J Clin Oncol 1988; 6: 338–43.
- *An important aspect of glioma imaging.*

Pleomorphic xanthoastrocytoma

Kepes JJ, Rubinstein LJ. Pleomorphic xanthoastrocytoma: a distinctive meningocerebral glioma of young subjects with relatively favorable prognosis. Cancer 1979; 44: 1839–52.
- *First description.*

Petropoulou K, Whiteman MLH, Altman NR, Bruce J, Morrison G. CT and MRI of pleomorphic xanthoastrocytoma: unusual biologic behavior. J Comput Assist Tomogr 1995; 19: 860–5.
- *Describes an unusually aggressive case.*

Subependymal giant-cell astrocytoma

Okuchi K, Hiramatsu K, Modimoto T, Tsunoda S, Sakaki T, Iwasaki S. Astrocytoma with widespread calcification along axonal fibres. Neuroradiology 1992; 34: 328–30.

Piepmeier JM. Tumors and approaches to the lateral ventricles: introduction and overview. J Neurooncol 1996; 30: 267–74.

Roszkowski M, Drabik K, Barszcz S, Jozwiak S. Surgical treatment of intraventricular tumors associated with tuberous sclerosis. Child's Nerv Syst 1995; 11: 335–9.

Ependymoma

Chang T, Teng MM, Lirng JF. Posterior cranial fossa tumors in childhood. Neuroradiology 1993; 35: 274–8.

Kim DG, Han MH, Lee SH, et al. MRI of intracranial subependymoma: report of a case. Neuroradiology 1993; 35: 185–6.

Nagib MG, O'Fallon MT. Posterior fossa lateral ependymoma in childhood. Pediatr Neurosurg 1996; 24: 299–305.

Neumann K, Schörner W, Hosten N, Iglesias JR, Bock JC. [Magnetic resonance tomography of intracranial ependymomas: their clinical appearance and comparison with computed tomography; in German]. RöFo Fortschr Geb Röntgenstr Neuen Bildgeb Verfahr 1992; 157: 111–7.

Piepmeier JM. Tumors and approaches to the lateral ventricles: introduction and overview. J Neurooncol 1996; 30: 267–74.

Subependymoma

Kim DG, Han MH, Lee SH, et al. MRI of intracranial subependymoma: report of a case. Neuroradiology 1993; 35: 185–6.

Plexus papilloma, carcinoma of choroid plexus

Coates TL, Hinshaw DB, Peckman N, et al. Pediatric choroid plexus neoplasm: MR, CT, and pathologic correlation. Radiology 189; 173: 81–8.
- *Report of four patients, including one with choroid plexus carcinoma.*

Kart BH, Reddy SC, Rao GR, Poveda H. Choroid plexus metastasis: CT appearance. J Comput Assist Tomogr 986; 10: 537–40.
- *Case report with discussion of differential diagnosis.*

Ken JG, Sobel DF, Copeland B, Davis J, Kortman KE. Choroid plexus papillomas of the foramen of Luschka: MR appearance. AJNR Am J Neuroradiol 1991; 12: 1201–3.
- *Rare site of occurrence, with CT findings.*

Gliomatosis cerebri

Kyritsis AP, Levin VA, Yung WK, Leeds NE. Imaging patterns of multifocal gliomas. Eur J Radiol 1993; 16: 163–70.

Onal C, Bayindir C, Siraneci R, et al. A serial CT scan and MRI verification of diffuse cerebrospinal gliomatosis: a case report with stereotactic diagnosis and radiological confirmation. Pediatr Neurosurg 1996; 25: 94–9.

Shin YM, Chang KH, Han MH, et al. Gliomatosis cerebri: comparison of MR and CT features. AJR Am J Roentgenol 1993; 161: 859–62.

Gangliocytoma

Altman NR. MR and CT characteristics of gangliocytoma: a rare cause of epilepsy in children. AJNR Am J Neu-

roradiol 1988; 9: 917–21.
● *Description of three examinations using MRI and CT.*
Armstrong EA, Harwood-Nash DC, Ritz CR, Chuang SH, Pettersson H, Martin DJ. CT of neuroblastomas and ganglioneuromas in children. AJR Am J Roentgenol 1982; 139: 571–6.
● *Deals mainly with tumors of the trunk.*
Ashley DG, Zee CS, Chandrasoma PT, Segall HD. Lhermitte–Duclos disease: CT and MR findings. J Comput Assist Tomogr 1990; 14: 984–7.
● *MRI description of a case, with CT findings.*

Ganglioglioma
Castillo M, Davis PC, Takei Y, Hoffman JC. Intracranial ganglioglioma: MR, CT, and clinical findings in 18 patients. AJNR Am J Neuroradiol 1990; 11: 109–14
● *Comparison of CT and unenhanced MRI.*
Martin DS, Levy B, Awwad EE, Pittman T. Desmoplastic infantile ganglioglioma: CT and MR features. AJNR Am J Neuroradiol 1991; 12: 1195–7.
● *Rare variant of this rare tumor.*
Tampieri D, Moumdjian R, Melanson D, Ethier R. Intracerebral gangliogliomas in patients with partial complex seizures. AJNR Am J Neuroradiol 1991; 12: 749–55.
● *Clinical preselection of patients.*
Tien RD, Tuori SL, Pulkingham N, Burger PC. Ganglioglioma with leptomeningeal and subarachnoid spread: results of CT, MR, and PET imaging. AJR Am J Roentgenol 1992; 159: 391–3.
● *Case report.*

Neurocytoma
Cheung YK. Central neurocytoma occurring in the thalamus: CT and MRI findings. Aust Radiol 1996; 40: 182–4.
● *Deals with an uncommon variant.*
Fukui M, Matsushima T, Fujii K, Nishio S, Takeshita I, Tashima T. Pineal and third ventricle tumors in the CT and MR eras. Acta Neurochir 1991; 53 (Suppl): 127–36.
● *Large neurosurgical review.*
Goergen SK, Gonzales MF, McLean CA. Interventricular neurocytoma: radiologic features and review of the literature. Radiology 1992; 182: 787–92.
● *Review of previously published cases, many with illustrations.*
Porter-Grenn LM, Silbergleit R, Stern HJ, Patel SC, Mehta B, Sanders WP. Intraventricular primary neuronal neoplasms: CT, MR, and angiographic findings. J Comput Assist Tomogr 1991; 15: 365–8.
● *Differentiation from neuroblastoma, includes angiography.*
Tomura N, Hirano H, Watanabe O, et al. Central neurocytoma with clinically malignant behavior. AJNR Am J Neuroradiol 1997; 18: 1175–8.
● *Two cases with postoperative dissemination.*

Esthesioneuroblastoma
Burker DP, Gabrielsen TO, Knake JE, et al. Radiology of olfactory neuroblastoma. Radiology 1980; 137: 367–72.
● *CT images outdated; informative angiograms.*
Feyerabend T. Role of radiotherapy in the treatment of esthesioneuroblastoma. HNO 1990; 38: 20–3.
● *Review of treatment with three case presentations.*
Regenbogen VS, Zinreich SJ, Kim KS, et al. Hyperostotic esthesioneuroblastoma: CT and MR findings. J Comput Assist Tomogr 1988; 12: 52–6.
● *Important for differentiation from meningioma.*

Vanhoenacker P, Hermans R, Sneyers W, et al. Atypical aesthesioneuroblastoma: CT and MRI findings. Neuroradiology 1993; 35: 466–7.
● *Case report.*

Pineocytoma, pineoblastoma, pineal cyst
Evanson EJ, Lewis PD, Colquhoun IR. Primary germinoma of the posterior cranial fossa: a case report. Neuroradiology 1997; 39: 716–8.
● *Very well-documented examinations.*
Neuhold A, Fezoulidis I, Frühwald F, Wicke K, Stiskal M. [Space-occupying lesions of the pineal region in magnetic resonance tomography; in German]. RöFo Fortschr Geb Röntgenstr Neuen Bildgeb Verfahr 1989; 151: 210–5.
● *Compares MRI and CT in 24 histologically confirmed lesions.*

Medulloepithelioma
Poot RD. Medulloepithelioma: first CT images. Neuroradiology 1986; 28: 286
● *Good illustration of CT finding, but with equivocal histology.*

Neuroblastoma
Goldberg RM, Keller IA, Schonfeld SM, Mezrich RS, Rosenfeld DL. Intracranial route of a cervical neuroblastoma through skull base foramina. Pediatr Radiol 1996; 26: 715–6.
● *Case report.*
Wiegel B, Harris TM, Edwards MK. Smith RR, Azzarelli B. MRI of intracranial neuroblastoma with dural sinus invasion and distant metastases. AJNR Am J Neuroradiol 1991; 12: 1198–200.
● *Addresses the important issue of sinus infiltration.*

Ependymoblastoma
Hanakita J, Handa H. [Clinical features and CT scan findings of supratentorial ependymomas and ependymoblastomas; in Japanese]. No Shinkei Geka 1984; 12: 253–60.
● *One of the rare descriptions; in Japanese, but with comprehensive English abstract.*

PNET/medulloblastoma
Kingsley DPE, Harwood-Nash DC. Parameters of infiltration in posterior fossa tumors of childhood using a high-resolution CT scanner. Neuroradiology 1984; 26: 347–50.
● *Comparison of tumor infiltration found at surgery with CT, for astrocytoma, medulloblastoma, and ependymoma; acceptable image quality.*
Lee YY, Tien RD, Bruner JM, DePena CA, Van Tassel P. Loculated intracranial leptomeningeal metastases: CT and MR characteristics. AJR Am J Roentgenol 1989; 10: 1171–9.
● *With CT scans of leptomeningeal metastases from various primary tumors.*
Pickuth D, Leutloff U. Computed tomography and magnetic resonance imaging findings in primitive neuroectodermal tumours in adults. Br J Neuroradiol 1996; 69: 1–5.
● *Findings in five adults.*
Tortori-Donati P, Fondelli MP, Rossi A, et al. Medulloblastoma in children: CT and MRI findings. Neuroradiology 1996; 38: 352–9.
● *Recent study using MRI as standard procedure.*

Schwannoma (neurinoma)

Balestri P, Calistri L, Vivarelli R, et al. Central nervous system imaging in reevaluation of patients with neurofibromatosis type 1. Child's Nerv Syst 1993; 9: 448–51.

Dalley RW, Robertson WD, Nugent RA, Durity FA. Computed tomography of anterior inferior cerebellar artery aneurysm mimicking an acoustic neuroma. J Comput Assist Tomogr 186; 10: 881–4.
- *Pitfall.*

Ebeling U, Huber P. Acute mass lesions of the posterior cranial fossa. Schweiz Med Wochenschr 1986; 116: 1394–1401.

Evanson EJ, Lewis PD, Colquhoun IR. Primary germinoma of the posterior cranial fossa: a case report. Neuroradiology 1997; 39: 716–8.
- *Description of an atypical case.*

Nakada T, St John JN, Knight RT. Solitary metastasis of systemic malignant lymphoma to the cerebellopontine angle. Neuroradiology 1983; 24: 225–8.
- *Deals with differential diagnosis.*

Paz-Fumagalli R, Daniels DL, Millen SJ, Meyer GA, Thieu TM. Dural "tail" associated with an acoustic schwannoma in MR imaging with gadopentetate dimeglumine. AJNR Am J Neuroradiol 1991; 12: 1206.
- *Important pitfall in MRI differential diagnosis.*

Sigal R, d'Anthouard F, David P, et al. Cystic schwannoma mimicking a brain tumor: MR features. J Comput Assist Tomogr 1990; 14: 662–4.
- *With CT image.*

Thron A, Bockenheimer S. Giant aneurysms of the posterior fossa suspected as neoplasms on computed tomography. Neuroradiology 1979; 18: 93–7.
- *Occasional source of error, even with present-day image quality.*

Tsuiki H, Kuratsu J, Ishimaru Y, et al. Intracranial intraparenchymal schwannoma: report of three cases. Acta Neurochir 1997; 139: 756–60.
- *With commentary noting the difficult differential diagnosis of ring-like lesions.*

Neurofibroma

Jacoby CG, Go RT, Beren RA. Cranial CT of neurofibromatosis. AJR Am J Roentgenol 1980; 135: 553–7.
- *With scan illustrating a malignant schwannoma of the orbit.*

Mayfrank L, Mohadjer M, Wullich B. Intracranial calcified deposits in neurofibromatosis. Neuroradiology 1990; 32: 33–7.
- *Very good documentation of imaging findings.*

Tegos S, Georgouli G, Gogos C, Polythothorakis J, Sanidas V, Mavrogiorgos C. Primary malignant schwannoma involving simultaneously the right Gasserian ganglion and the distal part of the right mandibular nerve: case report. J Neurosurg Sci 1997; 41: 293–7.
- *Case report of a malignant schwannoma.*

Meningioma

Flaschka G, Ebner F, Kleinert R. [A pitfall of neuroradiological diagnosis: a double intracerebral tumor in CT and MR (intraventricular meningioma and corpus callosum glioma—a case report; in German]. RöFo Fortschr Geb Röntgenstr Neuen Bildgeb Verfahr 1990; 152: 739–41.
- *Meningioma and glioma.*

Halpin SES, Britton J, Wilkins P, Uttley D. Intradiploic meningiomas: a radiological study of two cases confirmed histologically. Neuroradiology 1991; 33: 247–50
- *Two unusual cases.*

Lang FF, Macdonald OK, Fuller GN, DeMonte F. Primary extradural meningiomas: a report on nine cases and review of the literature from the era of computerized tomography scanning. /CLJ Neurosurg 2000; 93(6): 940–50 [Review]

Schörner W, Schubeus P, Henkes H, Rottacker C, Hamm B, Felix R. Intracranial meningiomas: comparison of plain and contrast-enhanced examinations in CT and MRI. Neuroradiology 1990; 32: 12–8.
- *Analysis of imaging findings in 50 patients.*

Schubeus P, Schörner W, Rottacker C, Sander B. Intracranial meningiomas: how frequent are indicative findings in CT and MRI? Neuroradiology 1990; 32: 4467–73.
- *Quantitative information on image interpretation.*

Schuknecht B, Müller J, Nadjmi M. [Malignant melanoma of the meninges: MR and CT diagnosis; in German]. RöFo Fortschr Geb Röntgenstr Neuen Bildgeb Verfahr 1990; 152: 80–6.
- *Rare form of meningeal tumor.*

Servo A, Porras M, Jaaskelainen J, Paetau A, Haltia M. Computed tomography and angiography do not reliably discriminate malignant meningiomas from benign ones. Neuroradiology 1990; 32: 94–7.
- *Based on a very large series.*

Lipoma

Maiuri F, Corriero G, Gallicchio B, Simonetti L. Lipoma of the ambient cistern causing obstructive hydrocephalus. J Neurosurg Sci 1987; 31: 53–8.
- *Deals with a possible complication.*

Fibrous histiocytoma

Schrader B, Holland BR, Friedrichsen C. Rare case of a primary malignant fibrous histiocytoma of the brain. Neuroradiology 1989; 31: 177–9.
- *Describes one case and reviews ten previously published cases.*

Hemangiopericytoma

Alpern MP, Thorsen MK, Kellman GM, Pojunas K, Lawson TL. CT appearance of hemangiopericytoma. J Comput Assist Tomogr 1986; 10: 264–7.
- *Hemangiopericytomas at various sites, including one in the posterior fossa.*

Chiechi MV, Smirniotopoulos JG, Mena H. Intracranial hemangiopericytomas: MR and CT features. AJNR Am J Neuroradiol 1996; 17: 1365–71.
- *Review of 34 confirmed cases, MRI and CT findings.*

Rhabdomyosarcoma

Cornell SH, Hibri NS, Menzes AH, Graf CF. The complimentary nature of computed tomography and angiography in the diagnosis of cerebellar hemangioblastoma. Neuroradiology 1979; 17: 201–5.

Lee JH, Lee MS, Lee BH, et al. Rhabdomyosarcoma of the head and neck in adults: MR and CT findings. AJNR Am J Neuroradiol 1996; 17: 1923–8.

Naidich TP, Lin JP, Leeds NE, Pudlowski RM, Naidich JB. Primary tumors and other masses of the cerebellum and fourth ventricle: differential diagnosis by computed tomography. Neuroradiology 1977; 14: 153–74.

Lymphoma

Fest T, Rozenbaum A, Cattin F, Chambers R, Carbillet JP, Bonneville JF. Neuroblastoma-like epidural localization in non-Hodgkin's lymphoma. Neuroradiology 1988; 30: 569–70.
- *Case report with differential diagnosis of the split-suture finding.*

Watanabe M, Tanaka R, Takeda N, Wakabayashi K, Takahashi H. Correlation of computed tomography with the histopathology of primary malignant lymphoma of the brain. Neuroradiology 1992; 34: 36–42.
● *Correlation of CT and autopsy findings in seven patients.*

Germinoma
Fujimaki T, Matsutani M, Funada N, et al. CT and MRI features of intracranial germ cell tumors. J Neurooncol 1994; 19: 217–26.
● *Large review.*

Teratoma
Ganti SR, Hilal SK, Stein BM, Silver AJ, Mawad M, Sane P. CT of pineal region tumors. AJR Am J Roentgenol 1986; 146: 451–8.
● *Presents 60 rare pineal tumors, acceptable image quality.*
Radkowski MA, Naidich TP, Tomita T, Byrd SE, McLone DG. Neonatal brain tumors: CT and MR findings. J Comput Assist Tomogr 1988; 12: 10–20.
● *A review of brain tumors occurring in newborns.*

Rathke cleft cyst
Nemoto Y, Inoue Y, Fukuda T, et al. MR appearance of Rathke's cleft cyst. Neuroradiology 1988; 30: 155–9.
● *Describes three symptomatic patients.*

Epidermoid
Gentry LR, Jacoby CG, Turski PA, Houston LW, Strother CM, Sackett JF. Cerebellopontine angle–petromastoid mass lesions: comparative study of diagnosis with MR imaging and CT. Radiology 1987; 162: 513–20.
● *Presents various pathologies based on CT and MRI in 75 patients.*
Kenneth RD, Roberson GH, Taveras JM, New PFJ, Trevor R. Diagnosis of epidermoid tumor by computed tomography. Radiology 1976; 119: 347–53.
● *Cited here as an example of a classic cranial CT study from the 1970 s. The differential-diagnostic considerations and histologic example are still of interest; first-generation CT images.*
Yuh WTC, Wright DC, Barloon TJ, Schultz DH, Sato Y, Cervantes CA. MR imaging of primary tumors of trigeminal nerve and Meckel's cave. AJR Am J Roentgenol 1988; 151: 577–82.
● *Review of Meckel cave masses that cause trigeminal neuralgia.*

Dermoid
Jamjoom AB, Cummins BH. The diagnosis of ruptured intracranial dermoid cysts. Br J Neurosurg 1989; 3: 609–12.
● *One case and review of the literature.*
Wilms G, Casselman J, Demaerel P, Plets C, DeHaene I, Baert AL. CT and MRI of ruptured intracranial dermoids. Neuroradiology 1991; 33: 149–51.
● *Two cases of this complication.*

Colloid cyst
Deinsberger W, Boker DK, Samii M. Flexible endoscopes in treatment of colloid cysts of the third ventricle. Minim Invasive Neurosurg 1994; 37: 12–6.
● *Deals with CT-guided endoscopy of colloid cysts.*
Maeder PP, Holtas SL, Basibuyuk LN, Salford LG, Tapper UA, Brun A. Colloid cysts of the third ventricle: correlation of MR and CT findings with histology and chemical analysis. AJR Am J Roentgenol 1990; 155: 135–41.

● *Eight patients, correlation of cyst contents with imaging features.*
Mamourian AC, Cromwell LD, Harbaugh RE. Colloid cyst of the third ventricle: sometimes more conspicuous on CT than MR. AJNR Am J Neuroradiol 1998; 19: 875–8.
● *Colloid cysts in two patients; better delineation with CT.*
Mohadjer M, Teshmar E, Mundinger F. CT-stereotaxic drainage of colloid cysts in the foramen of Monro and the third ventricle. J Neurosurg 1987; 67: 220–3.
● *CT-guided aspiration in 12 cases.*
Urso JA, Ross GJ, Parker RK, Patrizi JD, Stewart B. Colloid cyst of the third ventricle: radiologic-pathologic correlation. J Comput Assist Tomogr 1998; 22: 524–7.
● *Case report of a colloid cyst with a layered structure.*
Waggenspack GA, Guinto FC. MR and CT of masses of the anterosuperior third ventricle. AJR Am J Roentgenol 1989; 152: 609–14.
● *Five cysts, one astrocytoma; problems of differential diagnosis.*
Yuceer N, Baskaya M, Gokalp HZ. Huge colloid cyst of the third ventricle associated with calcification in the cyst wall. Neurosurg Rev 1996; 19: 131–3.
● *Case report of a calcified cyst.*

Pituitary adenoma
Kasperlik-Zaluska A, Walecki J, Brzezinski J, et al. MRI versus CT in the diagnosis of Nelson's syndrome. Eur Radiol 1997; 7: 106–9.
● *Comparison.*
Kersjes W, Allmendinger S, Stiebler H, Christ F, Bockisch A, Klingmuller D. [A comparison of the value of magnetic resonance tomography and computed tomography in Nelson syndrome patients; in German]. RöFo Fortschr Geb Röntgenstr Neuen Bildgeb Verfahr 1992; 156: 166–71.
● *Thirteen patients.*
Kuhn MJ, Swenson LC, Youssef HT. Absence of the septum pellucidum and related disorders. Comput Med Imaging Graph 1993; 17: 137–47.
● *Review based on 15 patients with various associated changes.*
Saito K, Takayasu M, Akabane A, Okabe H, Sugita K. Primary chronic intrasellar hematoma: a case report. Acta Neurochir 1992; 114: 147–50.
● *Case report.*
Sidhu PS, Kingdon CC, Strickland NH. Case report: CT scan appearances of a pituitary abscess. Clin Radiol 1994; 49: 427–8.
● *An unusual case.*
Stadnik T, Spruyt D, van Binst A, Luypaert R, d'Haens J, Osteaux M. Pituitary microadenomas: diagnosis with dynamic serial CT, conventional CT and T1-weighted MR imaging before and after injection of gadolinium. Eur J Radiol 1994; 18: 191–8.
● *Comparison of CT and MRI.*

Craniopharyngioma
Ebel H, Rieger A, Spies EH, Boker DK. Stereotactic cysto-ventricular shunting in diencephalic (arachnoid) cysts and failure in cystic craniopharyngioma. Minim Invasive Neurosurg 1995; 38: 41–7.
● *Stereotactic cyst drainage, includes craniopharyngioma.*

Hamburger C, Schonberger J, Lange M. Management and prognosis of intracranial giant aneurysms: a report on 58 cases. Neurosurg Rev 1992; 15: 97–103.
- *Misdiagnoses of giant aneurysm, including craniopharyngioma, meningioma, glioblastoma, and pituitary adenoma.*

Hellwig D, Bauer BL, List-Hellwig E, Mennel HD. Stereotactic–endoscopic procedures on processes of the cranial midline. Acta Neurochir 1991; 53 (Suppl): 23–32.
- *Deals with craniopharyngiomas and midline masses.*

Paraganglioma

Noble ER, Smoker WRK, Ghatak NR. Atypical skull base paragangliomas. AJNR Am J Neuroradiol 1997; 18: 986–90.
- *Very fine correlation of CT, MRI and angiography in two patients.*

Chordoma

Brown RV, Sage MR, Brophy BP. CT and MR findings in patients with chordomas of the petrous apex. AJNR Am J Neuroradiol 1990; 11: 121–4.
- *Presents three cases located off-midline, all with CT illustrations.*

Oot RF, Melville GE, New PFJ, et al. The role of MR and CT in evaluating clival chordomas and chondrosarcomas. AJR Am J Roentgenol 1988; 151: 567–75.

Probst EN, Zanella FE, Vortmeyer AO. Congenital clivus chordoma. AJNR Am J Neuroradiol 1993; 14: 537–9.
- *Well-documented case with CT, MRI, and ultrasound.*

Chondroma, chondrosarcoma

Steurer M, Kautzky M, Zrunek M. A chondrosarcoma of the nose and paranasal sinuses. HNO 1993; 41: 30–2.
- *Presents a case with CT and MRI interpretation.*

Tanohata K, Maehara T, Aida N, et al. Computed tomography of intracranial chondroma with emphasis on delayed contrast enhancement. J Comput Assist Tomogr 1987; 11: 820–3.
- *Presents two cases.*

Carcinoma

Chong VF, Fan YF, Khoo JB. Nasopharyngeal carcinoma with intracranial spread: CT and MR characteristics. J Comput Assist Tomogr 1996; 20: 563–9.
- *Compares CT and MRI in 114 patients; routes of spread are shown.*

Miura T, Hirabuki N, Nishiyama K, et al. Computed tomographic findings of nasopharyngeal carcinoma with skull base and intracranial involvement. Cancer 1990; 65: 29–37.
- *Capabilities for TNM staging in a small number of patients.*

Sham JS, Cheung YK, Choy D, Chan FL, Leong L. Nasopharyngeal carcinoma: CT evaluation of patterns of tumor spread. AJNR Am J Neuroradiol 1991; 12: 265–70.
- *Deals with skull base involvement.*

Metastases

Akeson P, Larsson EM, Kristoffersen DT, Jonsson E, Holtas S. Brain metastases: comparison of gadodiamide injection–enhanced MR imaging at standard and high dose, contrast-enhanced CT and non–contrast-enhanced MR imaging. Acta Radiol 1995; 36: 300–6.
- *Study of MRI contrast media, includes CT comparison.*

el-Sonbaty MR, Abdul-Ghaffar NU, Marafy AA. Multiple intracranial tuberculomas mimicking brain metastases. Tuber Lung Dis 1995; 76: 271–2.
- *One of the few studies on differential diagnosis.*

Guy RL, Benn JJ, Ayersetal AB. A comparison of CT and MRI in the assessment of the pituitary and parasellar region. Clin Radiol 1991; 43: 156–61.
- *In 40 patients; also cites several strengths of CT.*

Heinz R, Wiener D, Friedman H, Tien R. Detection of cerebrospinal fluid metastasis: CT myelography or MRI? AJNR Am J Neuroradiol 1995; 16: 1147–51.
- *Superiority of MRI.*

Kohno M, Matsutani M, Sasaki T, Takakura K. Solitary metastasis to the choroid plexus of the lateral ventricle: report of three cases and a review of the literature. J Neurooncol 1996; 27: 47–52.
- *Presents three original cases and reviews eight from the literature.*

Pedersen H, McConnell J, Harwood-Nash DC, Fitz CR, Chuang SH. Computed tomography in intracranial, supratentorial metastases in children. Neuroradiology 1989; 31: 19–23.
- *CT features of metastases vs. brain tumors in children.*

Reider-Groswasser I, Merimsky O, Karminsky N, Chaitchik S. Computed tomography features of cerebral spread of malignant melanoma. Am J Clin Oncol 1996; 19: 49–53.
- *Small study, but one of the few publications on cerebral metastases from melanoma.*

Ricke J, Baum K, Hosten N. Calcified brain metastases from ovarian carcinoma. Neuroradiology 1996; 38: 460–1.

Salvati M, Cervoni L, Raco A. Single brain metastases from unknown primary malignancies in CT era. J Neurooncol 1995; 23: 75–80.
- *100 patients.*

6 Degenerative and Demyelinating Diseases

Degenerative Diseases

Degenerative diseases of the brain (Tables 6.**1**, 6.**2**) are often referred for computed tomography (CT) scanning in patients undergoing evaluation for dementia. The most frequent cause of senile dementia is Alzheimer disease. The diagnosis of Alzheimer disease is based on specific clinical criteria, and cranial CT examination contributes to the diagnosis only by excluding other, potentially treatable causes such as intracranial masses (such as tumors or subdural hematoma) and normal-pressure hydrocephalus. This type of diagnosis is made with

Table 6.**1** Overview of the CT features of dementia diseases (after Tien et al., AJR Am J Roentgenol 1993; 161: 245–55)

Type	CT features
Cortical dementias	
● Alzheimer disease	Atrophy of temporal, parietal, and anterior frontal lobe cortices*
● Pick disease	Frontal and temporal cortical atrophy; the parietal and occipital lobes are relatively unaffected
Subcortical dementias	
● Parkinson disease	The midbrain is essentially normal on CT. MRI shows significant narrowing of the pars compacta of the substantia nigra
● Parkinsonian syndromes	CT normal. MRI shows iron deposition in the putamen
● Huntington disease	Caudate atrophy (bicaudate ratio). The putamen and globus pallidus are less affected. Frontal and temporal atrophy
● Wilson disease	Ventricular dilatation, cortical atrophy, and decreased density of the basal ganglia
● Normal-pressure hydrocephalus	Ventricular dilatation disproportionate to the degree of sulcal enlargement

Type	CT features
● Multiple sclerosis	Lesions in the periventricular white matter, cerebral atrophy
● HIV encephalopathy	Progressive diffuse leukoencephalopathy (symmetrical)
Combined cortical and subcortical dementias	
● Vascular dementia – Multi-infarct dementia – Binswanger disease – Cerebral lacunae	See p. 206
● Creutzfeldt–Jakob disease	Progressive, diffuse atrophy
● Hypoxic encephalopathy	Globus pallidus necrosis, with early hypodensities and calcifications in the late stage. Other basal ganglia may also be affected

HIV: human immunodeficiency virus.

* Distinguished from multi-infarct dementia, in which multiple infarcts of varying age are usually detected in both hemispheres.

6.2 Diseases that involve the basal ganglia

Disease	CT findings	MRI findings
Wilson disease	Generalized cerebral atrophy; rarely hypodensities in the caudate nucleus, lentiform nucleus, and thalamus	Increased T2-weighted signal intensity in caudate nucleus, lentiform nucleus, midbrain, and periaqueductal tissue; decreased T2-weighted signal intensity in the central putamen • MRI recommended
Huntington disease	Atrophy of the caudate nucleus, widening of the frontal horns, diffuse cerebral atrophy in the late stage	Like CT, T2-weighted MRI also shows hypointensity of these nuclei • MRI equivocal
Hallervorden–Spatz disease	Usually normal	High T2-weighted signal intensity in the pallidum, and low signal intensity in the globus pallidus
Leigh disease	Symmetrical hypodensities in the putamen and caudate nucleus, rarely in the pallidum or thalamus	Increased T1-weighted signal intensity, decreased T2-weighted signal intensity in these nuclei • MRI equivocal
Parkinson disease	Generalized cerebral atrophy	Generalized cerebral atrophy in multiple system atrophy (Parkinson plus), low T2-weighted signal intensity in the putamen • MRI recommended
Adrenoleukodystrophy	Bilateral hypodensity of the occipital white matter, advancing anteriorly; pseudogyral enhancement	Occipital-to-rostral progression of demyelination • MRI recommended
Alexander disease	Marked, diffuse white-matter hypodensity	White matter shows low T1-weighted signal intensity, high T2-weighted signal intensity from rostral to occipital; pseudogyral enhancement • MRI recommended
Canavan disease	Diffuse white-matter hypodensity	White matter hypointense in T1-weighted image, hyperintense in T2-weighted image • MRI recommended
Pelizaeus–Merzbacher disease	Normal	White matter hypointense in T1-weighted image, hyperintense in T2-weighted image • MRI recommended
Cockayne syndrome	Atrophy and calcification of basal ganglia	Periventricular contrast reversal, sharply marginated lesions
Progressive multifocal leukoencephalopathy (PML)	Subcortical hypodensities, sharply marginated	Increased T2-weighted signal intensity (FLAIR sequence) corresponding to CT • MRI recommended
Progressive diffuse leukoencephalopathy (PDL)	Bilateral, predominantly frontal hypodensities sparing the subcortical white matter	Increased T2-weighted signal intensity (FLAIR sequence) corresponding to CT • MRI recommended

CT in approximately 1–2 % of cases, depending on the patient selection. The percentage is higher in patients who have an immediate history of trauma, urinary incontinence, or gait disturbance.

The use of cranial CT in dementia patients depends on the diagnostic yield of treatable conditions, the patient's and family's need to know, and considerations of expense. As a rule, CT does not contribute to the differential diagnosis of dementias, beyond screening for potentially treatable causes.

Alzheimer Disease

Frequency: the most common form of dementia (6 % prevalence after age 65); makes up approximately 60 % of senile dementias.

Suggestive morphologic findings: CT can exclude multi-infarct dementia and other dementias. There are no specific CT features of Alzheimer disease, other than possible atrophy of the medial temporal lobe.

Procedure: Alzheimer disease is diagnosed clinically or by brain biopsy.

Other studies: functional imaging studies (nuclear medicine). Coronal magnetic resonance imaging (MRI) demonstrates changes in the medial temporal lobe.

Checklist for scan interpretation:
▶ Cerebral infarcts? White matter changes?
▶ Other causes of dementia such as normal-pressure hydrocephalus, frontal tumors, etc.?
▶ Cortical atrophy? Accentuated in certain areas?

■ Pathogenesis

Alzheimer disease is the leading cause of dementia. Its prevalence increases with aging, starting at about 60 years of age, and it affects an estimated 6 % of patients over the age of 65. It is believed to be caused by amyloid deposition in the neurons.

■ Frequency

Alzheimer's type dementia is the most common form, accounting for 50–60 % of cases.

■ Histology

Histologically, there is a widespread loss of neurons that is manifested grossly by cerebral atrophy chiefly affecting the temporal lobes and hippocampus. The parietal lobes and anterior frontal lobes are also affected. Microscopic pathology consists of senile plaques in the gray matter and neurofibrillary tangles in the neurons. The diagnosis is confirmed by autopsy or brain biopsy.

■ Clinical Manifestations

The early symptoms of the disease, which takes a progressive course, include personality changes and an inability to follow complex instructions or comprehend relationships. There is a progressive decline in cognitive functions. Memory impairment is very characteristic, but motor impairment is not an early feature. Other symptoms, such as loss of sphincter control, appear in later stages of the disease.

■ CT Morphology

The CT findings are nonspecific. Cortical atrophy predominantly affects the medial portion of the temporal lobe. The parietal and anterior frontal lobes are affected to a lesser degree.

Coronal T2-weighted MRI can demonstrate increased signal intensity of the hippocampus. Among the radionuclide imaging methods, positron-emission tomography (PET) findings are relatively characteristic, and consist of decreased uptake of ^{18}F-deoxyglucose in the parietal lobes. Generally, this finding is bilateral and symmetrical.

■ Differential Diagnosis

As noted above, the CT features of Alzheimer disease and other imaging findings are relatively nonspecific (Fig. 6.**1**). The best use of imaging procedures is to exclude less common but potentially treatable causes of senile or presenile dementia–most notably normal-pressure hydrocephalus, but also meningioma and other anterior fossa tumors. Pick disease

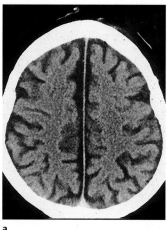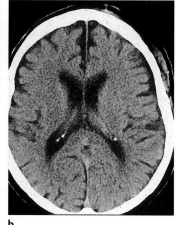

Fig. 6.**1 a, b Diffuse cortical atrophy in Alzheimer disease**. CT scans at the level of the centrum semiovale and ventricles in a 65-year-old man show marked sulcal enlargement and widening of the interhemispheric fissure. By contrast, the ventricular system shows only mild to moderate enlargement.

a   b

has similar clinical features, but a different CT appearance (see below).

Pick Disease

Frequency: 10–30 times less common than Alzheimer disease.

Suggestive morphologic findings: marked atrophy of the frontal and temporal lobes, with normal-appearing parietal and occipital lobes.

Other studies: MRI demonstrates gliotic changes in the frontal and temporal cortex. Functional nuclear medicine studies show bilateral frontal hypoperfusion.

Checklist for scan interpretation:
▶ Other causes of dementia such as tumors or normal-pressure hydrocephalus?
▶ Cortical sulci enlarged? Over which lobes?

■ Pathogenesis

Pick disease is included with Alzheimer disease in the category of cortical dementias.

■ Histology

Pick disease is characterized pathologically and radiologically by a focal atrophy affecting the frontal or temporal lobes. Microscopically, cytoplasmic inclusions (Pick bodies) are found in silver-stained sections from the affected cortex. The senile plaques and neurofibrillary tan-

gles of Alzheimer disease, as well as other neuropathologic signs, are absent in Pick disease.

■ Clinical Manifestations

Pick disease usually has an earlier clinical onset than Alzheimer disease, and initial changes often appear before age 65. Consistent with the morphologic findings, frontal lobe symptoms are common and consist of inappropriate social behavior (hyperorality, sexual disinhibition, etc.) and occasional depression or obsessive ideation.

■ CT Morphology

CT demonstrates focal cortical atrophy affecting the frontal lobes (Fig. 6.**2**) or temporal lobes and sparing the parietal and occipital lobes. The precentral gyrus forms the "watershed" for cortical changes, with sulcal enlargement occurring anterior but not posterior to the gyrus.

■ Differential Diagnosis

Pick disease should be considered in differential diagnosis whenever focal cortical atrophy is detected. Differentiation from Alzheimer disease is aided by the fact that atrophy of the caudate nucleus in Pick disease can lead to rounding of the frontal horns. Otherwise CT is used mainly to exclude other causes of dementia.

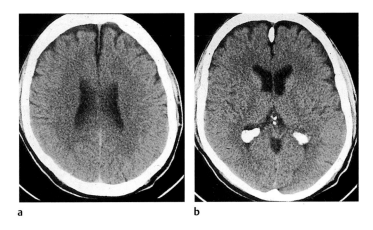

Fig. 6.**2 a, b** redominantly frontal cerebral atrophy. CT scans through the upper portion of the lateral ventricles and at the level of the frontal and occipital horns in a 49-year-old man demonstrate sulcal enlargement over both frontal lobes. The ventricular system is only mildly to moderately enlarged.

a   b

Creutzfeldt–Jakob Disease

CT and MRI of the brain in patients with prion-induced Creutzfeldt–Jakob disease is usually normal in the initial stage. CT may demonstrate cortical atrophy later in the disease.

Parkinson Disease

Frequency: Parkinson disease affects approximately 1% of the population over 50 years of age.

Suggestive morphologic findings: CT scans are normal.

Other studies: MRI may show enlargement of the interpeduncular cistern and changes in the substantia nigra.

Checklist for scan interpretation:
▶ Evidence of a parkinsonian syndrome (basal ganglia changes)?
▶ Atrophy?

■ Pathogenesis, Histology

Parkinson disease is characterized histologically by a degeneration of pigmented cells in the substantia nigra, leading to dysfunction of the nigrostriatal dopaminergic system. Cytoplasmic inclusions (Lewy bodies) are found in surviving neuronal cells.

■ Frequency

Parkinson disease and the parkinsonian syndromes are common disorders with a high prevalence.

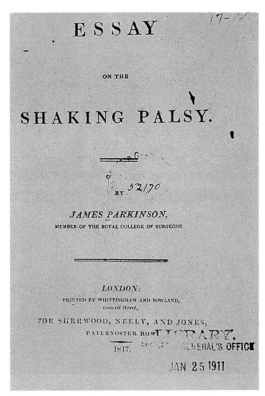

Fig. 6.**3** **Title page of the first publication on the condition now known as Parkinson disease** (courtesy of the National Library, Berlin).

■ Clinical Manifestations

The clinical manifestations of Parkinson disease (Fig. 6.**3**) and the parkinsonian syndromes chiefly involve the motor system. They occur in a classic triad:

- Bradykinesia
- Resting tremor
- Gait disturbance

Parkinson disease and the parkinsonian syndromes may be associated with dementia. Reports on incidence are highly variable.

■ CT Morphology

CT may demonstrate atrophic changes in Parkinson disease, but no characteristic CT features are observed. The parkinsonian syndromes are characterized by changes in the basal ganglia, which MRI demonstrates with much higher sensitivity. T2*-weighted images show a decrease in signal intensity caused by increased iron deposition.

Other imaging findings are reviewed in Fig. 6.**4.**

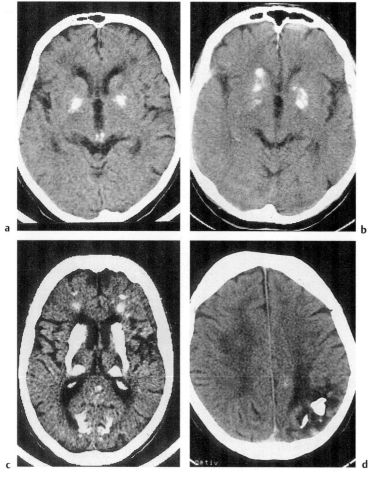

a

b

c

d

Fig. 6.**4 Calcifications of the basal ganglia.** Figures 6.**4 a–c** show varying degrees of calcification in the basal ganglia. The symmetrical distribution makes it unlikely that an oligodendroglioma or other tumor is the cause.

a Symmetrical calcifications of the globus pallidus.

b Asymmetrical calcifications additionally involving the head of the caudate nucleus on the right side.

  c Very pronounced calcifications in a scan from a 74-year-old woman. Besides extensive symmetrical calcifications of the basal ganglia including the thalamus, the scan shows corkscrew-like calcifications in the occipital white matter and patchy calcifications in the frontal white matter.

d Calcifications like those found in oligodendroglioma. These calcifications have a somewhat flocculent appearance, and are surrounded by hypodense tumor. Calcifications of the basal ganglia that are symmetrical, or almost symmetrical, are known as Fahr disease. It should be noted, however, that metabolic disorders (calcium metabolism) can lead to patterns like that shown in **c.**

■ Differential Diagnosis

Parkinson disease is distinguished from the parkinsonian syndromes, which are characterized by a poor response to antiparkinson medication. Another useful differentiating criterion is that, while CT and MRI are usually normal in Parkinson disease, at least MRI will show abnormalities in parkinsonian syndromes such as iron deposition. Olivopontocerebellar atrophy (OPCA) is usually associated with definite volume loss in the cerebellum and pons, and this is clearly demonstrable by CT and MRI.

Multiple System Atrophy

Frequency: rare.

Suggestive morphologic findings: trophy of the cerebellum, pons, and medulla oblongata.

Procedure: ame clinical features as Parkinson disease, with poorer response to medications.

Other studies: RI shows altered signal intensity in the basal ganglia.

Checklist for scan interpretation:
▶ Atrophy?
▶ Which parts of the brain are affected?

■ Pathogenesis

Multiple system atrophy (MSA) is a collective term applied to diseases that have Parkinson-like symptoms but respond poorly to antiparkinson medications. It was formerly referred to as "Parkinson plus syndrome."

The following diseases are included in this category:

● OPCA (known familial occurrence)
● Striatonigral degeneration
● Shy–Drager syndrome
● Steele–Richardson–Olszewski syndrome

■ Clinical Manifestations

OPCA is characterized by a combination of ataxia, dysarthria, and dysphagia. The disease can be fatal in middle age. As in striatonigral

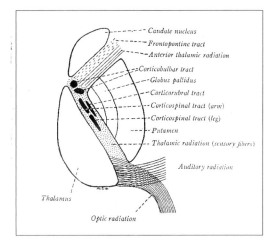

Fig. 6.**4e** Historical illustration detailing the anatomy of the basal ganglia, from Stephen W. Ranson, *The anatomy of the nervous system from the standpoint of development and function* (Philadelphia: Saunders, 1920).

degeneration, the symptoms overlap with those of Parkinson disease. Orthostatic hypotension may occur, especially in Shy–Drager syndrome.

Steele–Richardson–Olszewski syndrome is also associated with oculomotor disturbances, particularly vertical gaze palsy.

■ CT Morphology

The atrophic changes in MSA vary in their distribution (Figs. 6.**5**, 6.**6**).

The most prominent feature of OPCA is atrophy of the cerebellum and pons. The changes may be extreme, and are often strikingly disproportionate to the width of the supratentorial CSF spaces. Similar findings are noted in Shy–Drager syndrome. Supratentorial atrophy is additionally seen in striatonigral degeneration.

■ Differential Diagnosis

Normal findings on CT and MRI are virtually characteristic of Parkinson disease. At most, MRI may demonstrate altered signal intensity in the pars compacta of the substantia nigra.

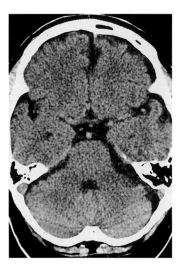

ig. 6.**5** **Isolated hemiatrophy of the left cerebellum.** While the extra-axial cerebrospinal fluid spaces show a normal width in the anterior and middle cranial fossae, the extra-axial spaces at the infratentorial level are markedly enlarged on the left side.

Huntington Disease and Wilson Disease

Frequency: rare.

Suggestive morphologic findings: CT findings are nonspecific.

Procedure: MRI is an essential adjunct to CT.

Other studies: MRI and functional imaging studies (nuclear medicine) may be more specific.

Checklist for scan interpretation:
▶ Atrophy of the basal ganglia, particularly affecting the putamen and caudate nucleus?

■ Pathogenesis

Both of these diseases primarily affect the basal ganglia, and both are clinically manifested more by motor symptoms than by dementia. Huntington disease presents with a typical choreiform motor disorder, while Wilson disease presents with dyskinesia. The CT findings are nonspecific, and rounding of the frontal horns due to caudate atrophy is occasionally observed. This feature appears to be more common in Huntington disease than in Wilson disease.

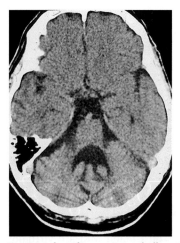

Fig. 6.**6 a, b** **Olivopontocerebellar atrophy.**
a Axial CT shows a massive infratentorial volume loss, with a slender pons and accentuated cerebellar gyri.

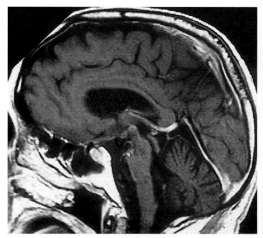

b The sagittal magnetic resonance image demonstrates loss of the rostral portions of the pons, along with cerebellar atrophy. The aqueduct is markedly enlarged due to the atrophy.

Clinical Manifestations

Huntington disease and Wilson disease should at least be mentioned among the potential causes of dementia. Both are congenital diseases with clinical manifestations including motor dysfunction and dementia. In Huntington disease, CT scans of the head are usually normal and circumscribed atrophy of the caudate nucleus and lentiform nucleus are seen only in advanced stages. In Wilson disease (hepatolenticular degeneration), an enzyme defect leads to excessive copper deposition in various body tissues. The condition may present clinically with focal neurologic signs or as a liver disease. Degenerative changes in the basal ganglia may be detected with CT.

CT Morphology

CT demonstrates marked atrophy of the basal ganglia, but the diagnosis of both diseases is the domain of MRI.

Differential Diagnosis

The differential diagnosis should include other potential causes of basal ganglia atrophy such as a prolonged hypoxic state or carbon monoxide poisoning.

Other Radiologic Findings in Dementia

Normal-Pressure Hydrocephalus

Frequency: prevalence is 30:100 000, with an approximately 2:1 preponderance of males.

Suggestive morphologic findings: predominantly intra-axial enlargement of supratentorial cerebrospinal fluid (CSF) spaces.

Procedure: trial of CSF drainage for 3–4 days, shunt insertion if required.

Other studies: functional MRI shows increased CSF flow in the aqueduct and fourth ventricle. Sagittal MRI may show volume loss in the corpus callosum.

Checklist for scan interpretation:
▶ Disproportion between ventricular dilatation and sulcal enlargement?
▶ Shape of ventricular system: ballooning of frontal horns?
▶ Pressure cones?
▶ Width of sulci in superior parietal region?

Pathogenesis

Contrary to the term "normal-pressure hydrocephalus," elevation of the CSF pressure can occur, but the pressure increase is intermittent rather than constant. Accordingly, periventricular hypodensities may be found as evidence of CSF diapedesis, though they are not always present.

Frequency

Normal-pressure hydrocephalus is not always "idiopathic," as was once believed. Some cases are secondary to subarachnoid hemorrhage, trauma, meningitis, or other causes of impaired CSF circulation.

Clinical Manifestations

The classic clinical triad consists of gait disturbance, dementia, and urinary incontinence. These symptoms justify a presumptive diagnosis of normal-pressure hydrocephalus, as the disease is one of the few treatable causes of dementia. Shunt insertion, if indicated, will be of at least some benefit. A test having both diagnostic and prognostic importance consists of draining CSF at a rate of approximately 10 mL/h for 3–4 days. If the patient's condition improves, it may be assumed that shunt insertion will be beneficial. The diagnosis of normal-pressure hydrocephalus is tentatively supported by imaging procedures (see below).

■ CT Morphology

The lateral ventricles and third ventricle may appear markedly enlarged on CT scans, while the fourth ventricle and cortical sulci are unchanged (Fig. 6.**7**).

The discrepancy between the dilated ventricles and normal sulci is often striking. Intermittent pressure peaks can cause CSF to extravasate from the ventricular system into the periventricular white matter. This causes loss of definition of the ventricular walls in that region, and decreased density of the periventricular white matter (periventricular lucencies). Patients who do not manifest sulcal enlargement in the superior parietal region are most likely to benefit from shunting.

■ Differential Diagnosis

Differentiation from hydrocephalus ex vacuo is not always easy, and functional MRI (CSF pulsation study) should be added. Flow through the aqueduct and fourth ventricle is frequently accelerated in normal-pressure hydrocephalus.

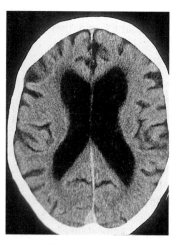

Fig. 6.7 Normal-pressure hydrocephalus. CT scan at the level of the lateral ventricles in a 58-year-old man shows a discrepancy between ventricular dilatation and sulcal enlargement. The lateral ventricles are greatly enlarged, and the ballooned frontal horns have lost their physiologic constriction. A faint white-matter hypodensity is visible anterior to the frontal horns.

Multi-Infarct Dementia

Frequency: the second most common cause of senile dementia.

Suggestive morphologic findings: bilateral infarcts.

Procedure: CT examination to exclude other treatable causes.

Other studies: MRI is more sensitive, but CT is preferred, to reduce costs.

Checklist for scan interpretation:
▶ Atrophy? Which parts of the brain are affected?
▶ Old or acute/subacute infarcts?

■ Pathogenesis

Cerebral infarcts may be causative of dementia or only an associated finding, given the frequent occurrence of both entities in the geriatric population. It is important to distinguish multi-infarct dementia from Parkinson disease. The diagnosis of multi-infarct dementia requires bilateral vascular lesions. If such lesions are absent, Parkinson disease is a more likely diagnosis.

Various forms of vascular disease may underlie multi-infarct dementia. Multiple cortical infarcts are found in typical cases, but purely lacunar infarcts and mixed patterns can also occur. Binswanger disease (subcortical atherosclerotic encephalopathy) is characterized by hypodensities in the superior white matter (centrum semiovale and corona radiata).

■ Clinical Manifestations

The vascular dementias generally affect both cortical and subcortical structures. The symptoms and history suggest a "stroke" with sudden onset, prior history of hypertension, etc. Clinical examination reveals pyramidal and extrapyramidal signs. Gait disturbance and incontinence may be present in addition to dementia.

■ CT Morphology

The CT appearance of the vascular changes is described fully in Chapter 3 (p. 61). It should be added that patients with multi-infarct syndrome exhibit bilateral, circumscribed sulcal enlargement as a result of cortical infarctions (Fig. 6.**8**).

Binswanger disease is associated with corresponding, somewhat patchy hypodensities in the white matter. Lacunar lesions are rounded, involve the gray matter in the basal ganglia region and the internal capsule, and appear as nodular hypodensities 5–15 mm in diameter.

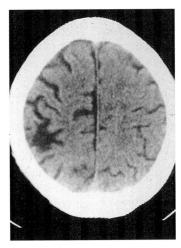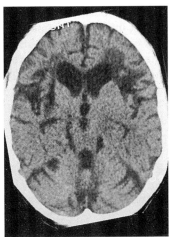

a   b

Fig. 6.**8 a, b Multi-infarct dementia.** CT shows global atrophy, accompanied by hypodensities high in the right parietal area (**a**) and in the outer basal ganglia on the right side (**b**).

Diseases of the White Matter

The following are included in the category of demyelinating diseases:

- Multiple sclerosis
- Acute disseminated encephalomyelitis (ADEM)
- Central pontine myelinolysis

Even today, these diseases are acutely evaluated by CT *before* they have been diagnosed, and it is important to offer at least a presumptive diagnosis. These *demyelinating* diseases, which involve a breakdown of healthy existing myelin, are distinguished from *dysmyelinating* diseases, based on abnormal myelin sheath formation. Dysmyelinating diseases are usually congenital, and they are no longer diagnosed by cerebral CT, owing to the superiority of MRI.

Multiple Sclerosis

Frequency: 30–80 per 100 000 in Europe, with a female predominance of 1.7 : .

Suggestive morphologic findings: a hypodense lesion with no mass effect; shows contrast enhancement in acute cases.

Procedure: CT is performed only before a diagnosis is made. If multiple sclerosis is considered in the differential diagnosis of ring-enhancing lesions with no mass effect, brain biopsy can occasionally be withheld in favor of noninvasive studies.

Other studies: MRI has become the imaging modality of choice.

Checklist for scan interpretation:
▶ When white-matter lesions are found in typical locations, a suspicion of multiple sclerosis should be raised and MRI recommended.

■ **Pathogenesis, Histology**

Multiple sclerosis is characterized by demyelination without significant axonal degeneration. It affects oligodendroglia and myelin, even in brain areas that are clinically silent. These silent brain lesions may, however, correlate with abnormalities on CT and especially on MRI. The histologic picture is characterized by macrophage activity (to remove myelin breakdown products) and perivascular inflammatory infiltrates. Complete demyelination occurs in late stages of the disease. Oligodendrocytes are absent, and perivascular inflammation is no longer apparent. On MRI, active and inactive plaques are clearly distinguished by their different signal characteristics on proton-density images (high and low signal intensity, respectively).

■ **Frequency**

Today, knowledge of the typical CT features of multiple sclerosis is mainly academic, since MRI provides a more sensitive technique for primary diagnosis and follow-up. Especially in patients with an initial diagnosis of optic neuritis, MRI of the head is performed to demonstrate typical periventricular signal changes before the initiation of cortisone therapy. It is important to be familiar with atypical imaging findings, which are seen in atypical primary manifestations with a peracute course.

■ **Clinical Manifestations**

Optic neuritis is a frequent initial presenting symptom of multiple sclerosis. The typical sensory and motor deficits correlate with a disturbance of various evoked potentials (visual, auditory, sensorimotor). Oligoclonal bands can be demonstrated in the CSF. The diagnosis is based on a scoring system for clinical findings and symptoms.

■ **CT Morphology**

CT demonstrates hypodense focal lesions, with no significant mass effect. These lesions show a predilection for the periventricular white matter and exhibit varying morphologic features (Figs. 6.**9**, 6.**10**).

It is common to find small to medium-sized nodular lesions. The individual lesions may coalesce to form various hypodense configurations, which may have somewhat indistinct scalloped margins. Contrast enhancement occurs in the acute stage.

Cases that present initially with a large ring-enhancing lesion are important in differential diagnosis. Because these cases often have atypical clinical features, it is very important to consider multiple sclerosis versus an intracranial tumor, for example.

A demyelinating disease that is distinct from multiple sclerosis and has peracute clinical features is acute disseminated encephalomyelitis (ADEM). This disease occurs in response to a previous viral infection or vaccination, and its imaging features are often similar to those of multiple sclerosis.

■ **Differential Diagnosis**

The initial differential diagnosis of nodular or ring-enhancing lesions consists of primary brain tumors and metastatic masses. With an atypical location at the gray–white matter junction, the differential diagnosis should also include infectious lesions and embolisms.

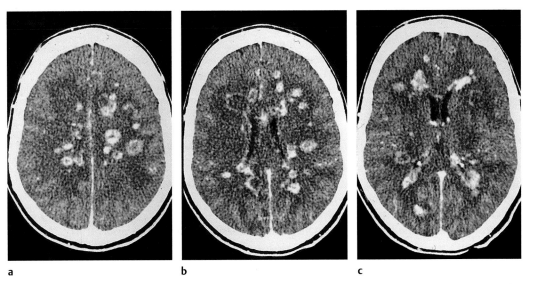

Fig. 6.**9 a–c** **Multiple sclerosis.** The typical CT appearance of multiple sclerosis after contrast administration: multiple nodular and ring-enhancing lesions in the periventricular white matter.

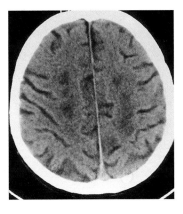

Fig. 6.**10** **End-zone infarcts,** as a differential diagnosis for Fig. 6.**9 a**. The scan shows bilateral hypodense lesions in the centrum semiovale, with the deeper layers having a normal appearance.

Central Pontine Myelinolysis

Frequency: rare.

Suggestive morphologic findings: ypodensity of the pons near the midline.

Procedure: diagnosis is based on imaging findings and typical clinical situation (alcoholic or intensive-care unit patient).

Other studies: MRI is more sensitive for defining the extent, but is not essential if CT is positive.

■ Pathogenesis

Central pontine myelinolysis is an acute demyelinating disease that occurs in typical clinical situations. It mainly affects alcoholics and patients with acid–base or electrolyte disorders. Hyponatremia, especially after rapid correction of the Na$^+$ level, is characteristic.

■ Frequency

The overall incidence is low. The history suggests the correct diagnosis.

■ Clinical Manifestations

Structures affected by demyelination include the long tracts, resulting in tetraparesis. Consciousness is impaired, perhaps partly due to the circumstances that surround the disease (see Fig. 3.**26**).

■ CT Morphology

Central pontine myelinolysis should be considered in the appropriate clinical setting when CT shows midline or near-midline hypodensity, often symmetrical and with sharp margins, located in the region of the pons.

■ Differential Diagnosis

Hypodensities of the pons are also seen in other demyelinating diseases, such as multiple sclerosis. However, the clinical situation (e.g., an intensive-care unit patient with alcohol-related disease or electrolyte imbalance) combined with a centrally located hypodense lesion in the pons will suggest the correct diagnosis.

■ References

Recommended for further study

Alzheimer disease
Erkinjuntti T, Ketonen L, Sulkava R, Vuorialho M, Palo J. CT in the differential diagnosis between Alzheimer's disease and vascular dementia. Acta Neurol Scand 1987; 75: 262–70.

Pick disease
Mendez MF, Selwood A, Mastri AR, Frey WH. Pick's disease versus Alzheimer's disease: a comparison of clinical characteristics. Neurology 1993; 43: 289–92.
Tien RD, Felsberg GJ, Ferris NJ, Osumi AK. The dementias: correlation of clinical features, pathophysiology, and neuroradiology. AJR Am J Roentgenol 1993; 161: 245–55.
● *Comprehensive review article.*

Parkinson disease
Rutledge JN, Hilal SK, Silver AJ, Defendini R, Fahn S. Study of movement disorders and brain iron by MR. AJR Am J Roentgenol 1987; 149: 365–79.
Tien RD, Felsberg GJ, Ferris NJ, Osumi AK. The dementias: correlation of clinical features, pathophysiology, and neuroradiology. AJR Am J Roentgenol 1993; 161: 245–55.

Multiple system atrophy
Gosset A, Pelissier JF, Delpeuch F, Khalil R. Striatonigral degeneration associated with olivopontocerebellar degeneration. Rev Neurol 1983; 139: 125–39.
● *Three cases with anatomic correlation.*

Huntington disease and Wilson disease
Harris GI, Pearlson GD, Peyser CE, et al. Putamen volume reduction on magnetic resonance imaging exceeds caudate changes in mild Huntington's disease. Ann Neurol 1992; 31: 69–75.
Starkstein SE, Folstein SE, Brandt J, Pearlson GD, McDonnell A, Folstein M. Brain atrophy in Huntington's disease: a CT-scan study. Neuroradiology 1989; 31: 156–9
● *Significance of the bicaudate index.*

Normal-pressure hydrocephalus
Wikkelsö C, Andersson H, Blomstrand C, Matousek M, Svendsen P. Computed tomography of the brain in the diagnosis of and prognosis in normal pressure hydrocephalus. Neuroradiology 1989; 31: 160–5.
● *Describes criteria useful in selecting patients for a ventriculoperitoneal shunt.*

Multi-infarct dementia
Erkinjuntti T, Ketonen L, Sulkava R, Vuorialho M, Palo J. CT in the differential diagnosis between Alzheimer's disease and vascular dementia. Acta Neurol Scand 1987; 75: 262–70.
Kohlmeyer K. [Problems in CT diagnosis of the aging brain; in German]. Radiologe 1989; 29: 584–91.
● *Detailed review.*

Multiple sclerosis
Nesbit GM, Forbes GS, Scheithauer BW, Okazaki H, Rodriguez M. Multiple sclerosis: histopathologic and MR and/or CT correlation in 37 cases at biopsy and three cases at autopsy. Radiology 1991; 180: 467–74.
● *The authors correlate histologic findings with CT and MR images in a significant number of patients; good presentation of basic principles.*

Central pontine myelinolysis
Adams RD, Victor M, Mancall EL. Central pontine myelinolysis. Arch Neurol Psychiatry 1959; 81: 38–56
● *First description.*

Recent and basic works

Alzheimer disease
Early B, Escalona PR, Boyko OB, et al. Interuncal distance measurements in healthy volunteers and in patients with Alzheimer disease. AJNR Am J Neuroradiol 1993; 14: 907–10.
George AE, de Leon MJ, Stylopoulos LA, et al. CT diagnostic features of Alzheimer disease: importance of the choroidal/hippocampal fissure complex. AJNR Am J Neuroradiol 1990; 11: 101–7.
Kido DK, Caine ED, LeMay M, et al. Temporal lobe atrophy in patients with Alzheimer disease: a CT study. AJNR Am J Neuroradiol 1989; 10: 551–5.
● *Also deals with quantitative aspects.*
de Leon MJ, George AE, Reisberg B, et al. Alzheimer's disease: longitudinal CT studies of ventricular change. AJR Am J Roentgenol 1989; 152: 1257–62.

Pick disease
Jakob H. [Clinical-anatomical aspects of "pure" temporal lobe seizures in Pick disease and the basal neocortex; in German]. Dtsch Z Nervenheilkd 1969; 196: 20–39.

Paris BE. The utility of CT scanning in diagnosing dementia. Mt Sinai J Med 1997; 64: 372–5.

Parkinson disease
Chida K, Goto N, Kamikura I, Takasu T. Quantitative evaluation of pontine atrophy using computer tomography. Neuroradiology 1989; 31: 13–5.
Chida K, Tamura M, Kamikura I, Takasu T. A quantitative evaluation of pontine volume by computed tomography in patients with cerebellar degeneration. Neurology 1990; 40: 1241–5.
Savoiardo M, Bracchi M, Passerini A, et al. Computed tomography of olivopontocerebellar degeneration. AJNR Am J Neuroradiol 1983; 4: 509–12.
  ● *Deals with the differential diagnosis of posterior fossa atrophy.*
Savoiardo M, Strada L, Girotti F, et al. Olivopontocerebellar atrophy: MR diagnosis and relationship to multisystem atrophy. Radiology 1990; 174: 693–6.
Wessel K, Huss GP, Bruckmann H, Kompf D. Follow-up of neurophysiological tests and CT in late-onset cerebellar ataxia and multiple system atrophy. J Neurol 1993; 240: 168–76.

Huntington disease and Wilson disease
Williams FJ, Walshe JM. Wilson's disease: an analysis of the cranial computerized tomographic appearances found in 60 patients and the changes in response to treatment with chelating agents. Brain 1981; 104: 735–52.
  ● *Reviews CT signs in a relatively large group of patients.*

Normal-pressure hydrocephalus
Huckman MS. Normal pressure hydrocephalus: evaluation of diagnostic and prognostic tests. AJNR Am J Neuroradiol 1981; 2: 385–95.

Multi-infarct dementia
Gorelick PB, Chatterjee A, Patel D, et al. Cranial computed tomographic observations in multi-infarct dementia: a controlled study. Stroke 1992; 23: 804–11.

Multiple sclerosis
Giang DW, Poduri KR, Eskin TA, et al. Multiple sclerosis masquerading as a mass lesion. Neuroradiology 1992; 34: 150–4.
  ● *Findings on this important pitfall in six patients.*
Mushlin AI, Detsky AS, Phelps CE, et al. The accuracy of magnetic resonance imaging in patients with suspected multiple sclerosis. JAMA J Am Med Assoc 1993; 269: 3146–51.
  ● *Sophisticated method of comparing CT and MRI (receiver operating characteristics curves).*
Plant GT, Kermode AG, Turano G, et al. Symptomatic retrochiasmal lesions in multiple sclerosis: clinical features, visual evoked potentials, and magnetic resonance imaging. Neurology 1992; 42: 68–76.
Thomas KG, Griffiths GJ. Case report: the vanishing ring sign—an unusual CT manifestation of multiple sclerosis. Clin Radiol 1992; 46: 213–5.

Central pontine myelinolysis
Koci TM, Chiang F, Chow P, et al. Thalamic extrapontine lesions in central pontine myelinolysis. AJNR Am J Neuroradiol 1990; 11: 1229–33.
Miller GM, Baker HL, Okazaki H, Whisnant JP: Central pontine myelinolysis and its imitators: MR findings. Radiology 1988; 168: 795–892.
  ● *Contains little on practical clinical CT, but generally informative.*

7 Congenital Brain Diseases

Phacomatoses

Neurofibromatosis (Figs. 7.1, 7.2)

Neurofibromatosis Type 1

Frequency: a common phacomatosis (with a prevalence of one in 3000 in Central Europe).

Suggestive morphologic findings: café-au-lait pigmentation, sphenoid wing dysplasia, gliomas (especially optic glioma), and neurofibromas.

Procedure: postcontrast examination is essential.

Other studies: magnetic resonance imaging (MRI) is the imaging modality of choice.

Checklist for scan interpretation:
▶ Multiple meningiomas?
▶ Acoustic schwannoma?
▶ Glioma?

■ Pathogenesis

Neurofibromatosis is a phacomatosis (neurocutaneous syndrome) with an autosomal-dominant mode of inheritance and approximately 100% penetrance. The mutated gene is located on chromosome 17, and the spontaneous mutation rate is high (approximately 50% of new somatic mutations).

■ Frequency

Neurofibromatosis type 1, formerly known as von Recklinghausen disease, is the most common phacomatosis.

■ Clinical Manifestations

A distinction is drawn between overt and abortive forms of the disease. The overt forms can be diagnosed from the presence of café-au-lait spots or neurofibromas. Optic nerve glioma is often the initial manifestation of the less overt forms.

■ CT Morphology

Computed tomography (CT) often demonstrates marked sphenoid wing dysplasia, which tends to be unilateral and can extend to complete absence of the bone. Optic glioma appears as a thickening of the optic nerve that extends into the optic chiasm. Intraorbital neurofibromas are common and can assume various forms. A series of masses several millimeters in diameter arranged in a string-of-beads pattern is a very characteristic finding. The frequent extracoronal location is clearly demonstrated by MRI and by special CT views.

■ Differential Diagnosis

Differentiation from neurofibromatosis type 2 is straightforward, owing to the distinctive character of the tumors. Craniosynostosis is another common setting in which sphenoid wing dysplasia may occur. Optic neuritis is often considered initially in patients with an isolated optic nerve glioma, but persistence or rapid enlargement of the lesion should raise suspicion of a glioma. Involvement of the optic chiasm further supports the diagnosis of optic glioma rather than neuritis. Sarcoidosis is a

a, c

b, d

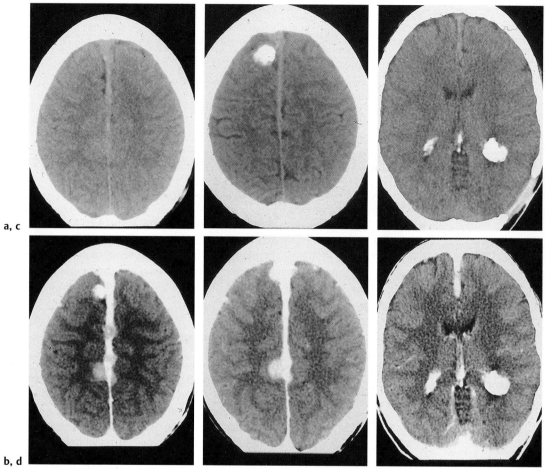

Fig. 7.**1 a–f Neurofibromatosis.** Neurofibromatosis can have a variety of imaging appearances. These scans are from a woman with multiple falx meningiomas (**a, c, e** precontrast; **b, d, f** postcontrast).

a, c Noncontrast CT shows calcification of the lesions.

b, d Postcontrast CT shows multiple enhancing tumors on the thickened falx.

e, f Large calcified tumors are visible in the occipital horns of both lateral ventricles. Even here, meningiomas and physiologic plexus calcification cannot be excluded as the cause.

potential source of confusion, but is very rare. With intraorbital neurofibromas, it is often necessary to consider numerous diagnostic possibilities. Multiple tumors in the same patient can show varying enhancement characteristics after contrast administration. Lesions at certain sites can even mimic cavernomas.

Fig. 7.**2** **Pontine glioma.** Pontine glioma also occurs in the setting of neurofibromatosis. Noncontrast CT shows extensive hypodensity of the brain stem on the left side. Significant enhancement does not occur on the postcontrast scan.
a Before contrast administration.
b fter contrast administration.

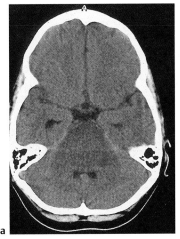
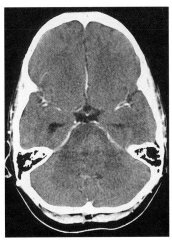

a
b

Neurofibromatosis Type 2

Frequency: less common than neurofibromatosis type 1.

Suggestive morphologic findings: bilateral acoustic schwannomas; may coexist with meningioma.

Procedure: obtain thin-slice bone-window CT scans to define the internal auditory canal.

Other studies: typical acoustic schwannomas are visible on CT only when a large extrameatal component is present.

Checklist for scan interpretation:
▶ Expansion of the internal auditory canal?
▶ Intrameatal contrast enhancement?

■ Pathogenesis

Neurofibromatosis type 2 has been recognized as a separate phacomatosis. The tumors in this disease arise from Schwann cells and from the meninges. Cutaneous neurofibromas are not observed. Neurofibromatosis type 2 results from a mutation on chromosome 22.

■ Frequency

The disease is less common than neurofibromatosis type 1, with an estimated incidence of approximately one in 50,000 births.

■ Clinical Manifestations

The characteristic acoustic schwannomas and meningiomas may be manifested at any age, but the third decade is typical. The symptoms are the same as those associated with acoustic schwannomas and meningiomas that occur outside the setting of neurofibromatosis.

■ CT Morphology

With acoustic schwannoma, expansion of the internal auditory canal on bone-window CT may signify an intrameatal acoustic schwannoma. Since the detection of this enlargement is often based on a side-to-side comparison, the bilateral acoustic schwannomas in neurofibromatosis type 2 can be misleading. Enlargement to more than 8 mm is very suspicious for an intrameatal tumor, and should be investigated by MRI. Large extrameatal tumors are visible as enhancing masses in the cerebellopontine angle. As expected, meningiomas are hyperdense on noncontrast CT, are broadly based on the calvarium, and enhance intensely after contrast administration.

■ Differential Diagnosis

Bilateral acoustic schwannomas, even when accompanied by meningiomas, establish the diagnosis of neurofibromatosis type 2.

Von Hippel–Lindau Syndrome

Frequency: rare (the prevalence is approximately one in 40 000).

Suggestive morphologic findings: hemangioblastoma combined with retinal hemangioma.

Procedure: surgical removal of the intracranial tumor.

Other studies: angiography and MRI are more sensitive than CT for detecting mural nodules.

Checklist for scan interpretation:
▶ One or more cystic masses with an enhancing nidus?

■ Pathogenesis

The von Hippel–Lindau syndrome is thought to have an autosomal-dominant mode of transmission, with incomplete penetrance. The genetic anomaly has recently been identified, and appears to involve a defective tumor-suppressor gene on chromosome 3.

■ Frequency

Rare (the prevalence is approximately one in 40,000).

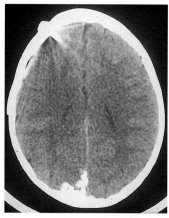

Fig. 7.3 Sturge–Weber syndrome. Sturge–Weber syndrome is characterized by angiomatosis of the cerebral surface. The diagnosis is suggested by corkscrew-like calcifications that follow the cerebral convolutions. This CT scan shows a corkscrew-like calcification on the surface of the right occipital lobe. The disease had been present for some time, prompting the insertion of a ventricular drain.

■ Clinical Manifestations

The two most common tumor entities that are observed in von Hippel–Lindau syndrome differ in their times of appearance: retinal hamartomas occur before puberty, while hemangioblastomas develop after puberty. Hemangioblastomas of the cerebellum lead to gait disturbance or the characteristic features of hydrocephalus. Retinal hamartomas often prompt referral for ophthalmologic examination.

■ CT Morphology

Retinal hamartomas are too small to be detected on CT scans. Hemangioblastomas appear as cystic masses with mural tumor nodules that enhance strongly after contrast administration.

■ Differential Diagnosis

Cystic posterior fossa masses in von Hippel–Lindau syndrome are sometimes difficult to distinguish from pilocytic astrocytomas or cystic metastases from carcinoma.

Sturge–Weber Syndrome (Fig. 7.3)

Frequency: rare.

Suggestive morphologic findings: xtensive vascular malformation projected in the subarachnoid space, appearing either as an enhancing mass or as calcification; tram-track pattern of calcifications.

Procedure: it is occasionally necessary to resect brain areas underlying angiomatous lesions.

Other studies: MRI demonstrates the effects on cerebral tissue.

Checklist for scan interpretation:
▶ Tram-track calcifications?
▶ Hemiatrophy?

■ Pathogenesis

Sturge–Weber syndrome, also known as encephalotrigeminal angiomatosis, is a congenital disease characterized by the development of superficial vascular malformations involving the face and brain.

The histologic features consist of angiomatous changes in the meninges, usually the pia mater. Both arterial and venous malformations can occur. Similar lesions are found in the face. The pathogenesis is not fully established, but presumably involves persistence of primordial vascular structures. Calcifications bordering the vascular malformations develop within the brain substance. Concomitant hemiatrophy of the affected hemisphere is often present.

■ Frequency

Rare.

■ Clinical Manifestations

The severity of symptoms correlates roughly with the extent of the vascular malformations on the brain surface. Consequently, the CT and MRI findings are useful in making a prognosis. Seizures are an early feature of Sturge–Weber syndrome. With passage of time, focal neurologic symptoms appear. Most patients show some form of developmental delay.

■ CT Morphology

Noncontrast CT may demonstrate gyral calcifications that follow the cortical band. The characteristic vascular malformations are located in the meninges, which follow the sulci. These lesions enhance intensely with intravenous contrast, creating a gyriform pattern of enhancement. The changes may be more or less extensive and may affect one or both hemispheres. Choroidal angiomas have been described, but generally are not detectable by CT. Vascular malformations in extracranial organs are not characteristic.

■ Differential Diagnosis

Facial angioma (port-wine stain) and other extracerebral changes, along with the age of the patient, should minimize problems of differential diagnosis. Posttraumatic calcifications, calcifications secondary to inflammatory disease, etc., may perhaps be considered.

Tuberous Sclerosis (Fig. 7.4)

Frequency: rare.

Suggestive morphologic findings: subependymal nodules, cortical tubers.

Procedure: MRI is required.

Other studies: MRI is more sensitive than CT for detecting cortical tubers.

Checklist for scan interpretation:
▸ Evidence of tuberous sclerosis?

■ Pathogenesis

Tuberous sclerosis is an inherited disease, but its mode of transmission is uncertain. An autosomal-dominant inheritance with low penetrance is assumed.

■ Frequency

Tuberous sclerosis is a rare phacomatosis. Its prevalence in Central Europe is estimated at one in 50,000.

■ Clinical Manifestations

The following triad characterizes the fully developed clinical picture of tuberous sclerosis:

- Adenoma sebaceum
- Seizures
- Developmental delay

The characteristic adenoma sebaceum consists of a papular facial rash involving the cheeks and the angle between the nose and lower eyelids.

■ CT Morphology

The spectrum of findings in tuberous sclerosis includes retinal hamartomas, which rarely are visible on CT as small calcifications. A more

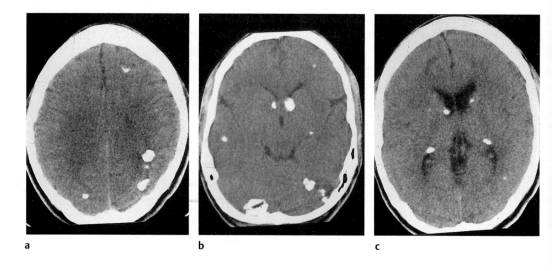

a   b   c

Fig. 7.**4 a–c Tuberous sclerosis.** Tuberous sclerosis is characterized by the presence of subependymal tumors and cortical tubers. The subependymal tumors are particularly apt to calcify. In the example shown, multiple calcified lesions are seen in the ventricular walls and cor- tical region. CT is excellent for detecting these calcific foci, but magnetic resonance imaging is preferred for showing contrast enhancement of the ventricular wall tumors, which may signify malignant transformation.

prominent feature is the characteristic subependymal tumors, which may consist of hamartomas or giant-cell astrocytomas. Other findings consist of cortical hamartomas (tubers) and white-matter lesions. Both the tubers and white-matter lesions are hypodense on noncontrast CT, although the tubers may calcify, and in very rare cases may enhance with contrast. The various tumors are differentiated by their location. The tubers are located in the cerebral cortex, and the other lesions occur in the white matter.

Subependymal hamartomas appear as nodular tumors in the ventricular wall. Their appearance changes with aging, and calcifications are increasingly observed. Contrast enhancement occurs in some cases.

Subependymal giant-cell astrocytomas are typically located near the foramen of Monro. These tumors produce a mass effect leading to hydrocephalus. The histologic features vary, and hamartomas are found in addition to actual tumors.

■ Differential Diagnosis

Nodular structures in the ventricular wall are occasionally found in heterotopias, which are fairly common in patients with tuberous sclerosis. Heterotopic nodules are isodense to the cortex, however, in accordance with their pathogenesis. Enhancing nodules are also found in rare cases of tuberculosis. Cortical tubers are more difficult to detect with CT, and other causes of cortical hypodensities (e.g., vascular lesions) should be considered in cases where the diagnosis of tuberous sclerosis has not yet been established.

Dandy–Walker Malformation (Fig. 7.5)

■ **Frequency:** rare.

Suggestive morphologic findings: absent or incomplete cerebellar vermis and cystic dilatation of the fourth ventricle.

Procedure: generally, treatment is not required.

Other studies: Dandy–Walker malformation requires differentiation from arachnoid cysts and large cerebellomedullary cistern. Borderline cases can be resolved by cerebrospinal fluid (CSF) pulsation study (MRI) or CT after intrathecal contrast administration.

Checklist for scan interpretation:
▶ Differentiation from large cerebellomedullary cistern.

■ **Pathogenesis**

Dandy–Walker malformation is based on a developmental anomaly that involves membranous occlusion of the fourth ventricle.

■ **Frequency**

Rare.

■ **Clinical Manifestations**

Besides hydrocephalus, the clinical picture is marked by associated anomalies:

● Spina bifida
● Syringomyelia
● Coloboma
● Cardiovascular anomalies

The principal neurologic symptoms are as follows:

● Ataxia
● Spasticity
● Decreased motor control
● Seizures

■ **CT Morphology**

Axial scans through the posterior fossa in Dandy–Walker malformation show an incomplete or absent cerebellar vermis and massive enlargement of the CSF spaces. The fourth ventricle communicates directly with the subarachnoid spaces. The posterior fossa is usually enlarged, and the tentorium is displaced upward. Associated intracerebral (callosal dysplasia) and extracranial anomalies (cardiac defects, etc.) may be found. Hydrocephalus is usually present.

Fig. 7.**5 a, b Dandy–Walker malformation.** A characteristic feature of this syndrome is an apparent splaying of the cerebellar hemispheres caused by congenital absence of the vermis.

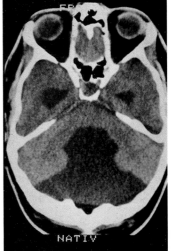

a
b

■ Differential Diagnosis

Dandy–Walker malformation can usually be readily distinguished from even a very large cerebellomedullary cistern. Infratentorial arachnoid cysts can mimic Dandy–Walker, but are distinguishable by their mass effect on surrounding structures, particularly their spherical impression on adjacent cerebellum and infratentorial ballooning of the calvarium with thinning of the bone. This calvarial change is also seen with arachnoid cysts at other locations.

Arachnoid Cysts (Fig. 7.6)

Frequency: a common CT finding.

Suggestive morphologic findings: an extra-axial mass of fluid density located between the inner table and brain surface, causing displacement of the brain structures and ballooning of the calvarium.

Procedure: generally, treatment is not required.

Other studies: CSF pulsation study (MRI) or CT with intrathecal contrast can confirm communication with the subarachnoid space.

■ Pathogenesis

Arachnoid cysts are cystic, fluid-filled dilatations of the arachnoid membrane. They may or may not communicate with the subarachnoid spaces.

■ Frequency

Arachnoid cysts are common findings, and are usually detected incidentally.

■ Clinical Manifestations

Arachnoid cysts are often discovered incidentally during sectional imaging investigation of nonspecific symptoms such as headache. Arachnoid cysts usually become clinically symptomatic due to impairment of CSF circulation.

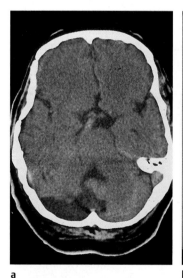 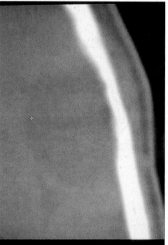 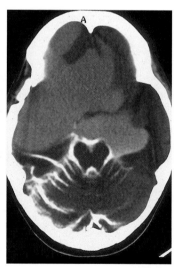

a   b   c

Fig. 7.6 a–c Arachnoid cyst.

a This arachnoid cyst of the right posterior cerebellar hemisphere is distinguishable from a large cerebellomedullary cistern by its eccentric location.

b Another common feature is local thinning of the calvarium in the bone-window scan.

c After intrathecal contrast administration, enhancement of the infratentorial cerebrospinal fluid spaces is observed. A broad communication with the basal portion of a large left-hemispheric arachnoid cyst is not definitely apparent, and the faint enhancement within the cyst may result from contrast permeation.

CT Morphology

Arachnoid cysts appear as extra-axial fluid-filled spaces located between the calvarium and brain surface. They can appear as discrete cystic masses, or as simple expansions of the arachnoid space. Communication with the subarachnoid space cannot be established on noncontrast CT scans. In rare cases, MRI flow studies of the CSF may demonstrate a jet or simultaneous pulsations. Delayed CT imaging after intrathecal contrast administration is still the most reliable study. If a communication exists, contrast medium will appear within the cyst.

A distinctive feature of arachnoid cysts is their tendency to produce some degree of mass effect. This may consist of a rounded indentation of adjacent brain structures. Ballooning and thinning of the adjacent calvarium may also occur.

Differential Diagnosis

The differential diagnosis may include various lesions, depending on the location. Middle-fossa arachnoid cysts are common and require differentiation from temporal lobe dysplasia. Arachnoid cysts in the posterior fossa may resemble Dandy–Walker malformation.

Corpus Callosum Dysplasia (Figs. 7.7, 7.8)

Frequency: not uncommon.

Suggestive morphologic findings: axial scans show ballooning of the occipital horns, parallel nonconverging lateral ventricles, and upward extension of the third ventricle.

Procedure: no treatment.

Other studies: the anomaly is well defined by sagittal MRI.

Checklist for scan interpretation:
▶ Other associated anomalies?

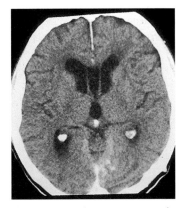

Fig. 7.**7** **Corpus callosum anomaly: Verga's ventricle.** The septum pellucidum in this CT slice appears as two separate layers between the frontal horns; the cavity between them is known as Verga's ventricle (cavum vergae). This differs from a septum pellucidum cyst, which does not extend the full length of the frontal horns. The term "cavum veli interpositi" refers to a cyst located posterior and inferior to the corpus callosum.

Pathogenesis

Dysplasia or dysgenesis of the corpus callosum can result from various disturbances occurring between 8 and 20 weeks of gestation. Different portions of the corpus callosum, normally composed of a rostrum, genu, body, and splenium, may be affected. Callosal dysgenesis is frequently associated with another malformation, corpus callosum lipoma. Associated central nervous system (CNS) anomalies may also occur.

CT Morphology

While sagittal MRI affords a direct view of the normal corpus callosum, dysplasia or aplasia of the corpus callosum is usually manifested on axial CT by secondary changes in the ventricular system. Scans generally show a larger-than-normal, high-riding third ventricle, ballooning of the occipital horns of the lateral ventricles,

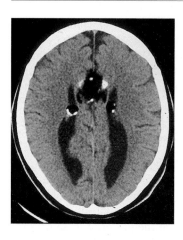

and narrow frontal horns that are parallel to the midline.

■ Differential Diagnosis

Generally, the findings are characteristic.

◁ Fig. 7.**8** **Corpus callosum lipoma.** Corpus callosum lipomas are frequently accompanied by other callosal anomalies, as shown here. The scan demonstrates a midline lipomatous mass bordered by cap-like calcifications on the lateral and occipital sides. The posterior portion of the corpus callosum is also hypoplastic, as indicated by the enlarged and elongated occipital horns.

Chiari Malformation (Fig. 7.9)

Frequency: not uncommon (approximately one in 25 000).

Suggestive morphologic findings: downward extension of the cerebellar tonsils, with or without lumbar myelomeningocele.

Procedure: correction of lumbar myelomeningocele; cranial anomalies are often left untreated.

Other studies: sagittal MRI clearly displays the features of the malformation.

Checklist for scan interpretation:
▶ Low-lying tonsils?
▶ Hydrocephalus?
▶ Other anomalies?

■ Pathogenesis

The following types of Chiari malformation can occur:

- *Chiari I malformation:* the main feature of the Chiari I malformation is inferior extension of the cerebellar tonsils. This may be accompanied by hydrocephalus and a narrow fourth ventricle.
- *Chiari II malformation:* this type is additionally characterized by kinking and inferior extension of the medulla oblongata. It is

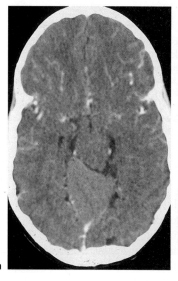

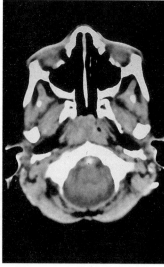

Fig. 7.**9 a, b** **Chiari malformation.** Inferior extension of the cerebellar tonsils is a feature common to all three types of Chiari malformation. The low-lying tonsils are directly visualized in sagittal or parasagittal images. The axial scans illustrate the appearance of the malformation at two different levels in the transverse plane.
a A scan at a higher level shows the typical "mass" located posterior to the brain stem.
b scan at the level of the foramen magnum shows the low-lying cerebellar tonsils on both sides of the medulla oblongata.

a

b

usually associated with lumbar myelo-meningocele.

- *Chiari III malformation:* this type consists of the features of Chiari II malformation (low-lying tonsils, lumbar myelomeningocele) combined with an encephalocele.

Frequency

Mild forms of Chiari malformation, characterized only by low-lying tonsils, are frequently encountered.

Clinical Manifestations

The clinical features are determined by the extent of the accompanying anomalies. The dominant features are usually due to spinal cord anomalies such as syringomyelia, or an associated tethered-cord syndrome.

CT Morphology

The low-lying cerebellar tonsils appear on axial CT scans as two rounded structures that flank the spinal cord within the foramen magnum.

Lumbar myelomeningocele, which is a feature of Chiari II malformation, appears as a protrusion of the spinal cord—a cystic expansion located dorsal to the spinal canal at the level of the lumbosacral junction. This anomaly is associated with dysplasia of local osseous structures. A tethered-cord syndrome is manifested by a low position of the cauda equina with tethering of the cord at the level of the myelomeningocele. Intrathecal contrast administration is usually necessary for CT visualization, but these features are more easily demonstrated by MRI, which is generally preferred. An intraspinal lipoma appears on CT as a mass of negative attenuation located in the dorsal part of the spinal canal.

Differential Diagnosis

Chiari I malformation is still detected incidentally in CT examinations. The diagnosis is established by sagittal MRI. The diagnosis of a Chiari I malformation by MRI or sagittal-reformatted CT requires that the cerebellar tonsils extend below a line connecting the hard palate with the caudal or anterior end of the occipital squama.

References

Recommended for further study

Neurofibromatosis type 1 and 2

Bilaniuk LT, Molloy PT, Zimmermann RA, et al. Neurofibromatosis type 1: brain stem tumors. Neuroradiology 1997; 39: 642–53.
- *Description of findings in 25 patients.*

Chen MC, Liu HM, Huang KM. Agenesis of the internal carotid artery associated with neurofibromatosis type II. AJNR Am J Neuroradiol 1994; 15: 1184–6.
- *Description of one case.*

Fukuta K, Jackson IT. Orbital neurofibromatosis with enophthalmos. Br J Plast Surg 1993; 46: 36–8.
- *Description of two cases, with an analysis of three-dimensional CT findings.*

Higgins JN, Valentine AR, Bradford R. CT-directed perineural infiltration in the localization of radicular pain in a patient with neurofibromatosis. Br J Neurosurg 1995; 9: 73–5.
- *Symptomatic CT-guided therapy.*

Jacoby CG, Go RT, Beren RA. Cranial CT of neurofibromatosis. AJR Am J Roentgenol 1980; 135: 553–7.
- *Early description of the spectrum of imaging features.*

Leisti EL, Pyhtinen J, Poyhonen M. Spontaneous decrease of a pilocytic astrocytoma in neurofibromatosis type 1. AJNR Am J Neuroradiol 1996; 17: 1691–4.
- *Describes one patient who was followed for 12 years.*

Lovblad KO, Remonda L, Ozdoba C, Huber P, Schroth G. Dural ectasia of the optic nerve sheath in neurofibromatosis type 1: CT and MR features. J Comput Assist Tomogr 1994; 18: 728–30.
- *Important differential diagnosis for optic glioma in patients with neurofibromatosis.*

Mayer JS, Kulkarni MV, Yeakley JW. Craniocervical manifestations of neurofibromatosis: MR versus CT studies. J Comput Assist Tomogr 1987; 11: 839–44.
- *Comparison of CT and MRI in three patients.*

Massry GG, Morgan CF, Chung SM. Evidence of optic pathway gliomas after previously negative neuroimaging. Ophthalmology 1997; 104: 930–5.
- *Two of 360 patients developed an optic glioma over a seven-year course.*

Mayfrank L, Mohadjer M, Wullich B. Intracranial calcified deposits in neurofibromatosis type 2: a CT study of 11 cases. Neuroradiology 1990; 32: 33–7.
- *Description of various nontumoral calcifications in the choroid plexus, cerebellum, and hemispheres.*

Molenkamp G, Riemann B, Kuwert T, et al. Monitoring tumor activity in low-grade glioma of childhood. Klin Pädiatr 1998; 210: 239–42.
- *Compares nuclear medicine and sectional imaging studies.*

Tien RD, Osumi A, Oakes JW, Madden JF, Burger PC. Meningioangiomatosis: CT and MR findings. J Comput Assist Tomogr 1992; 16: 361–5.

- *Description of two patients with this rare condition, which may be associated with neurofibromatosis.*

Tonsgard JH, Kwak SM, Short MP, Dachman AH. CT imaging in adults with neurofibromatosis 1: frequent asymptomatic plexiform lesions. Neurology 1998; 50: 1755–60.
- *Studied in 91 atients.*

Hippel–Lindau syndrome

Spetzger U, Bertalanffy H, Huffmann B, Mayfrank L, Reul J, Gilsbach JM. Hemangioblastomas of the spinal cord and the brain stem: diagnostic and therapeutic features. Neurosurg Rev 1996; 19: 147–51.
- *Neurosurgical study dealing mainly with spinal manifestations.*

Wilms G, Raaijmakers C, Goffin J, Plets C. MR features of intracranial hemangioblastomas. J Belge Radiol 1992; 75: 469–75.
- *Comparison of CT and MRI in 10 patients.*

Sturge–Weber syndrome

Gardeur D, Palmieri A, Mashaly R. Cranial computed tomography in the phakomatoses. Neuroradiology 1983; 25: 293–304.
- *Early review work in a large population.*

Henkes H, Bittner R, Huber G, et al. [Sturge–Weber syndrome: diagnostic imaging relative to neuropathology; in German.] Radiologe 1991; 31: 289–96.
- *Review article.*

Tuberous sclerosis

Inoue Y, Nemoto Y, Murata R, et al. CT and MR imaging of cerebral tuberous sclerosis. Brain Dev 1998; 20: 209–21.
- *Review.*

Dandy–Walker malformation

Byrd SE, Radkowski MA, Flannery A, McLone DG. The clinical and radiological evaluation of absence of the corpus callosum. Eur J Radiol 1990; 10: 65–73.
- *Symptoms in 83 of 105 children, with associated imaging abnormalities for most cases.*

Curnes JT, Laster DW, Koubek TD, Moody DM, Ball MR, Witcofski RL. MRI of corpus callosal syndromes. AJNR Am J Neuroradiol 1986; 7: 617–22.

Golden JA, Rorke LB, Bruce DA. Dandy–Walker syndrome and associated anomalies. Pediatr Neurosci 1987; 13: 38–44.

Groenhout CM, Gooskens RH, Veiga-Pires JA, et al. Value of sagittal sonography and direct sagittal CT of the Dandy–Walker syndrome. AJNR Am J Neuroradiol 1984; 5: 476–7.

Koyama T, Okudera H, Tada T, Wada N, Kobayashi S. Periventricular enhancement following intraoperative CT cisternography in a patient with Dandy–Walker syndrome: case report. Neurosurg Rev 1997; 20: 288–90.

Utsunomiya H, Takano K, Ogasawara T, Hashimoto T, Fukushima T, Okazaki M. Rhombencephalosynapsis: cerebellar embryogenesis. AJNR Am J Neuroradiol 1998; 19: 547–9.
- *Deals with issues of differential diagnosis.*

Arachnoid cyst

Awada A, Scherman B, Palkar V. Cystic meningiomas: a diagnostic and pathogenic challenge. Eur J Radiol 1997; 25: 26–9.
- *Unusual differential diagnosis: meningioma with a localized CSF collection.*

Briellmann RS, Jackson GD, Torn-Broers Y, Berkovic SF. Twins with different temporal lobe malformations: schizencephaly and arachnoid cyst. Neuropediatrics 1998; 29: 284–8.
- *Schizencephaly as an added differential diagnosis.*

Britz GW, Kim DK, Mayberg MR. Traumatic leptomeningeal cyst in an adult: a case report and review of the literature. Surg Neurol 1998; 50: 465–9.
- *Another differential diagnosis.*

Cheung SW, Broberg TG, Jackler RK. Petrous apex arachnoid cyst: radiographic confusion with primary cholesteatoma. Am J Otol 1995; 16: 690–4.
- *Deals with the differential diagnosis of cholesteatoma.*

Eustace S, Toland J, Stack J. CT and MRI of arachnoid cyst with complicating intracystic and subdural hemorrhage. J Comput Assist Tomogr 1992; 16: 995–7
- *Describes a rare complication.*

Ide C, De Coene B, Gilliard C, et al. Hemorrhagic arachnoid cyst with third nerve paresis: CT and MR findings. AJNR Am J Neuroradiol 1997; 18: 1407–10.
- *Describes a rare complication; similar to Pelletier et al.*

Koch CA, Moore JL, Voth D. Arachnoid cysts: how do postsurgical cyst size and seizure outcome correlate? Neurosurg Rev 1998; 21: 14–22.
- *Deals with treatment.*

Koga H, Mukawa J, Miyagi K, Kinjo T, Okuyama K. Symptomatic intraventricular arachnoid cyst in an elderly man. Acta Neurochir 1995; 137: 113–7.
- *Differential diagnosis of a rare location.*

Pelletier J, Milandre L, Peragut JC, Cronqvist S. Intraventricular choroid plexus "arachnoid" cyst: MRI findings. Neuroradiology 1990; 12: 523–5.

von Wild K. Arachnoid cysts of the middle cranial fossa. Neurochirurgia 1992; 35: 177–82.
- *Diagnosis and treatment in 18 patients.*

Corpus callosum dysplasia

Oba H, Barkovich AJ. Holoprosencephaly: an analysis of callosal formation and its relation to development of the interhemispheric fissure. AJNR Am J Neuroradiol 1995; 16: 453–60.
- *Fundamental work in 17 patients.*

Palmeri S, Battisti C, Federico A, Guazzi GC. Hypoplasia of the corpus callosum in Niemann–Pick type disease. Neuroradiology 1994; 36: 20–2.
- *Describes two patients with this rare abnormality.*

Recent and basic works

Neurofibromatosis type 1 and 2

Menor F, Marti-Bonmati L, Mulas F, Cortina H, Olague R. Imaging considerations of central nervous system manifestations in pediatric patients with neurofibromatosis type 1. Pediatr Radiol 1991; 21: 389–94.
- *Prospective comparison in 41 children, covering the spectrum of cerebral pathology.*

North KN. Neurofibromatosis 1 in childhood. Semin Pediatr Neurol 1998; 5: 231–42.
- *Review that is not oriented toward imaging.*

Zanella FE, Mödder U, Benz-Bohm G, Thun F. [Neurofibromatosis in childhood: computed tomographic findings in the skull and neck areas; in German]. RöFo Fortschr Geb Röntgenstr Nuklearmed 1984; 141: 498–504.
- *Introduction.*

Hippel–Lindau syndrome

Elster AD, Arthur DW. Intracranial hemangioblastomas: CT and MR findings. J Comput Assist Tomogr 1988; 12: 736–9.
- *Hemangioblastoma in eight patients, three of whom had Hippel–Lindau syndrome.*

Nelson DR, Yuh WT, Waziri MH, et al. MR imaging of Hippel–Lindau disease: value of gadopentetate dimeglumine. J Magn Reson Imaging 1991; 1: 469–76.
- *Comprehensive study comparing MRI and CT in seven patients.*

Otsuka F, Ogura T, Nakagawa M, et al. Normotensive bilateral pheochromocytoma with Lindau disease: case report. Endocr J 1996; 43: 719–23.
- *Informative report on a case with a familial incidence.*

Sturge–Weber syndrome

Chamberlain MC, Press GA, Hesselink JR. MR imaging and CT in three cases of Sturge–Weber syndrome: prospective comparison. AJNR Am J Neuroradiol 1989; 10: 491–6.
- *Comparison of CT and MRI in three patients.*

Griffiths PD, Boodram MB, Blaser S, et al. Abnormal ocular enhancement in Sturge–Weber syndrome: correlation of ocular MR and CT findings with clinical and intracranial imaging findings. AJNR Am J Neuroradiol 1996; 17: 749–54.
- *Ocular contrast enhancement in 15 atients with Sturge–Weber syndrome.*

Marti-Bonmati L, Menor F, Mulas F. The Sturge–Weber syndrome: correlation between the clinical status and radiological CT and MRI findings. Child's Nerv Syst 1993; 9: 107–9.
- *Comparison in 14 patients.*

Stimac GK, Solomon MA, Newton TH. CT and MR of angiomatous malformations of the choroid plexus in patients with Sturge–Weber disease. AJNR Am J Neuroradiol 1986; 7: 623–7.
- *Describes the observation of an additional Sturge–Weber feature.*

Wagner EJ, Rao KC, Knipp HC. CT–angiographic correlation in Sturge–Weber syndrome. J Comput Tomogr 1981; 5: 324–7.
- *Compares CT and angiography in one case.*

Yeakley JW, Woodside M, Fenstermacher MJ. Bilateral neonatal Sturge–Weber–Dimitri disease: CT and MR findings. AJNR Am J Neuroradiol 1992; 13: 1179–82.
- *Case report with a very early manifestation.*

Tuberous sclerosis

DiPaolo D, Zimmerman RA. Solitary cortical tubers. AJNR Am J Neuroradiol 1995; 16: 1360–4.
- *Deals with differential diagnosis.*

Kato T, Yamanouchi H, Sugai K, Takashima S. Improved detection of cortical and subcortical tubers in tuberous sclerosis by fluid-attenuated inversion recovery MRI. Neuroradiology 1997; 39: 378–80.
- *Superiority of MRI when a special CSF signal suppressing technique is used.*

Menor F, Marti-Bonmati L, Mulas F, Cortina H, Olague R. Imaging considerations of central nervous system manifestations in pediatric patients with neurofibromatosis type 1. Pediatr Radiol 1991; 21: 389–94.
- *Prospective comparison of CT and MRI in 27 children.*

Thibaut H, Parizel PM, Van Goethem J, De Schepper AM. Tuberous sclerosis: CT and MRI characteristics. Eur J Radiol 1993; 16: 176–9.
- *Mostly CT examinations.*

Torres OA, Roach ES, Delgado MR, et al. Early diagnosis of subependymal giant cell astrocytoma in patients with tuberous sclerosis. J Child Neurol 1998; 13: 173–7
- *Histologic correlation in 19 patients.*

Van Tassel P, Cure JK, K Holden R. Cystlike white matter lesions in tuberous sclerosis. AJNR Am J Neuroradiol 1997; 18: 1367–73.
- *Describes lesions found in 8 of 18 patients.*

Dandy–Walker malformation

Hart MN, Malamud N, Ellis WG. The Dandy–Walker syndrome: a clinicopathological study based on 28 cases. Neurology 1972; 22: 771–80.

Arachnoid cyst

Sze G. Diseases of the intracranial meninges: MR imaging features. AJR Am J Roentgenol 1993; 160: 727–33.
- *Comprehensive review article.*

Chiari malformation

Castillo M, Wilson JD. Spontaneous resolution of a Chiari I malformation: MR demonstration. AJNR Am J Neuroradiol 1995; 16: 1158–60.
- *Attributes the resolution to bone growth.*

Curnes JT, Oakes WJ, Boyko OB. MR imaging of hindbrain deformity in Chiari II patients with and without symptoms of brain stem compression. AJNR Am J Neuroradiol 1989; 10: 293–302.
- *MRI findings in these patients.*

Demaerel P, Kendall BE, Wilms G, Halpin SFS, Casaer P, Baert AL. Uncommon posterior cranial fossa anomalies: MRI with clinical correlation. Neuroradiology 1995; 37: 72–6.
- *Rare findings with differential diagnoses.*

Duffau H, Sahel M, Sichez JP, Marro B. Three-dimensional computerized tomography in the presurgical evaluation of Chiari malformations. Acta Neurochir 1998; 140: 429–36.
- *Advantages of three-dimensional analysis evaluated in 10 patients.*

Goldstein JH, Kaptain GI, Do HM, Cloft HJ, Jane JA, Phillips CD. CT-guided percutaneous drainage of syringomyelia. J Comput Assist Tomogr 1998; 22: 984–8.
- *Diagnostic and therapeutic importance of this procedure.*

Kan S, Fox AJ, Vinuela F. Delayed metrizamide CT enhancement of syringomyelia: postoperative observations. AJNR Am J Neuroradiol 1985; 6: 613–6.
- *Important contribution to understanding MRI flow dynamics.*

Klekamp J, Batzdorf U, Samii M, Bothe HW. The surgical treatment of Chiari I malformation. Acta Neurochir 1996; 138: 788–801.
- *Reviews surgical outcomes in 133 patients.*

8 Postoperative Findings and Follow-Up

Ventriculoperitoneal and Ventriculoatrial Shunts (Fig. 8.1)

Frequency: shunt malfunction is a common problem, with repeated failures reported to occur up to approximately every 18 months in a large group.

Suggestive morphologic findings: new occurrence of hydrocephalus (undershunting), bilateral subdural hygromas (overshunting).

Procedure: risk of irreversible brain damage; neurosurgical shunt revision.

Other studies: ultrasound when possible.

Checklist for scan interpretation:
▶ Evidence of shunt failure or slit ventricle?

- Congenital forms: aqueductal stenosis, Arnold–Chiari malformation, arachnoid cyst, and other cysts
- Acquired forms: postmeningitic, posthemorrhagic, tumor-associated

The causes of shunt malfunction include:

- Displacement of the shunt
- Proximal obstruction of the shunt by ingrowth of choroid plexus or distal obstruction by fluid collections, etc.

■ Pathogenesis

Ventriculoperitoneal and ventriculoatrial shunts are used for the treatment of hydrocephalus in children. The following forms can occur:

■ Clinical Manifestations

Shunt malfunction presents clinically with general signs of increased intracranial pressure, usually consisting of headache and impaired consciousness. Symptoms relating to the peritoneal or abdominal end of the shunt are also nonspecific.

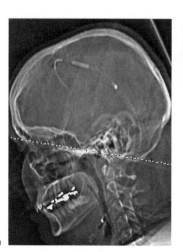
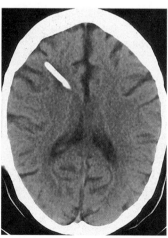

Fig. 8.**1 a, b** Ventriculoatrial shunt in a patient with hydrocephalus, caused by a pineal cyst (not shown).

a

b

■ CT Morphology

The hallmark of undershunting is dilatation of the ventricular system compared with the previous examination. This may be accompanied by sulcal effacement. Overshunting (valve malfunction) leads to hygroma formation.

Cranial computed tomography (CT) should be supplemented by thoracic or abdominal CT to evaluate the peripheral limb of the shunt.

■ Differential Diagnosis

Meningitic changes should be considered. They can be investigated by tapping the shunt, or other techniques.

Follow-Up after Tumor Resection

Frequency: one of the most common indications for CT.

Suggestive morphologic findings: early contrast enhancement at the resection site.

Procedure: imaging provides a baseline for further follow-up. The decision on the resection site is a neurosurgical one.

Other studies: magnetic resonance imaging (MRI) is more sensitive than CT for detecting contrast enhancement.

Checklist for scan interpretation:
▶ When enhancement occurs, is the pattern linear or nodular?

■ Pathogenesis

One of the most common indications for CT is to evaluate postsurgical tumor patients for residual or recurrent disease. This assessment is complicated by surgical induction of contrast enhancement at the intracranial operative site. It is also important to distinguish tumors that enhance postoperatively due to a defect in the blood–brain barrier (intra-axial) from tumors that show perfusion-related enhancement (extra-axial) and from nonenhancing tumors (i.e., tumors that did not enhance preoperatively).

■ Clinical Manifestations

Recurrent tumors that develop after the immediate postoperative period may present with a variety of clinical signs, depending on their lo-

cation. For example, infratentorial tumors that lead to hydrocephalus can present with general signs of increased intracranial pressure. Tumor recurrence may be manifested by new or recurrent seizures or by cranial nerve palsies, again depending on the tumor location.

■ CT Morphology

Despite some overlap, a residual tumor can be distinguished from surgery-induced changes if early contrast-enhanced images are available. Several key points should be emphasized:

● Residual tumor should be diagnosed at CT only if comparison with prior images shows that tissue of soft-tissue density has been left behind.
● It is normal for contrast medium to enter fluid-filled resection cavities on very early scans acquired during the initial hours after surgery.
● It is also normal to find a narrow enhancing rim surrounding a resection cavity.
● New perifocal edema and new mass effect are signs of recurrent tumor.

The CT findings will vary, depending on the type of tumor that has been removed.

With a higher-grade primary brain tumor that enhanced nonhomogeneously prior to surgery, residual tumor will display more than linear contrast enhancement at a site that enhanced before surgery. It is normal to find narrow rim enhancement of the resection margins, starting on about the third postoperative day. Early enhancement of a fluid-filled resection cavity is also normal.

With a low-grade primary brain tumor that did not enhance preoperatively, an enhancing rim may be seen around the resection cavity a few days after surgery. Thus, new enhancement does not necessarily signify malignant transformation.

Extra-axial brain tumors such as meningiomas show a different pattern of postoperative development. There is no true resection cavity, and brain tissue previously displaced by the tumor will soon reexpand to fill the subarachnoid space. Foci of contrast enhancement may be found on the meninges or cerebral surface, and do not indicate residual tumor.

■ Differential Diagnosis

Radiation necrosis is an important differential diagnosis, especially in patients who have received postoperative radiotherapy for a brain malignancy. Areas of radiation necrosis may show nodular or irregular ring enhancement that mimics the enhancement pattern of brain tumors. Nuclear medicine imaging techniques (such as positron-emission tomography) appear to be particularly useful in making this differentiation.

■ References

Recommended for further study

Ventriculoperitoneal and ventriculoatrial shunts
Langen HJ, Alzen G, Avenarius R, Mayfrank L, Thron A, Kotlarek E. [Diagnosis of complications of ventriculoperitoneal and ventriculoatrial shunts; in German.] Radiologe 1992; 32: 333–9.
  • *Comprehensive discussion; includes flowchart for diagnostic assessment.*

Follow-up after tumor resections
Forsting M, Albert FK, Kunze S, Adams HP, Zenner D, Sartor K. Extirpation of glioblastomas: MR and CT follow-up of residual tumor and regrowth patterns. AJNR Am J Neuroradiol 1993; 14: 77–87.
  • *Examinations performed during the first postoperative days; differentiation of enhancement patterns.*
Recent and basic works

Follow-up after tumor resections
Spetzger U, Thron A, Gilsbach JM. Immediate postoperative CT contrast enhancement following surgery of cerebral tumoral lesions. J Comput Assist Tomogr 1998; 22: 120–5.
  • *Describes findings during the initial hours after surgery.*

9 Facial Skeleton and Skull Base

Fundamentals

Clinical Aspects

Computed tomography (CT), with its high spatial resolution and detailed portrayal of bony anatomy, plays a special role in the diagnosis of diseases of the skull base, maxillofacial skeleton, and especially the petrous bone. The high-contrast visualization of soft-tissue structures that is possible with CT, combined with the use of densitometry for tissue discrimination, can often provide a definitive diagnosis even without the use of additional modalities such as magnetic resonance imaging (MRI). CT is the method of choice in examinations of the petrous pyramid, especially its osseous structures, and in screening for craniofacial fractures. Conventional tomography has become largely obsolete for this application.

If the patient has adequate flexibility of the cervical spine, direct coronal or even sagittal CT head images can be acquired in addition to axial scans. In other body regions, these views can be obtained only with MRI.

Common Indications

Inflammatory sinus diseases are among the most common indications for CT imaging of the midfacial region. Mucosal swelling, retained secretions, polyps, or bony abnormalities (erosion due to chronic sinusitis or bony deformities) may be responsible for the obstruction of sinus drainage. Coronal scanning is ideal for detecting these lesions, and it is better than axial scans for defining the relationship of sinus lesions to the orbit and excluding involvement of the skull base and neurocranium. Axial scans are preferred only for evaluating the pterygopalatine fossa and in cases in which coronal scans are difficult to interpret due to beam-hardening artifacts from nonremovable denture material or fillings. If necessary, the axial scans can be processed to generate reformatted images. The choice of slice thickness is governed by the general principles of CT imaging. Thin slices allow detailed evaluation of osseous structures, particularly by reducing partial volume effects, while somewhat thicker slices are often better for detecting soft-tissue abnormalities.

Another important indication for CT is in evaluating for osseous involvement or penetration of the bony skull base by a primary intracranial or extracranial tumor, such as meningioma or sinus carcinoma. CT is often performed as an adjunct to existing magnetic resonance images in this type of investigation.

In addition to showing bone destruction, CT can also demonstrate invasion through the foramina of the skull base. This is best appreciated on direct coronal scans or images reformatted from thin axial slices. Intravenous contrast administration will sometimes detect intracranial involvement by demonstrating enhancement of the meninges.

CT is an important tool for three-dimensional planning of surgical procedures, the planning of corrective or reconstructive procedures, and the fabrication of prosthetic bone implants and appliances used in oromaxillofacial surgery. Another application in this context is the use of CT data sets to carry out virtual endoscopy of the paranasal sinuses and image-guided surgical navigation.

The ability to generate suitable two-dimensional reformatted images of the maxilla and mandible is particularly useful for planning implantation procedures in oral surgery. The nonsuperimposed images provided by "dental CT" can be used to determine the dimensions of the alveolar crest and the cortical bone thickness with very high accuracy. Lesions can also be localized to specific dental regions with greater confidence, making it easier to compare CT findings with standard panoramic radiographs (Figs. 9.**1**, 9.**2**).

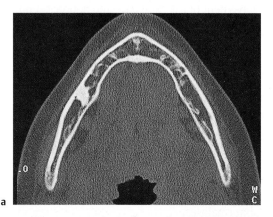

a

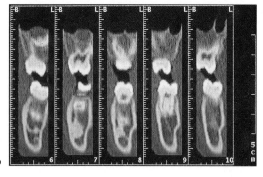

b

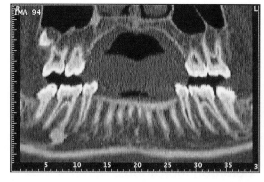

Fig. 9.**1 a–c** **Osteoma of the mandible.**
a Conventional axial CT scan of a woman with a mandibular osteoma.
b, c Semiautomated software is used to generate reformatted images perpendicular (**b**) and tangential (**c**) to the mandibular ramus. This technique, called dental CT, can document the precise relationship of the osteoma to the root of the right first molar using a scale at the bottom of the image (L: lingual; B: buccal).

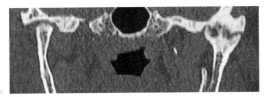

Fig. 9.**2 a, b Degenerative disease of the temporo-mandibular joint.** Axial and especially coronal CT can provide clear, nonsuperimposed views of degenerative changes in the temporomandibular joint, as in the severe case pictured here. Magnetic resonance imaging is better for visualizing the articular disk.

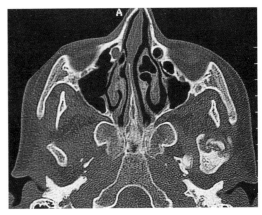

b

Malformations and Functional Disturbances

The nasal cavity, and the paranasal sinuses in particular, are subject to such extensive anatomic variation that diagnostic evaluations have to center on the question of whether demonstrable sinonasal changes have functional significance. Particularly in patients with chronic inflammatory sinus disease, CT can significantly advance the diagnosis by detecting impairment of sinus drainage due to normal anatomic variants or abnormal masses. These changes are best appreciated on direct coronal scans, although sagittal images reformatted from thin-slice axial data sets are helpful or necessary for some indications.

■ Pathogenesis

Inflammatory sinus disease is perhaps the most frequent indication for midfacial CT examinations. Direct coronal scanning (coronal sinus CT) is generally best for this purpose. It may be possible to reduce radiation exposure by acquiring noncontiguous thin slices, depending on the requirements of the referring physician. For presurgical assessment, however, contiguous thin-slice coverage should be obtained. The essential role of sinus CT is to define the ostia of the paranasal sinuses and identify possible outflow obstructions.

Inflammatory Sinus Disease (Fig. 9.3)

Frequency: very common.

Suggestive morphologic findings: mucosal thickening, retained secretions, possible bone erosion.

Procedure: coronal imaging. Some cases may require sagittal images reformatted from axial data.

Other studies: conventional radiographs.

Checklist for scan interpretation:
▶ Osteomeatal complex?
▶ Outflow obstruction due to normal anatomic variant?
▶ Bone destruction?
▶ Mucocele formation?

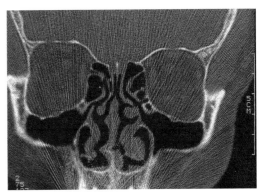

Fig. 9.**3 Coronal sinus CT scan** at the level of the osteomeatal complex defines the drainage tract of the maxillary sinus, frontal sinus, and anterior ethmoid cells.

Today we know that the drainage of sinus secretions depends on mucociliary clearance. The surgical creation of an unphysiologic ostium in the floor of a sinus has no effect on ciliary clearance, and the mucous film will simply be transported over or past the artificial orifice. Optimum clearance can occur when the width of the natural ostia just permits the opposing mucosal surfaces to come into contact. Narrowing of the ostia disrupts ciliary motility, resulting in stasis of secretions and colonization by bacteria.

Based on these discoveries, the concept of treating chronic inflammatory sinus disease with an old-fashioned fenestration procedure has given way to minimally invasive techniques in which the goal is to restore the natural routes of sinus drainage. Some of these techniques are already using image-guided navigation, in which an instrument is manipulated within a CT-based stereotactic space while its position is visualized in real time within the data set.

■ **Frequency**

Very common.

■ **Clinical Manifestations**

Inflammatory sinus disease presents with facial pain and headache that are aggravated by activities causing increased sinonasal pressure (e.g., coughing). Other symptoms are a feeling of pressure and nasal or postnasal drainage.

■ **CT Morphology**

In addition to the detection of mucosal thickening and accumulated secretions, special attention should be given to the sinus drainage routes, in view of the pathophysiology described above. Of key interest is the "osteomeatal complex," which is the route by which the anterior ethmoid cells, frontal sinus, and maxillary sinus are drained. As a result, anything causing obstruction of the osteomeatal complex can cause obstruction and disease in these three sinuses. (The drainage route of the sphenoid sinus and possible constrictions of the frontal sinus are best displayed in sagittal images reformatted from thin axial data sets.) Causes of obstruction in the osteomeatal complex include normal anatomic variants such as concha bullosa, ethmoid bullae, Haller cells of the maxillary sinus, and deviation of the bony nasal septum.

Choanal Atresia (Figs. 9.4, 9.5)

Frequency: the incidence of choanal atresia is one in 5000–8000 live births, with a female preponderance.

Suggestive morphologic findings: obstruction of the choanae by bone or connective tissue.

Procedure: evaluate with thin CT slices (2–3 mm) angled at approximately 5° to the hard palate.

Other studies: CT is the imaging procedure of choice.

Checklist for scan interpretation:
▶ Bony atresia?
▶ Membranous atresia?

■ **Pathogenesis**

Choanal atresia is a congenital anomaly in which one or both choanae are obstructed by bone or connective tissue. It occurs when a mesenchymal tissue membrane between the neurocranium and viscerocranium fails to disappear during embryonic development. Bilateral choanal atresia can be life-threatening in neonates, because the relatively high position of the larynx impedes oral breathing. These cases require immediate intervention to establish a nasal airway.

Choanal atresia sometimes occurs in association with other anomalies, which have been designated with the acronym CHARGE (coloboma, heart disease, atresia choanae, retarded growth, genital hypoplasia, ear anomalies).

Frequency

Females are more commonly affected. Hereditary factors have been identified. In approximately 75% of cases, choanal atresia is associated with other congenital defects or anomalies of the facial skeleton. The incidence is estimated at one in 5000–8000 births.

Clinical Manifestations

Nasal airway obstruction in the neonate, which can be life-threatening.

CT Morphology

CT is the imaging modality of choice, and the CT results direct the choice of surgical treatment. While a membranous obstruction can be perforated endoscopically, bony atresia usually requires a partial transpalatal resection of the vomer, which appears thickened posteriorly on axial CT scans (Fig. 9.**4**). Sagittal reformatted images can also help to define the choanal obstruction (Fig. 9.**5**). Choanal width should be at least 3.7 mm by 2 years of age and at least 3.4 mm by 8 years of age.

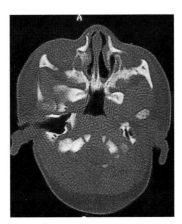

Fig. 9.**4 Bilateral bony choanal atresia.** Posterior thickening of the vomer is clearly visible in this axial CT scan.

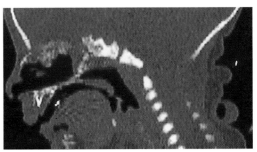

Fig. 9.**5 Bilateral bony choanal atresia.** Sagittal image reconstructed from the axial data set clearly demonstrates the obstructing bony membrane.

Tornwaldt Cyst

Frequency: a relatively common incidental finding.

Suggestive morphologic findings: midline cystic mass in the upper nasopharynx.

Procedure: may require thin-slice scanning.

Other studies: sagittal T2-weighted MRI is the method of choice.

Checklist for scan interpretation:
▶ Differentiation is required from other nasopharyngeal masses, especially neoplasms.

Pathogenesis

Known also as pharyngeal bursitis, this anomaly results from persistence of the median fissure of the pharyngeal tonsil, which may close secondarily, leading to the formation of a pouch or cyst known as a Tornwaldt cyst. The cyst is filled with secretions and debris, and can produce a foul-smelling discharge when not completely closed. Inflammation of surrounding tissues is common.

Frequency

Tornwaldt cyst is a relatively common incidental finding.

■ **Clinical Manifestations**

Foul-smelling discharge, surrounding inflammatory reaction.

■ **CT Morphology**

CT demonstrates a midline cystic mass arising from the pharyngeal tonsil.

Otosclerosis

Frequency: the clinically overt form is somewhat rare, but otosclerotic lesions are found in up to 8 % of autopsies. Women predominate by a ratio of about 2: 1.

Suggestive morphologic findings: thickening of the stapes footplate, low-density resorption halo surrounding the cochlea.

Procedure: high-resolution CT, if necessary combined with densitometry; follow-ups.

Other studies: thin-slice MRI with intravenous contrast medium. Radionuclide bone scanning shows increased bone turnover during the active phase of otosclerosis.

Checklist for scan interpretation:
▶ Acuteness of the disease.
▶ Differentiate from focal manifestations of other systemic skeletal diseases with petrous bone involvement.

■ **Pathogenesis**

Otosclerosis is a primary focal disease of the bony otic capsule. Its etiology is unknown, but its familial occurrence and tendency to progress during pregnancy suggest a multifactorial etiology based on a combination of genetic and hormonal factors. Histologically, the active phase of the disease is characterized by abnormally increased activity of histiocytes and osteocytes in the otic capsule. This leads to resorption of the dense capsular bone, which is subsequently replaced by more vascularized spongy bone. This is followed by a reparative phase in which the spongy bone is replaced by dense, relatively avascular and acellular bone. The foci may progressively increase in size and eventually project into the middle ear cavity.

The most common site of occurrence is the otic capsule near the oval window. Usually, the sclerotic lesions cause fixation of the stapes footplate, and CT will often demonstrate thickening of the footplate in the oval window. The result is progressive conductive hearing loss. Involvement of the cochlea by otosclerotic foci can lead to sensorineural hearing loss.

The disease usually takes an undulating course, marked by alternating periods of remission and exacerbation. Early manifestation generally implies a poor prognosis.

Involvement of the middle ear and inner ear by Paget disease, osteogenesis imperfecta, or manifestations of other skeletal diseases are important differential diagnoses that may require further imaging studies or even laboratory tests, to distinguish them from otosclerosis.

■ **Frequency**

Otosclerosis is a relatively rare disease with an obscure, multifactorial etiology that appears to involve both genetic and hormonal causes. Women predominate by a ratio of about 2: 1, and Europeans are affected more often than Japanese and Africans. The clinically overt form is relatively rare, but otosclerotic foci are discovered in up to 8 % of autopsies.

■ **Clinical Manifestations**

Otosclerosis presents clinically with conductive hearing loss, sometimes accompanied by a sensorineural component. The pure-tone audiogram usually indicates pure conductive hearing loss, and the stapedius reflex may be abolished. The treatment of choice consists of stapedectomy with stapes reconstruction.

■ **CT Morphology**

There are two characteristic CT findings in otosclerosis. With fenestral otosclerosis, the oval window may be narrowed from its normal size of approximately 3 × 2 mm, and there may be appreciable thickening of the stapes footplate. With cochlear otosclerosis, a low-density resorption halo can be seen surrounding the cochlea during the active phase of the disease. Both findings can be seen only with high-resolution CT.

High-resolution CT can also be used to perform densitometry of the cochlear capsule. This is done by measuring the attenuation values at a number of defined points and comparing them with measurements in a normal population. Densitometry is also useful for following the progression of the disease and assessing its response to treatment.

Another important role for CT lies in documenting the postoperative findings after stapes reconstruction.

Tumors and Other Mass Lesions

This section deals with tumors of the skull base, petrous bone, and midfacial region that are important because of their frequency, imaging features, or potential importance in CT differential diagnosis. This listing is by no means complete. Several entities, such as meningioma and acoustic schwannoma, are discussed in Chapter 5 above, and are mentioned here only for completeness.

Odontogenic Tumors

Odontogenic tumors are mostly neoplasms that develop from the dental lamina. Generally, they are benign and rarely undergo malignant transformation. Because of their initial paucity of symptoms, these tumors are usually diagnosed only after they have produced significant facial deformity or asymmetry. The most important odontogenic tumors include ameloblastoma and odontoma, both of epithelial origin, and cementoma, which has a mesodermal origin. There are also numerous mixed forms, for which the varying proportions of tissue components are usually designated by the prefix "fibro-" or "myxo-," depending on whether the tumor has a high content of fibrous or connective tissue, or is mucus-forming. Conventional radiography is still the best method for the detection and differential diagnosis of lesions.

Ameloblastoma (Fig. 9.**6**)

Frequency: the most common jaw tumor. Most prevalent in the fourth and fifth decades of life, with no predilection for either sex.

Suggestive morphologic findings: CT shows an expansile mass associated with thinning of the cortex. The mass is occasionally multilocular and may contain a tooth bud. An extraosseous mass may develop.

Procedure: evaluate with thin-slice bone-window CT scans.

Other studies: MRI, panoramic radiograph.

Checklist for scan interpretation:
▶ Consider range of differential diagnoses.
▶ Risk of fracture?
▶ Degree of destruction?

■ Pathogenesis

Ameloblastoma is the most common jaw tumor. It is slow-growing, but locally destructive. The solid forms tend to be locally invasive, while the cystic forms show a more benign growth pattern. Recurrence is common after surgical removal, and up to 2% undergo malignant transformation. Approximately one-third are associated with a follicular cyst.

■ Frequency

Ameloblastoma is the most common tumor of the maxillomandibular region. It usually occurs in the fourth or fifth decade of life, and shows no predilection for either sex. The mandible is affected in 75% of cases, the maxilla in 25%.

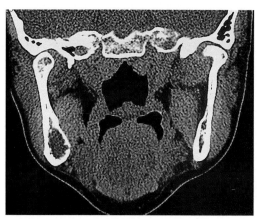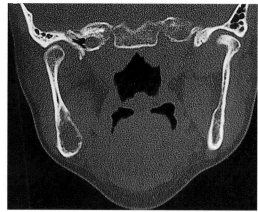

a

Fig. 9.**6 a, b   Ameloblastoma.** Soft-tissue and bone-window views of an ameloblastoma of the right mandible. Note the typical honeycomb appearance of the mass.

■ Clinical Manifestations

Ameloblastomas often grow for some time without causing symptoms, and are usually diagnosed only after causing appreciable jaw deformity.

■ CT Morphology

CT shows a unilocular or multilocular "honeycomb" lytic lesion with expansile margins. Because ameloblastomas are sometimes derived from a follicular cyst, they may contain a rudimentary or complete tooth. Their tendency to erode through the cortex can produce an extraosseous soft-tissue mass (Fig. 9.**6**).

Odontoma

Frequency: rare.

Suggestive morphologic findings: amorphous calcified mass or malformed tooth bud.

Procedure: evaluate with thin-slice CT scans. Dental CT may also be used.

Other studies: conventional panoramic radiograph.

Checklist for scan interpretation:
▶ Differential-diagnostic classification.

■ Pathogenesis

Odontomas contain all the tissue elements of a complete tooth: enamel, dentine, cement, and pulp. Consequently, they are more accurately described as malformations rather than tumors. There are numerous mixed forms, however, such as ameloblastic fibro-odontoma. Odontomas are of two basic types: complex odontomas, in which all the dental tissues occur in a disorderly pattern, and compound odontomas, in which the dental tissues show a high degree of differentiation. Numerous transitional forms also occur.

■ Frequency

Rare.

■ Clinical Manifestations

Nonspecific.

■ CT Morphology

There are no specific CT features of odontomas. They may appear as amorphous calcified masses or as malformed tooth buds.

Cementoma

> **Frequency:** rare.
>
> **Suggestive morphologic findings:** apical densities, usually located in the mandible. Mixed lytic–sclerotic patterns may occur.
>
> **Procedure:** evaluate with thin-slice bone-window scans. Dental CT may also be used.
>
> **Other studies:** panoramic radiograph.
>
> **Checklist for scan interpretation:**
> ▶ Differentiate from ossifying fibroma and fibrous dysplasia.

■ Pathogenesis

Cementoma is a collective term for a number of lesions that cannot be distinguished from one another by imaging studies, particularly CT. These lesions include:

- Cementoblastoma
- Cement-forming fibroma
- Periapical cemental dysplasia

Although cementomas are usually sclerotic, imaging may show periapical or even cystic hypodensities, depending on the specific entity and the stage of the disease.

■ Frequency

Rare.

■ Clinical Manifestations

Nonspecific.

■ CT Morphology

The typical CT appearance is that of an apical density, which may be quite small and is usually located in the mandible. Multicentric lesions are common. Mixed patterns with a combination of lytic and sclerotic features are also seen. Differentiation is required from ossifying fibroma and, with extensive involvement, from fibrous dysplasia.

Cystic Lesions of the Maxilla and Mandible

> **Frequency:** small, clinically insignificant lesions are common.
>
> **Suggestive morphologic findings:** cystic lesions in the maxilla or mandible, often developing around a single devitalized tooth, but occasionally involving a whole quadrant. Follicular cysts with tooth buds have a CT attenuation of approximately 5–15 HU. Odontogenic cysts have a peripheral calcified rim.
>
> **Procedure:** evaluate with thin CT slices. Use dental CT as required.
>
> **Other studies:** panoramic radiograph. Dental spot films are useful for smaller lesions. Other options: dental CT, MRI.
>
> **Checklist for scan interpretation:**
> ▶ Differentiate from other entities.

■ Pathogenesis

Since the majority of these lesions are not distinguishable by CT, and as differential diagnosis usually requires a panoramic radiograph or dental spot films, we shall briefly review only the most important entities.

True cysts, which have an epithelial lining, are distinguished from *pseudocysts,* which lack this lining. Their imaging appearance is marked by a slow, expansile growth pattern, usually resulting in well-defined margins or even a sclerotic rim if there is no inflammatory component inciting a perifocal reaction.

A further distinction is made between *odontogenic* and *nonodontogenic* cysts.

Odontogenic cysts. These include the following:

- Radicular cysts, which form around the apex of a diseased tooth, and lateral cysts, which project into the bone from lateral pulpal defects.
- Follicular cysts, which result from aberrant differentiation of the dental lamina. A primordial cyst can develop at the site of a supernumerary tooth bud. The primordial cyst can subsequently develop into a keratocyst through active keratinization of its epithelial lining. Other follicular cysts develop around the crown of an impacted or unerupted tooth (e.g., an eruption cyst around a wisdom tooth). The mandibular angle is a frequent site of occurrence (Figs. 9.**7**, 9.**8**).

Nonodontogenic cysts. Often located on the midline, nonodontogenic cysts develop from epithelial rests of the nasopalatine duct or from heterotopic elements of the palatine suture. In a broader sense, the nonodontogenic cysts include mucocele, aneurysmal bone cyst, and solitary bone cyst. While aneurysmal and solitary bone cysts are indistinguishable by conventional radiography, CT can sometimes demonstrate heterogeneous densities within an aneurysmal bone cyst, caused by blood-filled spaces within the lesion. In addition, internal portions of an aneurysmal bone cyst may enhance after intravenous contrast administration.

■ Frequency

The most common cystic jaw lesions are radicular cysts that develop around a devitalized tooth. The other entities are somewhat rare.

■ Clinical Manifestations

Besides their direct effects on involved teeth, cystic jaw lesions produce symptoms by their local mass effects on adjacent structures. These include mandibular nerve compression within the alveolar canal or involvement of the paranasal sinuses.

■ CT Morphology

CT demonstrates cystic lesions in the maxilla or mandible, which may surround individual tooth roots (often devitalized teeth), or may affect a whole quadrant. Follicular cysts may contain partial or complete tooth buds. Internal attenuation values range from 5 to 15 HU. Different types of cyst are indistinguishable by CT. Keratocysts can grow very large, expanding into the maxillary sinus. These large cysts are often septated or lobulated.

Odontogenic cysts frequently have a typical peripheral calcified rim along with central tooth buds.

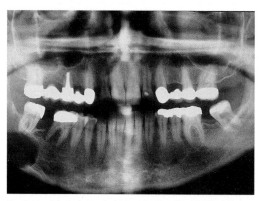

Fig. 9.**7** **Cystic lucency.** Panoramic radiograph demonstrates a cystic lucency of the right mandibular angle with no visible tooth bud. Radicular cyst.

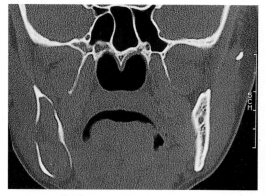

Fig. 9.**8** **Follicular cyst (keratocyst).** Coronal bone-window CT shows the typical appearance of a follicular cyst at its most common site of occurrence.

Contrast enhancement usually does not occur on CT scans, but may be seen with gadolinium-enhanced MRI, which is a much more sensitive study. It is often difficult to distinguish a keratocyst from ameloblastoma by CT.

Mucocele, Pyocele (Fig. 9.**9**)

Frequency: the most common cause of an expansile paranasal sinus mass; frequent in cystic fibrosis.

Suggestive morphologic findings: expansile soft-tissue mass of the paranasal sinuses; may be associated with bone erosion and ingrowth (e.g., into the orbit).

Procedure: evaluate with thin-slice axial scans or coronal bone-window CT.

Other studies: the lesions display a high signal intensity on T1-weighted and T2-weighted MRI. Conventional radiographs show extensive bone erosion.

Checklist for scan interpretation:
▶ Degree of expansion?
▶ Compression of important structures (e.g., optic nerve) or central nervous sytem (CNS) pathways?
▶ Signs of superinfection?

■ Pathogenesis

Mucoceles and pyoceles result from obstruction of the excretory duct of a paranasal sinus and from the retention of secretions within the sinus. The obstruction may be caused by an inflammatory process, trauma, or neoplasm. Rising intrasinus pressure tends to erode the bony wall, eventually transforming it into a fibrous capsule. Various mass effects can develop, such as exophthalmos caused by a mucocele in the frontal sinus (Fig. 9.**9**).

The most commonly affected sinuses are as follows (in descending order of frequency):

- Frontal sinus
- Ethmoid sinus
- Maxillary sinus

The sphenoid sinus is very rarely affected. A special form is a mucocele of the lacrimal sac, which is sometimes bilateral.

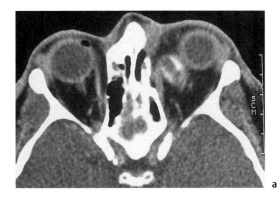

a

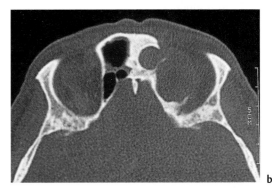

b

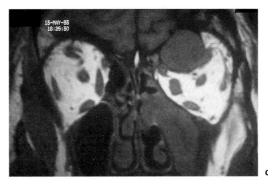

c

Fig. 9.**9 a–c Mucocele.** These images show a mucocele that arose from the anterior ethmoid cells and has invaded the orbit secondarily, presenting clinically as exophthalmos. The lesion is particularly well demonstrated by coronal magnetic resonance imaging (**c**).

■ Frequency

Mucocele is the most frequent cause of an expansile paranasal sinus mass. Its incidence is increased in cystic fibrosis.

■ Clinical Manifestations

The clinical features of a mucocele depend mainly on its location. Most mucoceles are initially asymptomatic and are diagnosed only after causing compression of important structure or forming an expansile mass leading to exophthalmos or another deformity. Serious complications include optic or oculomotor nerve compression and destruction of the bony sella.

■ CT Morphology

CT demonstrates a soft-tissue mass that may be associated with paranasal sinus expansion or bone erosion. Usually the mass does not enhance after contrast administration, but a mucocele may cause an accompanying inflammatory reaction that appears as a peripheral enhancing ring. Internal attenuation values depend on the degree of inspissation of the contents, and usually range from 40 to 50 HU.

Papilloma

Frequency: relatively rare. The two forms (inverted and exophytic) are about equally common.

Suggestive morphologic findings: *inverted papilloma:* lobulated surface, projects into paranasal sinus from nasal cavity; always unilateral. *Exophytic papilloma:* wart-like mass arising from the septum.

Procedure: coronal and axial scans.

Other studies: MRI is better than CT for distinguishing the papillomatous component from possible squamous-cell carcinoma located within the papilloma.

Checklist for scan interpretation:
▶ Surface structure? Extent of destruction?
▶ Compression of CNS pathways?
▶ Malignant transformation?

■ Pathogenesis

Papillomas are masses that arise from the mucosa lining the nasal cavity or paranasal sinuses. Several types are distinguished:

- Exophytic papilloma
- Inverted papilloma
- Cylindrical cell papilloma (rare)

Exophytic papillomas almost always arise from the nasal septum and have a wart-like gross appearance. Generally, they do not undergo malignant change.

Inverted papillomas arise from the lateral nasal wall and typically project into the ethmoid cells or maxillary sinus. They consist of a hyperplastic epithelium that is "inverted" into the underlying stroma. Inverted papillomas are always unilateral and have an extremely high recurrence rate after excision. Up to 15% of these lesions are associated with squamous-cell carcinoma, underscoring the importance of early detection and complete surgical removal.

■ Frequency

Inverted papilloma is the most common of all epithelial papillomas. Men are predominantly affected. The most common site of occurrence is the lateral nasal wall, from which the lesion projects into the paranasal sinuses. Some sources state that inverted and exophytic papillomas occur with approximately equal frequency.

■ Clinical Manifestations

Besides local symptoms, progressive nasal airway obstruction is the dominant feature in most patients.

■ CT Morphology

Exophytic papilloma arises from the nasal septum, while inverted papilloma arises from the lateral wall of the nasal cavity and projects into the paranasal sinuses. A lobulated surface structure is considered typical of inverted papilloma.

Fibrous Dysplasia (Fig. 9.**10**)

Frequency: the neurocranium or viscerocranium is involved in 15–20% of cases.

Suggestive morphologic findings: unilateral involvement, ground-glass density in the frontal skull base and midfacial region, cystic lucency in the mandible and calvarium, craniofacial asymmetry. Usually the lesions do not enhance after contrast administration.

Procedure: evaluate with axial and coronal thin-slice CT.

Other studies: conventional radiographs, radionuclide bone scan to screen for polyostotic disease.

Checklist for scan interpretation:
▶ Include in differential diagnosis other mass lesions such as Paget disease, neurofibromatosis, nonossifying fibroma, giant-cell tumor, and aneurysmal bone cyst.
▶ Compression of nerve pathways or vital structures?

■ Pathogenesis

Fibrous dysplasia (Jaffé–Lichtenstein disease) is a benign fibro-osseous lesion of unknown etiology. It is characterized histologically by an interwoven pattern of fibromyxoid tissue, spindle cells, cysts, and bony trabeculae within the medullary cavity.

Two major patterns of fibrous dysplasia are recognized:

● Monostotic form (85% of cases)
● Polyostotic form (15% of cases)

These special forms have also been described:

● An autosomal-dominant hereditary form with symmetrical involvement of the mandible and maxilla—known as cherubism, because the bilateral mandibular swellings impart a cherubic appearance.
● McCune–Albright syndrome, in which unilateral polyostotic fibrous dysplasia coexists with endocrine dysfunction and café-au-lait spots.

With involvement of the skull, two basic patterns are observed. Cystic expansile lesions predominate in the mandible and calvarium, while ground-glass density of the medullary cavity occurs in the skull base, petrous bone, and midfacial region (Fig. 9.**10**). Usually the involvement is unilateral, and over time it leads to craniofacial asymmetry. Narrowing of skull base foramina with compression of cranial nerves or the involvement of inner ear structures eventually leads to corresponding deficits.

Differentiation is mainly required from Paget disease, but this is sometimes difficult. A ground-glass appearance and asymmetrical, unilateral involvement are definite indications of fibrous dysplasia. Also, involvement of the calvarium by fibrous dysplasia tends to spare the inner table, whereas Paget disease affects both the inner and outer tables.

Another differential diagnosis is primary interosseous meningioma of the frontal skull base.

■ Frequency

The bones of the neurocranium and viscerocranium are affected in approximately 20% of patients with monostotic fibrous dysplasia and in approximately 15% of patients with polyostotic disease.

■ Clinical Manifestations

The dominant clinical feature, besides facial asymmetry, is the cranial nerve deficits caused by the narrowing of neural foramina, predominantly optic nerve compression. Involvement of middle-ear and inner-ear structures can cause hearing loss.

■ CT Morphology

The CT features of fibrous dysplasia are craniofacial asymmetry, a cystic expansile pattern in the mandible or calvarium, and ground-glass expansion in the skull base and midfacial region. Contrast enhancement usually does not occur.

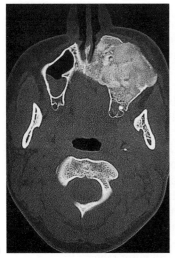

a

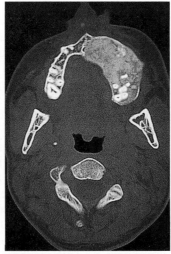

b

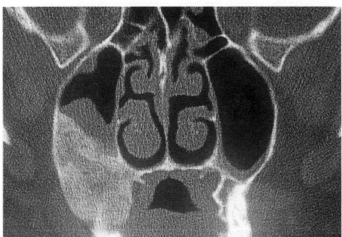

c

Fig. 9.**10 a–c Fibrous dysplasia.** Classic CT appearance of fibrous dysplasia of the left maxilla (**a, b**) and of the right maxilla in a different patient (**c**). Note the ground-glass opacity and expansion of the medullary cavity with an intact cortex. The marked facial asymmetry and displacement of maxillary teeth in scans **a** and **b** suggest the correct diagnosis.

Paget Disease

Frequency: the prevalence is approximately 3 %. Men are predominantly affected.

Suggestive morphologic findings: imaging findings are phase-dependent, and consist of circumscribed hypodensity or sclerosis, with a predominantly symmetrical pattern of involvement. With involvement of the petrous bone, the otic capsule is initially spared; later, the petrous bone takes on a washed-out appearance.

Procedure: evaluate with coronal and axial thin-slice CT.

Other studies: conventional radiographs, radionuclide bone scan.

Checklist for scan interpretation:
▶ Consider important differential diagnoses.
▶ Impending compression of CNS pathways?
▶ Involvement of petrous pyramids?

■ Pathogenesis

Paget disease is a disease of the osteoclasts that is believed to have a viral etiology. It is characterized by an increased rate of bone resorption, with reactive osteoblastic hyperactivity. The newly formed bone is not lamellar but has a soft, disordered structure. The initial (active) phase is marked by predominant osteoclastic activity within a vascular stroma that later regresses. Reactive hyperactivity of the osteoblasts leaves behind a very dense, sclerotic bone (inactive phase). Mixed patterns are also common. In approximately 1% of cases, the reactive osteoblasts undergo malignant transformation, giving rise to osteosarcoma, fibrosarcoma, or chondrosarcoma.

■ Frequency

The prevalence of Paget disease is approximately 3%, but the great majority of cases are asymptomatic. A familial incidence is noted in approximately 15% of cases. Males predominate by a ratio of 3:2. Most cases occur between 55 and 80 years of age.

■ Clinical Manifestations

Symptoms are location-dependent, and the dominant features are caused by compression of cranial nerves and CNS pathways.

■ CT Morphology

Paget disease of the cranium typically affects both the inner and outer tables. This can distinguish Paget disease from fibrous dysplasia, which generally spares the inner table. The CT findings depend on the phase of the disease. Scans may show a circumscribed hypodensity (osteoporosis), expansion of the diploë, or circumscribed sclerosis that may also affect the petrous bone and inner ear. Advanced cases may show basilar invagination with narrowing of the foramen magnum.

Involvement of the petrous pyramids typically starts at the apex and progresses laterally. Typically, there is an early prominence of the otic capsule, which subsequently demineralizes. General demineralization of the petrous pyramid gives the bone a "washed-out" appearance on CT scans. This finding is typical of Paget disease, and helps differentiate it from conditions such as otosclerosis.

Skull Base Meningioma (Figs. 9.11–9.13)

Frequency: relatively common.

Suggestive morphologic findings: bone infiltration with "reactive hyperostosis."

Procedure: thin-slice bone-window CT scans.

Other studies: MRI. Angiography may be useful for surgical planning.

Checklist for scan interpretation:
▶ Consider a range of differential diagnoses.
▶ Invasion of critical structures with compression of nerve pathways (orbital fissure, optic canal, cavernous sinus, sella, etc.)?

■ Pathogenesis

As meningiomas are discussed in some detail in Chapter 5, we shall consider them only briefly here. Common sites of occurrence besides the falx and convexity are the bony ridges of the medial and lateral sphenoid wing, the clivus, the crista galli, the planum sphenoidale, the sella turcica, and the cerebellopontine angle area. Like meningiomas at other sites, these tumors may penetrate the skull base by growing along fine vascular channels or cranial nerves (e.g., the penetrating fibers of the olfactory nerve). They may also infiltrate the bone itself, frequently leading to bone expansion (Figs. 9.11, 9.12). While this is often called "reactive hyperostosis," it is actually caused by infiltration. This pattern of spread results in a combination of intracranial and extracranial masses. Purely intraosseous meningioma is a rare special form that can be difficult to distinguish from other lesions (e.g., fibrous dysplasia).

■ Frequency

Relatively common.

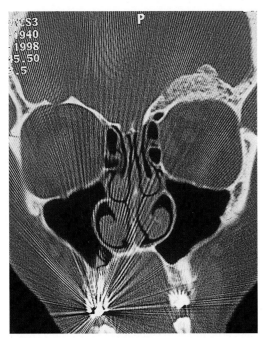

Fig. 9.**11** **Meningioma.** This frontobasal meningioma is associated with marked bone thickening that signifies intraosseous growth.

■ Clinical Manifestations

Besides nonspecific local symptoms, the clinical presentation is determined by the degree of compression of cranial nerves and vascular structures. Intrasellar tumors can cause hormonal disturbances.

■ CT Morphology

The typical features of skull base meningiomas on contrast-enhanced CT will generally suggest the correct diagnosis. Purely intraosseous meningiomas are rare and can be distinguished from fibrous dysplasia only by their intense contrast enhancement—assuming that enhancement is discernible within the intrinsic high density of the bone.

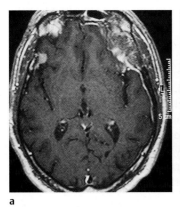

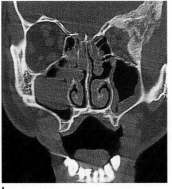

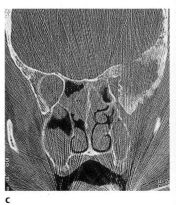

a   b   c

Fig. 9.**12 a–c** **Meningioma.** These images show another frontobasal meningioma that has infiltrated the medial and lateral sphenoid wing, orbital roof, and lateral orbital wall, producing an intraorbital mass effect.

a   Axial magnetic resonance imaging.
b, c Bone-window CT scans.

Fig. 9.**13 a, b** **Hyperostosis frontalis interna.** The symmetry of the thickening and the preservation of bone architecture are not consistent with intraosseous meningioma, fibrous dysplasia, or Paget disease. Nevertheless, the circumscribed variant of this benign bony hypertrophy, which mainly affects women, can lead to problems of differential diagnosis.

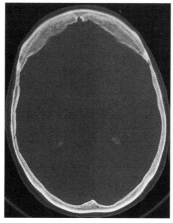
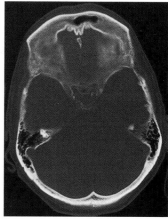

a

b

Esthesioneuroblastoma

Frequency: extremely rare.

Suggestive morphologic findings: mass located in the upper nasal cavity and ethmoid cells; homogeneous density, intense contrast enhancement; may have intracranial and extracranial components.

Procedure: contrast-enhanced coronal scans.

Other studies: coronal and sagittal MRI is the imaging procedure of choice.

Checklist for scan interpretation:
▶ Intracranial component?

This extremely rare tumor is discussed earlier (p. 141). It arises from the epithelial cells of the olfactory bulb, can have both intracranial and extracranial components, and may infiltrate the orbits.

Dermoids and epidermoids are benign congenital tumors that develop from the inclusion of ectodermal elements during neural closure. Epidermoids are unilocular or multilocular masses, usually cystic, that contain only epidermal cells. Dermoids additionally contain dermal appendages such as hair follicles, sweat glands, sebaceous glands, and fat.

Epidermoids are usually of water density. They are more homogeneous than dermoids, which appear isodense to hypodense on CT depending on their fat or sebum content. Consistent with their pathogenesis, epidermoids are most commonly located in the cerebellopontine angle and parasellar cisterns. Dermoids tend to be located near the midline. Contrast enhancement is not typical of epidermoids and dermoids and signifies infection of the cyst.

Dermoid, Epidermoid (Fig. 9.**14**)

Frequency: 1–2% of intracranial tumors. Epidermoids make up about 7% of cerebellopontine angle tumors.

Suggestive morphologic findings: epidermoids—water density, located in the cerebellopontine angle; dermoids—isodense or hypodense, located on the midline.

Procedure: standard CT; intravenous contrast administration as required.

Other studies: MRI.

Checklist for scan interpretation:
▶ Other differential diagnoses.

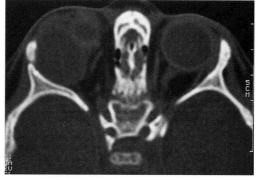

Fig. 9.**14** **Dermoid of the right orbit.**

Aneurysmal Bone Cyst (Fig. 9.**15**)

Frequency: rarely involves the facial skeleton or calvarium.

Suggestive morphologic findings: expansion of the bone with an intact cortex, fluid levels of varying density.

Procedure: thin-slice bone-window CT scans.

Other studies: MRI.

Checklist for scan interpretation:
▶ Differential diagnosis.
▶ Risk of pathologic fracture?

■ Pathogenesis

Aneurysmal bone cyst is a benign osteolytic bone lesion that most commonly affects the spine and long bones. It sometimes occurs in the calvarium or skull base. As noted, the lesion is not primary but develops in response to previous bone damage. It may also accompany a giant-cell tumor or fibrous dysplasia.

■ Frequency

Aneurysmal bone cyst is the second most common benign tumor of the spine. Craniofacial involvement is rare.

■ Clinical Manifestations

Painful swelling or local pain without swelling.

■ CT Morphology

CT usually demonstrates expansion of the affected bone, with intact cortical boundaries. It is common for the cyst to contain a fluid level of varying density, which can result from intracystic hemorrhage (Fig. 9.**15**).

Giant-Cell Tumor

Frequency: rare.

Suggestive morphologic findings: a homogeneous mass of soft-tissue density, sometimes associated with extensive bone erosion.

Procedure: maxillary lesions are evaluated on coronal scans. Mandibular lesions can be evaluated by dental CT.

Other studies: conventional radiographs. Panoramic radiograph for mandibular tumors.

Checklist for scan interpretation:
▶ Differential diagnosis.

■ Pathogenesis

Giant-cell tumors can occur in the maxillofacial skeleton, affecting predominantly the paranasal sinuses and mandible. They develop as an expansile mass causing local destruction. Giant-cell tumors are considered benign, and are usually treated by local excision. Most lesions occur in the mandible.

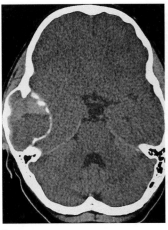 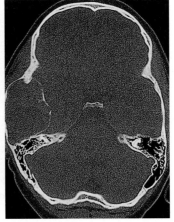

Fig. 9.**15 a, b Aneurysmal bone cyst of the right temporal bone.** The inner and outer tables of the cortex are separated by a cystic lesion containing a fluid level. The differential diagnosis at this location includes fibrous dysplasia, which often produces cystic calvarial lesions.

a   b

Frequency

Young women are most commonly affected. The site of predilection in the maxillofacial skeleton is the premolar region of the mandible.

Clinical Manifestations

Nonspecific.

CT Morphology

CT demonstrates a soft-tissue mass with no significant internal structures. The lesion has a locally erosive growth pattern that causes bone destruction.

Frequency

Relatively rare.

Clinical Manifestations

Pain on mastication, facial asymmetry.

CT Morphology

CT shows an exophytic bone tumor, frequently arising from the mandibular condyle, which apparently does not violate the continuity of the medullary cavity and cortex between the osteochondroma and the mandible (Figs. 9.**16**, 9.**17**).

Osteochondroma (Figs. 9.**16**, 9.**17**)

Frequency: relatively rare.

Suggestive morphologic findings: exophytic growth, often involving the mandibular condyle, with continuity of the medullary cavity.

Procedure: thin-slice CT scans, dental CT as required.

Other studies: panoramic radiograph.

Checklist for scan interpretation:
▶ Differential diagnosis.
▶ Assess degree of temporomandibular joint degeneration or deformity (if possible).

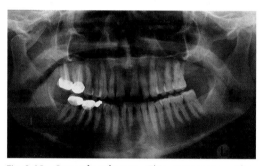

Fig. 9.**16** **Osteochondroma.** This panoramic radiograph in a woman with chronic, progressive symptoms in the right temporomandibular joint demonstrates an exophytic bone spur arising from the neck of the mandible.

Pathogenesis

Osteochondroma is a common benign tumor of the juvenile skeletal system. The mandibular condyle is a site of predilection where large osteochondromas can develop, particularly in young women. Located anterior to the actual articular surface of the temporomandibular joint, these tumors can obstruct movements of the joint and lead to facial deformity. In very advanced cases, a kind of neoarticulation may form between the osteochondroma and skull base. Small osteochondromas often lead to traumatic articular disk lesions and arthrotic changes in the temporomandibular joint.

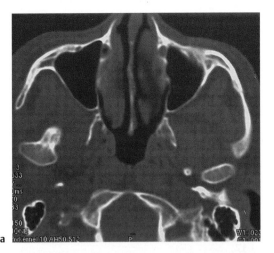

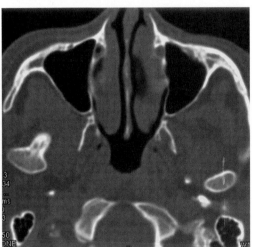

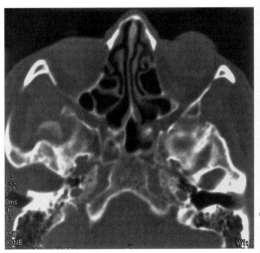

Fig. 9.**17 a–c Osteochondroma.** Typical appearance of osteochondroma on axial bone-window CT scans. Note the continuity of the cortex and medullary cavity. Note also the marked indentation at the skull base representing a neoarticulation.

Ossifying Fibroma (Figs. 9.**18**, 9.**19**)

Frequency: rare.

Suggestive morphologic findings: homogeneous tumor matrix with an intact cortex, resembles fibrous dysplasia.

Procedure: coronal thin-slice CT scans. Dental CT may be helpful for mandibular lesions.

Other studies: MRI may demonstrate contrast enhancement.

Checklist for scan interpretation:
▶ Differential diagnosis.
▶ Signs of temporomandibular osteoarthritis?

■ Pathogenesis

This entity is histologically related to fibrous dysplasia and adamantinoma. It is composed of maturing spindle cells with osteoblastic activity surrounded by a network of cartilaginous and osseous structures. The facial skeleton is a common site of occurrence. Maxillary lesions can grow within the maxillary sinus for some time without producing symptoms (Fig. 9.**18**).

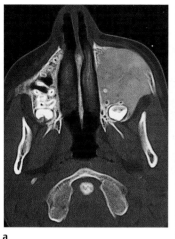
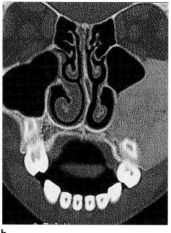
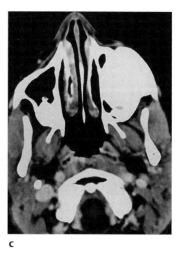

a   b   c

Fig. 9.**18 a–c   Ossifying fibroma.** The maxillary sinus is almost completely filled with a homogeneous mass of fibrous tissue, whose only clinical manifestation was facial deformity. **c** This scan, obtained after intravenous contrast administration, shows no further density increase, owing to the inherently faint enhancement pattern of these tumors on CT.

■ Frequency

Ossifying fibroma is relatively rare. Women are predominantly affected, and the peak occurrence is in the second to fourth decades of life.

■ Clinical Manifestations

Usually presents as a painless expansion of dentulous segments of the maxilla or mandible.

■ CT Morphology

Ossifying fibroma may be indistinguishable from fibrous dysplasia in its CT features, and even histologically. A key feature that distinguishes ossifying fibroma is its enhancement after intravenous contrast administration (Fig. 9.**19**). This does usually not occur in fibrous dysplasia.

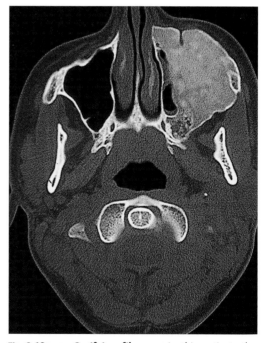

Fig. 9.**19 a–c   Ossifying fibroma.** In this patient, the CT examination (**a**) was supplemented by gadolinium-enhanced magnetic resonance imaging (MRI) to help differentiate between ossifying fibroma and fibrous dysplasia. T1-weighted MRI after contrast administration (**c**) shows a conspicuous increase in signal intensity compared with the precontrast image (**b**).

Fig. 9.**19 a–c** ▷

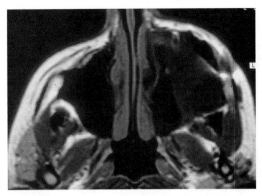

Fig. 9.**19 b**

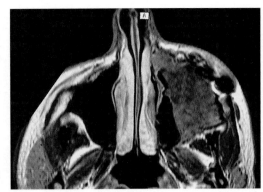

Fig. 9.**19 c**

Cholesterol Granuloma (Figs. 9.**20**, 9.**21**)

Frequency: the most common lesion of the petrous apex.

Suggestive morphologic findings: petrous apex mass of soft-tissue density; may show faint ring enhancement after contrast administration.

Procedure: thin-slice bone-window CT.

Other studies: MRI to differentiate from cholesteatoma and mucocele.

Checklist for scan interpretation:
▶ Degree of erosion.
▶ If significant, refer for MRI.

■ Pathogenesis

Cholesterol granuloma is a nonspecific, chronic inflammatory lesion of the middle ear and mastoid. Histologically, it consists of cholesterol crystals surrounded by foreign-body giant cells and embedded in a fibrous connective tissue containing hemosiderin-laden macrophages, inflammatory cells, and blood vessels. If the tympanic membrane is intact, cholesterol granuloma may be indistinguishable from a glomus tumor by otoscopic inspection.

■ Frequency

Cholesterol granuloma is the most common primary lesion of the petrous apex.

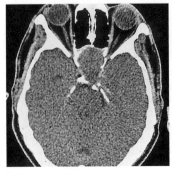

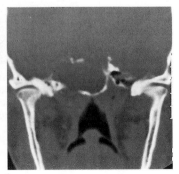

Fig. 9.**20 a, b Cholesterol granuloma.** Axial and coronal thin-slice CT scans demonstrate a destructive soft-tissue lesion of the petrous apex with involvement of the sella.

a   b

■ **Clinical Manifestations**

The chronic inflammatory process sometimes leads to erosion of the small auditory ossicles.

■ **CT Morphology**

Cholesterol granuloma appears on CT as a sharply circumscribed mass of soft-tissue or fat attenuation usually located in the petrous apex (Fig. 9.**20**). By its CT features alone, cholesterol granuloma may be indistinguishable from a cholesteatoma or mucocele of this region. A faint ring of enhancement sometimes appears around the lesion following contrast administration. MRI is necessary for differential diagnosis (Fig. 9.**21**).

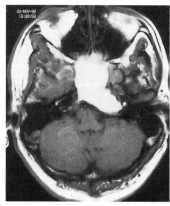

Fig. 9.**21 Cholesterol granuloma.** Due to its cholesterol content, the mass shows very high signal intensity on unenhanced T1-weighted magnetic resonance imaging.

Cholesteatoma

> **Frequency:** primary cholesteatoma is less common (approximately 2%) than the acquired form (98%).
>
> **Suggestive morphologic findings:** a mass of soft-tissue density eroding the bony structures in the middle ear cavity, bordering the tympanic membrane; does not enhance after contrast administration.
>
> **Procedure:** thin-slice CT, high-resolution CT, coronal and axial scans.
>
> **Other studies:** CT is the method of choice.
>
> **Checklist for scan interpretation:**
> ▶ Differentiate from other neoplastic lesions and from cholesterol granuloma.
> ▶ Ossicular erosion?

■ **Pathogenesis**

Two types of cholesteatoma are recognized:

• Congenital or primary cholesteatoma (rare)
• Acquired cholesteatoma (more common)

Congenital (primary) cholesteatoma. Congenital cholesteatomas are derived from embryonic ectodermal cell rests. By definition, they are associated with an intact tympanic membrane, and occur in the absence of antecedent otitis media. Cholesteatomas have the histologic characteristics of an epidermoid cyst. They are most commonly located in the anterior superior quadrant of the middle ear with involvement of the internal auditory canal, but they may occur anywhere in the petrous bone, in the cerebellopontine angle meninges, or in the jugular fossa. A special form of cholesteatoma involving the pars flaccida of the tympanic membrane, known as "occult cholesteatoma," is often indistinguishable from primary cholesteatoma. It leaves the tympanic membrane intact and shows a predominantly papillary growth pattern in the attic of the middle ear.

Acquired cholesteatoma. Acquired cholesteatoma is not a tumor in the true sense but a chronic inflammatory process leading to the progressive erosion of adjacent structures. For an acquired cholesteatoma to develop, keratinizing squamous epithelium from the external auditory canal has to come into direct contact with the mucoperiosteum of the middle ear. Various theories have been advanced to explain these lesions, including ingrowth of squamous epithelium through a retraction pocket in the tympanic membrane caused by chronic negative pressure in the middle ear cavity; ingrowth through a defect in the tympanic membrane; metaplastic transformation of the mucosa secondary to chronic otitis media; and deep penetration by papillary tissue growth. It has also been suggested that cholesteatoma results from a petrous bone fracture, causing the displacement of keratinizing squamous epithelium.

Regardless of the etiology, CT demonstrates signs of a slow-growing erosive mass lesion.

■ Frequency

Primary cholesteatoma accounts for only about 2% of cases. The remaining 98% are acquired lesions that develop in association with otitis media.

■ Clinical Manifestations

Besides the sequelae of chronic otitis media, the clinical manifestations of cholesteatoma are determined by its erosive effects on surrounding bone. Hearing loss can result from destruction of the cochlea or compression of the vestibulocochlear nerve. A labyrinthine fistula can lead to vertiginous symptoms, and facial nerve compression can lead to peripheral facial nerve palsy.

■ CT Morphology

CT is the imaging modality of choice, as it is better than MRI for demonstrating both the soft-tissue mass and the associated bone erosion. Accurate imaging requires thin-section, high-resolution axial and coronal CT scans. A mass of soft-tissue attenuation accompanied by bony erosion in the middle ear cavity adjacent to the tympanic membrane confirms the diagnosis. Ossicular destruction or displacement may also be observed. The lesions do not show contrast enhancement on CT or MRI.

Glomus Tumor (Paraganglioma)

■ **Frequency:** rare.

Suggestive morphologic findings: glomus tympanicum tumor—soft-tissue mass in the middle ear cavity; *glomus jugulare tumor*—erosion or enlargement of the jugular fossa, erosion of the petrous bone. Typical density curve after bolus contrast injection.

Procedure: thin-slice bone-window CT, dynamic contrast examination.

Other studies: MRI, angiography to establish the diagnosis, identify feeding vessels, and if necessary guide preoperative embolization.

Checklist for scan interpretation:
▶ Differentiate from other masses in the region.
▶ Degree of bone erosion?

■ Pathogenesis

Glomus tumors are of neuroectodermal origin and arise from nonchromaffin cells of the sympathetic paraganglia. They are among the most common masses of the middle ear. Glomus tumors of the skull base region are classified as follows, according to their pattern of spread:

- Glomus jugulare tumor
- Glomus vagale tumor
- Glomus tympanicum tumor
- Glomus hypotympanicum tumor

Glomus jugulare tumor leads to expansion and destruction of the jugular fossa and hypoglossal canal, and erodes the undersurface of the petrous pyramid. Glomus tympanicum tumor can usually be diagnosed clinically from the presence of a bluish retrotympanic mass. Glomus vagale tumor develops near the ganglion nodosum at the skull base and then usually spreads downward into the parapharyngeal space. Combined intracranial and extracranial growth, resulting in an hourglass-shaped mass, is rare.

All glomus tumors have a rich blood supply that can be demonstrated angiographically and by dynamic imaging after bolus contrast infusion. Glomus tumors are often classified into four types to facilitate surgical planning. This classification is based mainly on the tumor location, and secondarily on tumor size and extent:

- Type A: glomus tympanicum tumor.
- Type B: glomus hypotympanicum tumor.
- Type C: purely extracranial glomus jugulare tumor. Four subtypes are distinguished, depending on the degree of skull base erosion.
- Type D: glomus jugulare tumor with intracranial involvement.

■ Frequency

Glomus tumors are rare, making up approximately 0.6 % of head and neck tumors. Nevertheless, glomus tympanicum tumor is the most common neoplasm of the middle ear. Women predominate by a 6 : 1 ratio.

■ Clinical Manifestations

The symptoms depend on tumor location and size. Conductive hearing loss or cranial nerve deficits are usually the dominant features. Involvement of the labyrinth can lead to tinnitus, vertigo, and sensorineural hearing loss. Because of their neuroectodermal origin, glomus tumors have the capacity to secrete catecholamines, serotonin, histamine, and kallikrein. The resulting systemic symptoms as well as hazardous peri-interventional blood pressure peaks can be treated with alpha and beta blockers. The effects of serotonin and histamine secretion can be treated with alpha agonists or somatostatin analogs.

■ CT Morphology

The bone erosion and destruction caused by glomus tumors are manifested on noncontrast CT by expansion of the jugular foramen or the destruction of petrous bone structures. These changes are best appreciated on bone-window scans. When the findings suggest a glomus tumor, the diagnosis can be supported by performing a dynamic examination after bolus contrast injection. Glomus tumors that have not been embolized or thrombosed show a characteristic attenuation curve, with an immediate sharp upslope to an initial peak fol-

lowed by a brief decline and then another rise to a plateau. Several minutes later, the attenuation shows a gradual decline. This pattern is useful in differentiating small tumor masses from a high jugular bulb. While the initial peak in a glomus tumor results from early arterial perfusion, a high bulb will show a delayed peak caused purely by venous flow.

MRI sometimes provides better delineation of the tumor, which often shows a typical "salt-and-pepper" heterogeneous appearance caused by numerous flow voids. Diagnostic angiography confirms the diagnosis and is used preoperatively to identify the main feeding arteries. It can also be used to direct preoperative tumor embolization to minimize the risk of severe bleeding. MRI has largely replaced retrograde venography to demonstrate tumor growth within the jugular vein.

Glomus tympanicum tumor. CT demonstrates a soft-tissue mass in the middle ear cavity that may create a bulge in the tympanic membrane. Smaller tumors accompanied by inflammation and fluid accumulation in the middle ear cavity may be missed on CT, and MRI is definitely superior for this indication.

Glomus jugulare tumor. CT demonstrates erosion and enlargement of the jugular fossa. Larger tumors may cause posteroinferior erosion of the petrous bone.

Tumors of the Pharynx, Nasal Cavity, and Paranasal Sinuses: Squamous-Cell Carcinoma, Lymphoepithelial and Adenoid Cystic Carcinoma, Adenocarcinoma, Juvenile Angiofibroma
(Figs. 9.**22**–9.**28**)

Frequency: squamous-cell carcinoma is the most common tumor in this region.

Suggestive morphologic findings: a soft-tissue mass with associated inflammation and possible bone infiltration.

Procedure: axial scans are used for staging and evaluating lymph-node status. Coronal scans are used to exclude intracranial involvement.

Other studies: MRI generally provides better tumor delineation from surrounding tissues, inflammatory changes, and accumulated secretions. The added capacity for multiplanar imaging makes MRI superior to CT.

Checklist for scan interpretation:
▶ In most cases, the various tumor types that occur in this region are indistinguishable by CT.
▶ Assess the extent of infiltration (especially of structures inaccessible to direct or indirect endoscopic inspection—e.g., intracranial involvement or encasement of major neck vessels).
▶ Stage determination.
▶ Lymph-node status.

■ Pathogenesis

Squamous-cell carcinoma. Squamous-cell carcinoma is the most common pharyngeal tumor, accounting for 90 % of tumors of the nasopharynx. Although rare, squamous-cell carcinoma is becoming increasingly important, as it is one of the neoplastic diseases for which the incidence has been rising in recent years. Smoking and alcohol abuse have been cited as prime risk factors. Squamous-cell carcinoma of the nasopharynx has a strong predilection for skull base involvement and intracranial extension. Approximately 75 % originate from the pharyngeal recess, and about 50 % of these tumors spread toward the cranium and infiltrate the sphenoid sinus or invade the cranial cavity through the jugular foramen, foramen ovale, and foramen rotundum. The evaluation of tumor extent in these cases relies on thin-slice coronal scans acquired before and after contrast administration. The tumor itself often shows only moderate enhancement. Axial scans should also be obtained to evaluate nodal involvement.

The nasal cavity and paranasal sinuses are also sites of predilection for squamous-cell carcinoma, which makes up approximately 80 % of sinonasal malignancies. The maxillary sinus is the most frequent site of occurrence (about 80 % of cases), followed by the nasal cavity and ethmoid cells. The frontal and sphenoid sinuses are very rarely affected.

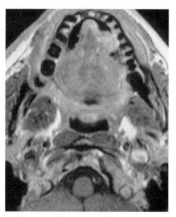

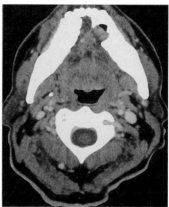

Fig. 9.**22 a, b** **Squamous-cell carcinoma of the anterior oral floor with erosion of the mandible.** T1-weighted magnetic resonance image (**a**) and CT (**b**) after intravenous contrast administration.

a

b

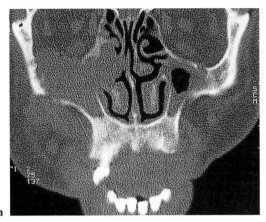

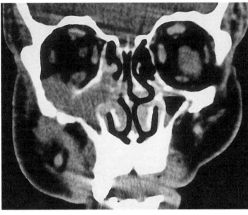

Fig. 9.**23 a, b   Tumor of the right maxillary sinus.** This tumor has led to destruction of the orbital floor and the medial wall of the maxillary sinus. Histologic examina-

tion identified the lesion as non-Hodgkin lymphoma, which is indistinguishable by CT from the far more common squamous-cell carcinoma.

CT contributes little to the differential diagnosis, due both to the marked predominance of squamous-cell carcinoma and to the lack of morphologic differentiating criteria. We shall therefore mention only briefly the most important differential diagnoses that should be considered.

Lymphoepithelial carcinoma and adenoid cystic carcinoma. Lymphoepithelial and adenoid cystic carcinomas are distinguished by their relatively aggressive behavior, with early invasion of adjacent structures, marked signs of bone erosion, and intracranial extension from a relatively small primary tumor.

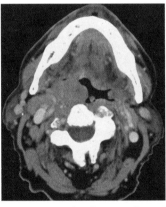

Fig. 9.**24   Involvement of the right pharyngeal tonsil by non-Hodgkin lymphoma.** There is concomitant involvement of a jugulodigastric lymph node on the right side.

Fig. 9.**25 a, b   Nasopharyngeal carcinoma.** This tumor completely fills both choanae, and has already infiltrated and eroded the bony skull base.

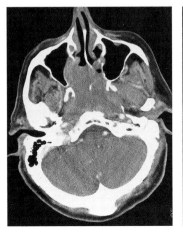

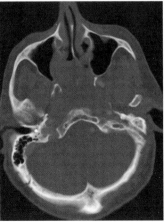

a

b

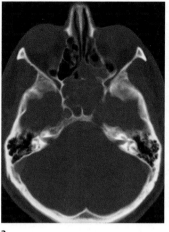
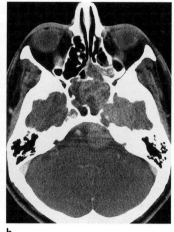

a   b

Fig. 9.**26 a, b Nasopharyngeal carcinoma.** This carcinoma has filled the sphenoid sinus and portions of the ethmoid sinus and has spread intracranially through the medial sphenoid wing. Tumor components are visible at intrasellar and perisellar sites and in the middle and posterior fossae, where tumor is already compressing the brain stem.

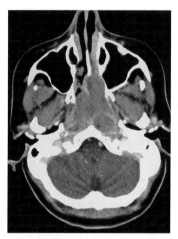
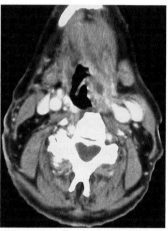

Fig. 9.**27 Nasopharyngeal carcinoma.** This tumor is obstructing the choanae and has started to erode and infiltrate the petrous bone from the jugular fossa.

Fig. 9.**28 Central hypodense mass of the left hypopharynx at the level of the epiglottis.** Visual inspection, clinical parameters, and rapid response to antibiotics indicated a suppurative inflammatory process. Biopsy was still performed to exclude malignant disease. The CT features alone cannot rule out a degenerating tumor with central necrosis.

Juvenile angiofibroma. Juvenile angiofibroma is a histologically benign but locally invasive hypervascular tumor that occurs almost exclusively in teenage boys. These tumors almost always arise from the nasopharynx and infiltrate the maxillary sinus, nasal cavity, and sphenoid and ethmoid sinuses. They may extend into the orbit through the inferior orbital fissure, and intracranial extension can occur through the skull base foramina. Because of their hypervascularity, these tumors enhance intensely following contrast administration. This distinguishes them from other common nasopharyngeal tumors, and provides an aid to differential diagnosis. Juvenile angiofibromas often present clinically with recurrent, intractable epistaxis.

■ Frequency

Squamous-cell carcinomas are the most common tumors of the pharynx, nasal cavity, and paranasal sinuses. The peak incidence is after 40 years of age (50–60), although the average age at initial presentation has declined in recent years. Men are still affected about twice as frequently as women, but the incidence among women has been rising.

■ Clinical Manifestations

The symptoms of sinonasal tumors are location-dependent, and include dull unilateral pain, purulent nasal discharge, swelling, olfactory impairment, and nasal airway obstruction. Local pain is usually the most common early symptom of nasopharyngeal, hypopharyngeal and oropharyngeal tumors, and may result from inflammation due to tumor-associated ulceration.

■ CT Morphology

The CT findings are nonspecific in terms of distinguishing malignant tumors from one another or from benign lesions. Contrast administration is not always helpful, since most tumors and surrounding inflammatory changes show only moderate enhancement. CT cannot accurate define the extent of tumor infiltration.

Intravenous contrast administration can, however, detect intracranial extension by demonstrating enhancement of the meninges or parenchyma. Solid and cystic tumor components, which may contain necrotic areas, can be distinguished from each other by their enhancement patterns. Contrast administration also aids tumor differentiation from vessels, especially in the evaluation of lymph-node status.

Schwannoma (Fig. 9.**29**)

Frequency: common.

Suggestive morphologic findings: a mass showing intense enhancement, regardless of its location. Acoustic schwannoma may cause expansion of the internal auditory canal.

Procedure: thin-slice high-resolution CT is used to define the internal auditory canal, semicircular canals, and jugular bulb. Scanning is repeated after intravenous contrast injection.

Other studies: MRI is the study of first choice for demonstrating small acoustic schwannomas owing to its higher sensitivity for contrast enhancement.

Checklist for scan interpretation:
▶ Degree of compression of vital structures—e.g., displacement of the brain stem and extent of bone erosion?
▶ Detect or exclude other mass lesions (e.g., that might suggest neurofibromatosis).
▶ Exclude meningiomas and intra-axial brain tumors.
▶ Surgical planning: relationship of the semicircular canals and jugular bulb to the tumor and route of surgical approach (a high bulb should definitely be noted).

■ Pathogenesis

Schwannomas are the most common tumors of the skull base region. They may arise from the trigeminal nerve, facial nerve, and especially from the vestibular portion of the vestibulocochlear nerve. The clinical presentation offers essential clues to the location and classification of neurogenic tumors. For example, trigeminal neuromas alter the sensation of the facial skin and can cause severe pain. Schwannomas of the hypoglossal nerve can lead to unilateral palsy of the lingual muscles with dysphagia, speech impediment, and fatty degeneration of the lingual muscles.

Although schwannomas are benign, they can cause erosion of surrounding bony structures (Fig. 9.**29**).

Differentiation is mainly required from meningiomas, glomus tumors, epidermoids, and other rare masses.

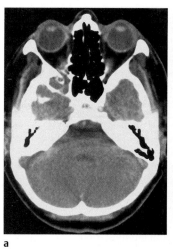
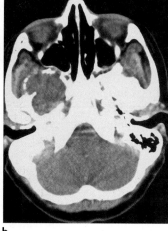
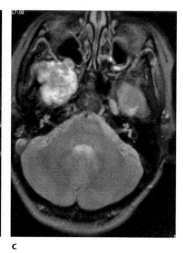

a   b   c

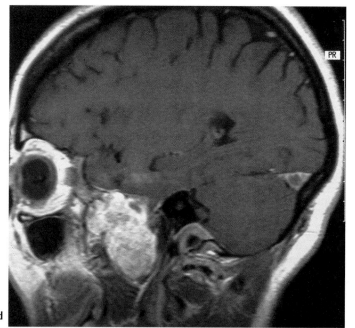

Fig. 9.29 a–d Classic imaging appearance of a schwannoma.

a, b CT scans in a patient with nonspecific headaches demonstrate a large mass in the pterygopalatine fossa that has eroded the pterygoid processes and the lateral wall of the maxillary sinus.

c The mass shows high signal intensity on T2-weighted magnetic resonance imaging.

d The tumor enhances very strongly after contrast administration. A small nodular extension is also seen projecting into the maxillary sinus.

d

Acoustic schwannoma. Acoustic schwannomas are classified as intrameatal or extrameatal, depending on whether they are located inside or outside the internal auditory canal. The earlier term "acoustic neurinoma" was a misnomer, as the tumor arises almost exclusively from the vestibular portion of the auditory nerve at the junction of the central and peripheral myelin sheaths. "Vestibular schwannoma" would be a more accurate term.

Approximately 95% of acoustic schwannomas arise from the intrameatal junction of the central, glial nerve sheath with the peripheral sheaths. Because of this location, they initially cause expansion of the internal auditory canal and extend from there toward the cerebellopontine angle. Only about 5% arise from the cerebellopontine angle and invade the canal secondarily. Acoustic schwannomas are histologically benign tumors based on a genetic defect. Approximately 95% are unilateral. Bilateral acoustic schwannomas are pathognomonic for neurofibromatosis type 2. This diagnosis should also be considered in patients under 40 years of age.

■ Frequency

Acoustic schwannomas make up approximately 5–7% (or up to 10%) of all intracranial tumors, 85% of intracranial schwannomas, and 80–90% of cerebellopontine angle tumors. Trigeminal neuromas are much less common, accounting for just 0.26% of brain tumors. The peak age incidence for both forms is between 35 and 60 years, and women predominate by a ratio of 2 : 1.

■ Clinical Manifestations

Clinical symptoms are determined mainly by cranial nerve deficits. The dominant features of acoustic schwannoma are hearing loss, dysequilibrium, and ipsilateral cerebellar hemispheric signs.

■ CT Morphology

Even with small acoustic schwannomas, CT often demonstrates expansion of the internal auditory canal, although lack of expansion does not exclude acoustic schwannoma in patients with clinical signs of an intrameatal mass. Like schwannomas of other cranial nerves, acoustic schwannomas usually show intense contrast enhancement, but this is more difficult to appreciate on thin-slice CT scans than on MRI, especially with smaller tumors. Large acoustic schwannomas sometimes have a lobulated, cystic appearance.

Intrathecal administration of 3–4 mL of air, followed by radiographic examination with the patient in the lateral decubitus position with the affected side up, can demonstrate an intrameatal mass indirectly as an air-filling defect in the internal auditory canal. This technique, known as pneumocysternography, is mainly of historical interest and is used only if MRI is unavailable.

A Stenvers radiograph is often sufficient to demonstrate a right–left disparity in the width of the internal auditory canal. In positive cases, the disparity should exceed 2 mm, or the canal lumen should be expanded to more than 8 mm.

However, MRI is the imaging procedure of choice for demonstrating acoustic schwannomas and trigeminal neuromas, especially when the lesions are small. The best technique consists of thin coronal and axial T1-weighted sequences after intravenous contrast administration.

Midfacial and Skull Base Fractures

Frequency: a common associated injury in trauma patients.

Suggestive morphologic findings: a linear hypodensity without sclerotic margins, possible intracranial or intraorbital air, air–fluid level in the paranasal sinus (hematosinus).

Procedure: thin CT slices, coronal if possible, otherwise reformatted. Use the bone-window setting.

Other studies: conventional radiographs.

Checklist for scan interpretation:
▶ Fracture classification: open skull fracture with intracranial air? Orbital blow-out fracture with herniation of fat or extraocular muscle entrapment?

■ Pathogenesis

The incidence of skull fractures increases with the severity of the trauma. In one series of 151 patients with fatal head injuries, skull fractures were found in 81% at autopsy. Severe comminuted midfacial fractures are a common steering-wheel injury sustained in motor-vehicle accidents. Moreover, any kind of traumatic impact to the midfacial region can produce typical fracture patterns, determined by the severity and location of the traumatizing force. CT is the diagnostic method of first choice for this type of injury. In particular, it can accurately define the extent of fractures involving the skull base and determine whether the patient has sustained an open or closed head injury. Less severe impacts that occur during sports or fist fights often lead to more localized fracture patterns, such as blow-out fractures of the orbital floor and lamina papyracea, or a "tripod fracture" of the zygoma.

The principal fracture patterns are reviewed below.

Tripod fracture (Figs. 9.30, 9.31). This fracture derives its name from the fact that essentially three pillars ("feet") are involved. The fracture line passes through the lateral orbital wall (frequently involving the frontozygomatic su-

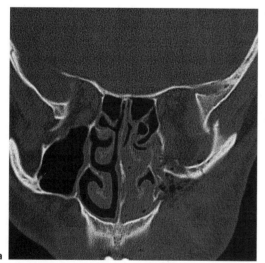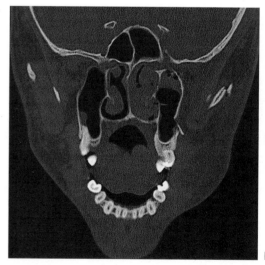

a

b

Fig. 9.**30 a, b   Tripod fracture.** Coronal CT views of a classic tripod fracture caused by a fall onto the left zygoma. The fracture extends through the zygomatic arch, the inferior wall of the maxillary sinus, and the floor and lateral wall of the orbit. Secondary fracture signs are blood in the maxillary sinus and intraorbital air.

ture), the zygomatic arch, the inferior orbital wall, and part of the lateral wall of the maxillary sinus. Maxillary hematosinus is almost always present.

Le Fort fractures (Fig. 9.32). Le Fort classified midfacial fractures into three basic types. All of the Le Fort fractures have a fairly symmetrical pattern:

- The Le Fort I fracture is a transmaxillary fracture that separates the maxilla from the rest of the midface. The fracture line runs through the alveolar process of the maxilla, the bony nasal aperture, and the inferior wall of the maxillary sinus.
- The Le Fort II fracture, sometimes called a zygomaticomaxillary fracture, starts at the nasal dorsum and extends laterally and obliquely to the nasal cavity, passing through the medial orbital wall, orbital floor, and inferior orbital rim.
- A Le Fort III fracture is one that creates a disjunction between the neurocranium and viscerocranium. The fracture line usually passes through the nasal dorsum, frontal sinus, frontozygomatic suture, lateral orbital wall, and zygomatic arch.

Orbital fractures (Figs. 9.33, 9.34). Isolated orbital fractures usually result from a direct impact to the globe, causing an abrupt rise of intraorbital pressure. Often this creates a "blow-out" mechanism that fractures the orbital floor and the thin lamina papyracea in the medial wall. Blow-out fractures may be complicated by the herniation of orbital fat and of extraocular muscles, particularly the inferior rectus and inferior oblique. This often results in impaired ocular motility or enophthalmos. Since the outcome of orbital blow-out fractures depends on the extent of herniation and on the early operative treatment of larger defects, particular attention should be given to these complications during imaging evaluation.

It is interest to note that some authors have advocated CT volumetry of the orbit in the planning of reconstructive surgery to correct posttraumatic enophthalmos.

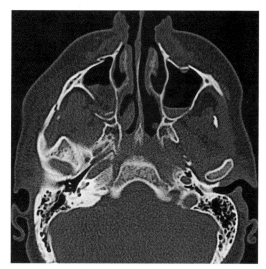

Fig. 9.**31 Tripod fracture.** Axial CT scan of a tripod fracture in a different patient, caused by a fist blow to the right zygoma. The depressed position of the fragment clearly indicates the mechanism of the fracture. There is blood in both maxillary sinuses, that on the left side having been caused by a concomitant fracture of the orbital floor and anterior sinus wall.

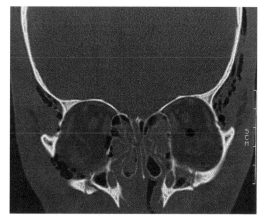

Fig. 9.**32 Le Fort fracture.** The Le Fort II fracture extends through the orbital floor, the anterior wall of the maxillary sinus, and the ethmoid cells. Air is visible inside and outside the orbital cone.

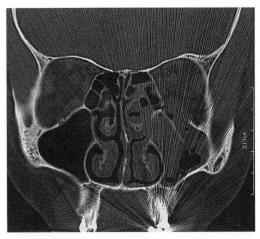

Fig. 9.**33** **Left orbital blow-out fracture.** A fist blow to the zygoma caused a sudden increase in intraorbital pressure, producing a blow-out fracture in the orbital floor and the lamina papyracea of the medial orbital wall. Secondary fracture signs consist of blood in the maxillary sinus and ethmoid cells and intraorbital extraconal air. There is no sign of entrapment of the inferior rectus and inferior oblique muscles, although the patient did have impaired ocular motility, with decreased upward gaze and mild diplopia.

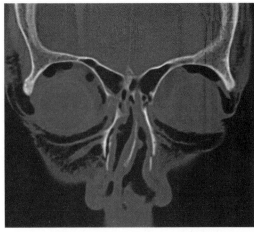

Fig. 9.**34** **Extensive intraorbital and periorbital soft-tissue emphysema resulting from a midfacial fracture involving the nasal bone and medial orbital wall.** Even in the absence of visible fracture lines, an intraorbital air collection after trauma is considered proof of a fracture. A phlegmonous infection with gas-forming bacteria is easily excluded by clinical examination.

Frontobasal fractures (Fig. 9.35). A blow to the frontal pillar or a very localized frontal impact can produce a frontobasal fracture involving the orbital roof and frontal sinus. Involvement of the posterior wall of the frontal sinus is likely to produce complications, as it constitutes an open fracture with risk of ascending infection.

Blunt trauma can produce various combinations of frontobasal fractures that include the following patterns.

- High frontobasal fracture with involvement of the frontal bone, posterior frontal sinus wall, and crista galli.
- Midbasal fracture with involvement of the frontal sinus, ethmoid cells, and cribriform plate.
- Low frontobasal fracture with involvement of the maxillary sinuses, ethmoid cells, orbit, and sphenoid sinus.

Petrous bone fractures (Figs. 9.36–9.38). In addition to various mixed forms, two main types of petrous bone fracture are recognized. Each is associated with a particular set of symptoms and potential complications:

- Longitudinal fractures are by far the more common type (70–90%). They usually extend through the suture between the squamous and petrous parts of the temporal bone and run parallel to or through the external auditory canal. They continue between the cochlea and semicircular canals, sparing cranial nerves VII and VIII but frequently disrupting the ossicular chain.
- Transverse fractures of the petrous bone run perpendicular to the external auditory canal and cross the cochlea, and may cause stretching, shearing, or tearing of cranial nerves VII and VIII or the geniculate ganglion. Longitudinal petrous bone fractures mainly cause middle ear involvement with

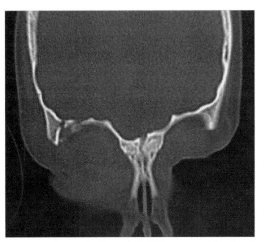

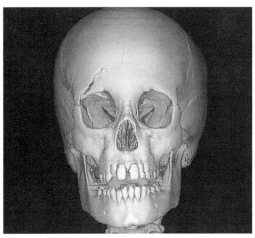

b

Fig. 9.**35 a, b** **Right frontal skull fracture with orbital roof involvement caused by a localized impact to the right frontal pillar.** The shaded surface reconstruction in **a** clearly demonstrates the depressed area and the fracture line through the orbital roof.

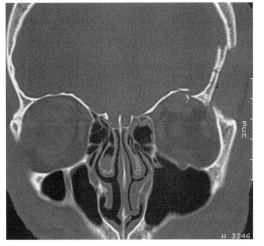

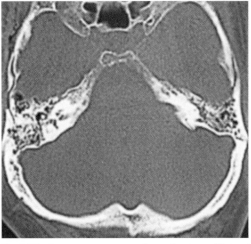

Fig. 9.**36** **Depressed fracture of the left frontal pillar.** This fracture was caused by severe blunt trauma sustained during a fall. It involves the calvarium, orbital roof, and left orbital wall. Small subcutaneous and subgaleal air collections are a result of concomitant soft-tissue injury.

Fig. 9.**37** **Transverse petrous bone fracture.** Bilateral petrous bone fractures with extension into the mastoid cells and hemorrhagic foci.

hematotympanum, rupture of the tympanic membrane, bleeding from the external auditory canal, conductive hearing loss, occasional facial nerve palsy (ca. 20%), and rarely cerebrospinal fluid (CSF) otorrhea. Transverse fractures, on the other hand, are characterized by inner ear involvement with an intact external auditory canal and tym-panic membrane, deafness, vertigo, nystagmus, and facial nerve palsy in approximately 50% of cases. Since the tympanic membrane is intact, CSF leakage usually occurs through the eustachian tube into the pharyngeal space. Besides the initial effects of the injury, an ascending infection from the pharynx can lead to meningitis or encephalitis.

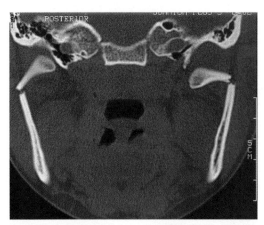

Fig. 9.**38** **Bilateral condylar neck fractures,** with medial displacement of the condyles due to muscular traction.

■ Frequency

Trauma patients are frequently evaluated for midfacial and basal skull fractures.

■ Clinical Manifestations

Clinical symptoms are determined by the location and extent of the injury and the functional impairment of nerve pathways, such as facial nerve palsy due to transverse petrous bone fractures or impaired ocular motility following an orbital blow-out fracture.

■ CT Morphology

CT scans are evaluated for fracture signs using the same technique previously described for identifying isolated calvarial fractures. The fracture lines usually appear as linear or hairline hypodensities that do not have sclerotic margins. Indirect radiographic signs are helpful and sometimes conclusive in disclosing the presence of an otherwise occult fracture. The detection of intraorbital or intracranial air or an air–fluid level caused by maxillary hematosinus can direct attention to the presence of an open skull fracture or maxillary fracture.

Two basic technical strategies are followed in imaging evaluation. First, evaluation of the bony skull base is hampered by partial volume

effects, especially in axial scans parallel to the skull base. For most frontobasal and midfacial fractures, therefore, it is better to start with direct coronal scans if the patient can tolerate and maintain the necessary position. Injuries to the cervical spine in trauma patients should be excluded radiographically. Otherwise, thin axial CT slices can be acquired and used to create reformatted coronal images. The risk of this approach in restless patients is that motion artifacts during volume acquisition will reduce the image quality.

Direct coronal scanning is helpful for evaluating the orbital floor.

■ References

Recommended for further study

Inflammatory sinus disease
Zeifer B. Update on sinonasal imaging: anatomy and inflammatory disease. Neuroimaging Clin N Am 1998; 8: 607–30.
  ● *Describes anatomic details that are important in planning endoscopic operations.*

Choanal atresia
Castillo M. Congenital abnormalities of the nose: CT and MR findings. AJR Am J Roentgenol 1994; 162: 1211–7.
  ● *Detailed look at the CT evaluation of cleft anomalies.*

Otosclerosis
Valvassori GE, Dobben GD. CT densitometry of the cochlear capsule in otosclerosis. AJNR Am J Neuroradiol 1985; 6: 661–7.
  ● *Early approach.*

Ameloblastoma
Minami M, Kaneda T, Ozawa K, Yamamoto H. Cystic lesions of the maxillomandibular region: MR imaging distinction of odontogenic keratocysts and ameloblastomas from other cysts. AJR Am J Roentgenol 1996; 166: 943–9.
  ● *Comprehensive, but the focus is on MRI.*

Odontoma
Sumi M, Yonetsu K, Nakamura T. CT of ameloblastic fibroodontoma. AJR Am J Roentgenol 1997; 169: 599–600.

Cystic lesions of the maxilla and mandible
Minami M, Kaneda T, Ozawa K, Yamamoto H. Cystic lesions of the maxillomandibular region: MR imaging distinction of odontogenic keratocysts and ameloblastomas from other cysts. AJR Am J Roentgenol 1996; 166: 943–9.
  ● *Comprehensive, but the focus is on MRI.*
Yoshiura K, Tabata O, Miwa K, et al. Computed tomographic features of calcifying odontogenic cysts. Dentomaxillofac Radiol 1998; 27: 12–6.
  ● *Four cases, with commentary on examination technique.*

Mucocele, pyocele

Mafee MF, Dobben GD, Valvassori GE. Computed tomography assessment of paraorbital pathology. In: Gonzales CA, Becker MH, Flanagan JC, editors. Diagnostic imaging in ophthalmology. Berlin: Springer, 1985: 281–302.
- *Review.*

Papilloma

Dammann F, Pereira P, Laniado M, Plinkert P, Lowenheim H, Claussen CD. Inverted papilloma of the nasal cavity and the paranasal sinuses: using CT for primary diagnosis and follow-up. AJR Am J Roentgenol 1999; 172: 534–8.
- *Comprehensive analysis of a relatively large number of cases.*

Fibrous dysplasia, Paget disease

Tehranzadeh J, Fung Y, Donohue M, Anavim A, Pribram HW. Computed tomography of Paget disease of the skull versus fibrous dysplasia. Skeletal Radiol 1998; 27: 664–72.
- *Analyzes the importance of roentgen signs for this differential diagnosis.*

Meningioma of the skull base

Tokumaru A, O'uchi T, Eguchi T, et al. Prominent meningeal enhancement adjacent to meningioma on Gd-DTPA–enhanced MR images: histopathologic correlation. Radiology 1990; 175: 431–3.

Aneurysmal bone cyst

Revel MP, Vanel D, Sigal R, et al. Aneurysmal bone cysts of the jaws: CT and MR findings. J Comput Assist Tomogr 1992; 16: 84–6.
- *Description of two cases.*

Giant-cell tumor

Lee HJ, Lum C. Giant cell tumor of the skull base. Neuroradiology 1999; 41: 305–7.

Ossifying fibroma

Han MH, Chang KH, Lee CH, Seo JW, Han MC, Kim CW. Sinonasal psammomatoid ossifying fibromas: CT and MR manifestations. AJNR Am J Neuroradiol 1991; 12: 25–30.
- *Description of cases; points out different enhancement features on CT and MRI.*

Cholesteatoma

Maffe MF. MRI and CT in the evaluation of acquired and congenital cholesteatomas of the temporal bone. J Otolaryngol 1993; 22: 239–48.

Glomus tumor (paraganglioma)

Maffe MH, Valvassori GE, Shugar MA. High-resolution and dynamic sequential computed tomography: use in the evaluation of glomus complex tumors. Arch Otolaryngol 1983; 109: 691–6.

Tumors of the pharyngeal region, nasal cavity, and paranasal sinuses

Silver AJ, Mawad ME, Hilal SK, Sane P, Ganti SR. Computed tomography of the nasopharynx and related spaces, 1: anatomy; 2: pathology. Radiology 1983; 147: 725–31, 733–8.

Schwannoma

Lidov M, Som PM, Stacy C, Catalano P. Eccentric cystic facial schwannoma: CT and MR features. J Comput Assist Tomogr 1991; 15: 1065–7.

Midfacial and skull base fractures

Ali QM, Dietrich B, Becker H. Patterns of skull base fractures: a three-dimensional computed tomography study. Neuroradiology 1994; 36: 622–4.
- *Still of interest, owing to the advanced technique.*

Recent and basic works

Common indications

Alexander AE, Caldemeyer KS, Rigby P. Clinical and surgical application of reformatted high-resolution CT of the temporal bone. Neuroimaging Clin N Am 1998; 8: 631–50.
- *Illustrates the continued superiority of CT over MRI for petrous bone imaging.*

Naito T, Hosokawa R, Yokota M. Three-dimensional alveolar bone morphology analysis using computed tomography. J Periodontol 1998; 69: 584–9.
- *Deals with dental CT.*

Venema HW, Phoa SSKS, Mirck PGB, Hulsmans FJH, Majoie CBLM, Verbeeten B, Jr. /CLPetrosal bone: coronal reconstructions from axial spiral CT data obtained with 0.5-mm collimation can replace direct coronal sequential CT scans. Radiology 1999; 213: 375–82.
- *Replacing direct coronal scans by multiplanar reconstructions without a loss of quality*

Weber AL. Computed tomography and magnetic resonance imaging of the nasopharynx. Isr J Med Sci 1992; 28: 161–8.

Weber AL. History of head and neck radiology: past, present, and future. Radiology 2001; 218: 15–24.
- *Historical overview of improvements and developments in radiologic methods*

Youssefzadeh S, Gahleitner A, Dorffner R, Bernhart T, Kainberger FM. Dental vertical root fractures: value of CT in detection. Radiology 1999; 210: 545–9.

Inflammatory sinus disease

Mason JD, Jones NS, Hughes RJ, Holland IM. A systematic approach to the interpretation of computed tomography scans prior to endoscopic sinus surgery. J Laryngol Otol 1998; 112: 986–90.

Choanal atresia

Admiraal RJ, Joosten FB, Huygen PL. Temporal bone CT findings in the CHARGE association. Int J Pediatr Otorhinolaryngol 1998; 45: 151–62.

Chinwuba C, Wallman J, Strand R. Nasal airway obstruction: CT assessment. Radiology 1986; 159: 503–6.

Jones JE, Young E, Heier L. Congenital bony nasal cavity deformities. Am J Rhinol 1998; 12: 81–6.
- *Review with illustrations based on five cases.*

Otosclerosis

Weissman JL. Hearing loss. Radiology 1996; 199: 593–611.

Ziyeh S, Berlis A, Ross UH, Reinhardt MJ, Schumacher M. MRI of active otosclerosis. Neuroradiology 1997; 39: 453–7.

Ameloblastoma

Kawai T, Murakami S, Kishino M, Matsuya T, Sakuda M, Fuchihata H. Diagnostic imaging in two cases of recurrent maxillary ameloblastoma: comparative evaluation of plain radiographs, CT and MR images. Br J Oral Maxillofac Surg 1998; 36: 304–10.
- *Two cases, with description of contrast enhancement problems in this region.*

Cystic lesions of the maxilla and mandible

Han MH, Chang KH, Lee CH, Na DG, Yeon KM, Han MC. Cystic expansile masses of the maxilla: differential diagnosis with CT and MR. AJNR Am J Neuroradiol 1995; 16: 333–8.

Weber AL, Easter K. Cysts and odontogenic tumors of the mandible and maxilla, 1 and 2. Contemp Diagn Radiol 1982; 5: 1–5.

Mucocele, pyocele

Driben JS, Bolger WE, Robles HA, Cable B, Zinreich SJ. The reliability of computerized tomographic detection of the Onodi (sphenoethmoid) cell. Am J Rhinol 1998; 12: 105–11.

- *Deals with the Onodi cell.*

Lim CC, Dillon WP, McDermott MW. Mucocele involving the anterior clinoid process: MR and CT findings. AJNR Am J Neuroradiol 1999; 20: 287–90.

Stackpole SA, Edelstein DR. The anatomic relevance of the Haller cell in sinusitis. Am J Rhinol 1997; 11: 219–23.

Papilloma

Woodruff WW, Vrabec DP. Inverted papilloma of the nasal vault and paranasal sinuses: spectrum of CT findings. AJR Am J Roentgenol 1994; 162: 419–23.

Fibrous dysplasia

Wenig BM, Mafee MF, Ghosh L. Fibro-osseous, osseous, and cartilaginous lesions of the orbit and paraorbital region: correlative clinicopathologic and radiographic features, including the diagnostic role of CT and MR imaging. Radiol Clin North Am 1998; 36: 241–59.

- *Comprehensive and informative review.*

Paget disease

Khetarpal U, Schuknecht HF. In search of pathologic correlates for hearing loss and vertigo in Paget's disease: a clinical and histopathologic study of 26 temporal bones. Ann Otol Rhinol Laryngol Suppl 1990; 145: 1–16

Meningioma of the skull base

Lang FF, Macdonald OK, Fuller GN, DeMonte F. Primary extradural meningiomas: a report on nine cases and review of the literature from the era of computerized tomography scanning. J Neurosurg 2000; 93(6): 940–50 [Review]

Moulin G, Coatrieux A, Gillot JC. Plaque-like meningioma involving the temporal bone, sinonasal cavities and both parapharyngeal spaces: CT and MRI. Neuroradiology 1994; 36: 629–31.

Aneurysmal bone cyst

Chateil JF, Dousset V, Meyer P, et al. Cranial aneurysmal bone cysts presenting with raised intracranial pressure: report of two cases. Neuroradiology 1997; 39: 490–4.

- *Compares CT and MRI findings in two cases.*

Giant-cell tumor

Rimmelin A, Roth T, George B, Dias P, Clouet PL, Dietemann JL. Giant cell tumor of the sphenoid bone: case report. Neuroradiology 1996; 38: 650–3.

Silvers AR, Som PM, Brandwein M, Chong JL, Shah D. The role of imaging in the diagnosis of giant cell tumor of the skull base. Am J Neuroradiol 1996; 17: 1392–5.

- *Case report.*

Uchino A, Kato A, Yonemitsu N, Hirctsu T, Kudo S. Giant cell reparative granuloma of the cranial vault. Am J Neuroradiol 1996; 17: 1791–3.

Ossifying fibroma

Sterling KM, Stollman A, Sacher M, Som PM. Ossifying fibroma of sphenoid bone with coexistent mucocele: CT and MRI. J Comput Assist Tomogr 1993; 17: 492–4.

Cholesteatoma

Valvassori GE, Buckingham RA. Cholesteatoma of the middle ear and mastoid. In: Valvassori GE, Maffe MF, Carter BL, editors. Imaging of the head and neck. New York: Thieme Medical, 1995: 83–100.

Glomus tumor (paraganglioma)

Vogl TJ, Mack MG, Juergens M, et al. Skull base tumors: gadodiamide injection-enhanced MR-imaging: dropout effect in the early enhancement pattern of paragangliomas versus different tumors. Radiology 1993; 188: 339–46.

Midfacial and skull base fractures

Harris GJ, Garcia GH, Logani SC, et al. Orbital blow-out fractures: correlation of preoperative computed tomography and postoperative ocular motility. Trans Am Ophthalmol Soc 1998; 96: 329–47.

- *Informative article written from a surgical perspective.*

Harris JH, Jr. The cervicocranium: its radiographic assessment. Radiology 2001; 218: 337–51.

Ng P, Chu C, Young N, Soo M. Imaging of orbital floor fractures. Aust Radiol 1996; 40: 264–8.

Schuhknecht B, Carls F, Valavanis A, Sailer HF. CT assessment of orbital volume in late posttraumatic enophthalmos. Neuroradiology 1996; 38: 470–5.

Computed Tomography
of the Spine

Anatomy of the Spine

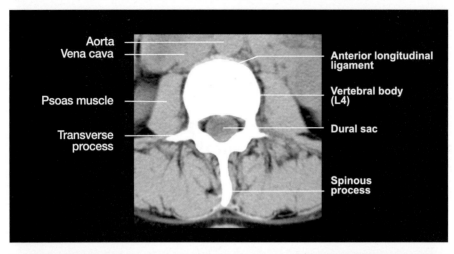

1

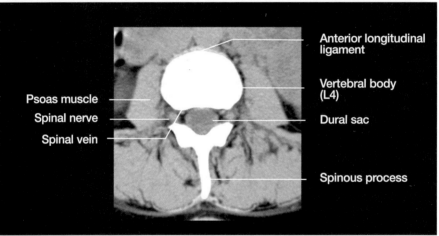

2

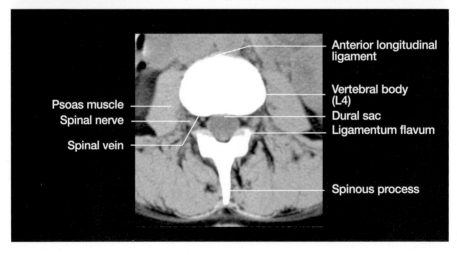

3

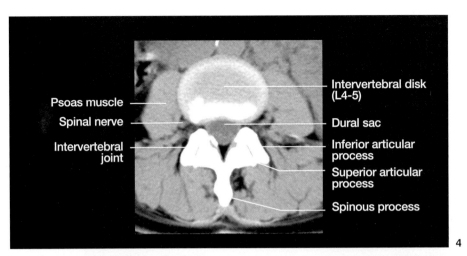

Psoas muscle ——

Spinal nerve ——

Intervertebral joint ——

Intervertebral disk (L4-5)

Dural sac

Inferior articular process

Superior articular process

Spinous process

4

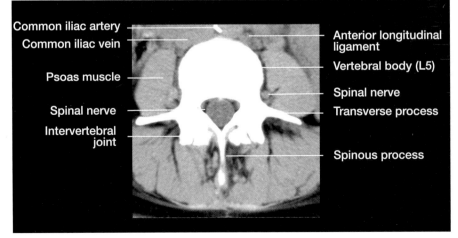

Psoas muscle ——

Spinal nerve ——

Intervertebral joint ——

Anterior longitudinal ligament

Dural sac

Transverse process

Ligamentum flavum

Spinous process

5

Common iliac artery ——

Common iliac vein ——

Psoas muscle ——

Spinal nerve ——

Intervertebral joint ——

Anterior longitudinal ligament

Vertebral body (L5)

Spinal nerve

Transverse process

Spinous process

6

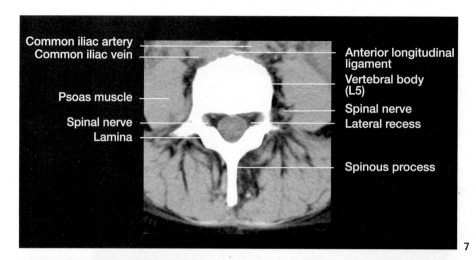

Common iliac artery
Common iliac vein

Psoas muscle

Spinal nerve
Lamina

Anterior longitudinal ligament
Vertebral body (L5)
Spinal nerve
Lateral recess

Spinous process

7

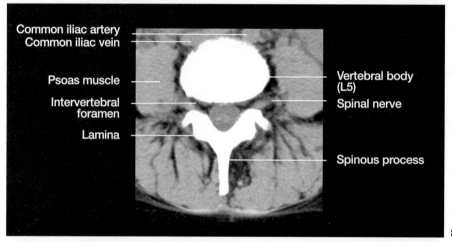

Common iliac artery
Common iliac vein

Psoas muscle

Intervertebral foramen

Lamina

Vertebral body (L5)
Spinal nerve

Spinous process

8

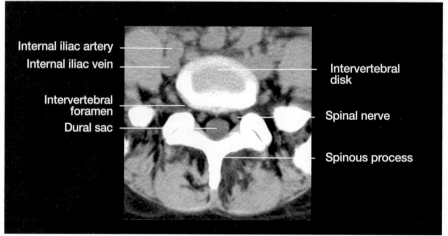

Internal iliac artery
Internal iliac vein

Intervertebral foramen
Dural sac

Intervertebral disk

Spinal nerve

Spinous process

9

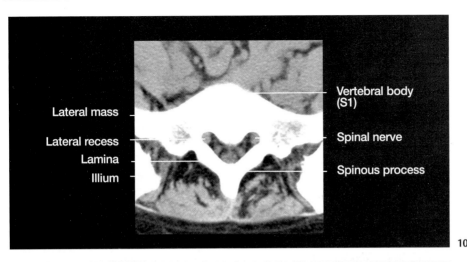

Lateral mass

Lateral recess
Lamina
Illium

Vertebral body
(S1)

Spinal nerve

Spinous process

10

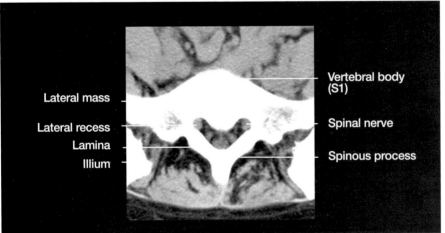

Lateral mass

Lateral recess
Lamina
Illium

Vertebral body
(S1)

Spinal nerve

Spinous process

11

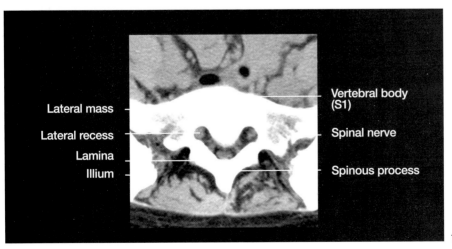

Lateral mass

Lateral recess
Lamina
Illium

Vertebral body
(S1)

Spinal nerve

Spinous process

12

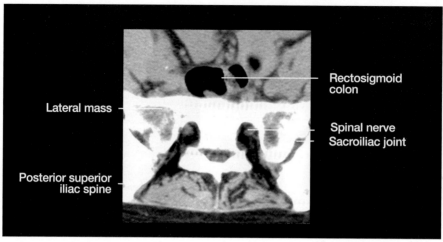

13

Fig. **1–13**   Axial scans parallel to vertebral endplates depicted in soft tissue window-setting

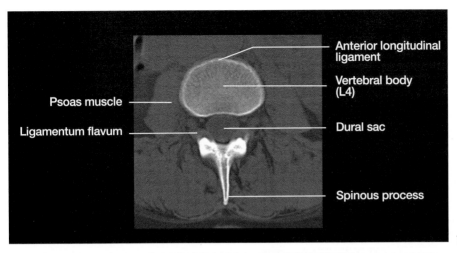

Anterior longitudinal ligament

Vertebral body (L4)

Psoas muscle

Dural sac

Ligamentum flavum

Spinous process

14

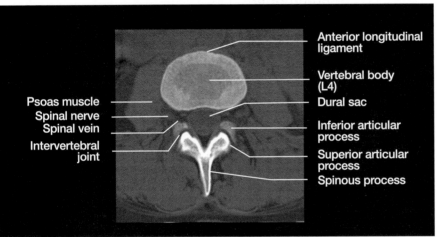

Anterior longitudinal ligament

Vertebral body (L4)

Psoas muscle

Dural sac

Spinal nerve

Spinal vein

Inferior articular process

Intervertebral joint

Superior articular process

Spinous process

15

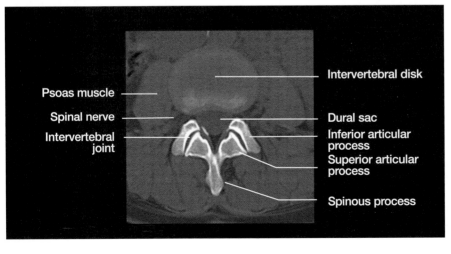

Intervertebral disk

Psoas muscle

Spinal nerve

Dural sac

Intervertebral joint

Inferior articular process

Superior articular process

Spinous process

16

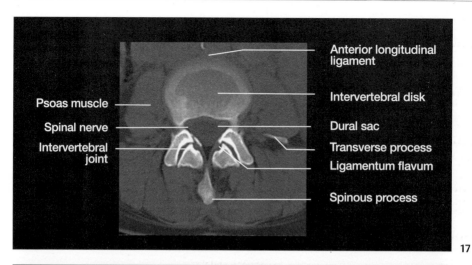

Anterior longitudinal ligament

Intervertebral disk

Psoas muscle

Spinal nerve

Intervertebral joint

Dural sac

Transverse process

Ligamentum flavum

Spinous process

17

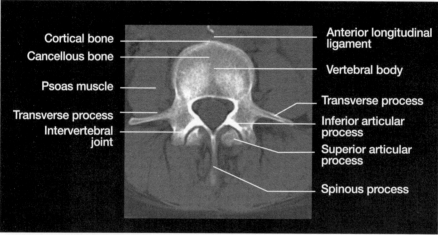

Cortical bone

Cancellous bone

Psoas muscle

Transverse process

Intervertebral joint

Anterior longitudinal ligament

Vertebral body

Transverse process

Inferior articular process

Superior articular process

Spinous process

18

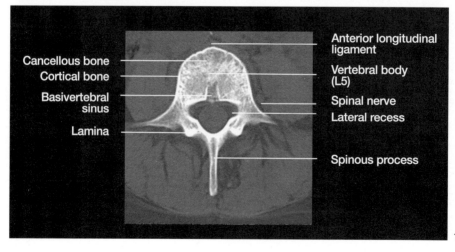

Cancellous bone

Cortical bone

Basivertebral sinus

Lamina

Anterior longitudinal ligament

Vertebral body (L5)

Spinal nerve

Lateral recess

Spinous process

19

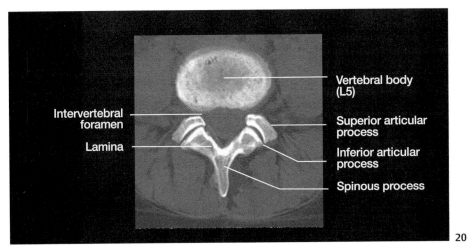

20

Fig. **14–20**   Axial scans of the lumbar spine, parallel to vertebral endplates—bone window

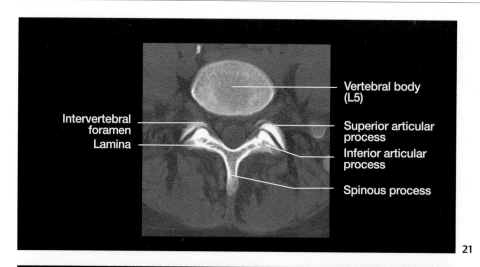

Intervertebral foramen
Lamina

Vertebral body (L5)
Superior articular process
Inferior articular process
Spinous process

21

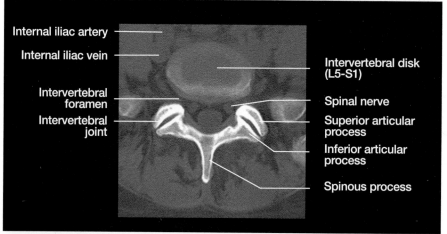

Internal iliac artery
Internal iliac vein
Intervertebral foramen
Intervertebral joint

Intervertebral disk (L5-S1)
Spinal nerve
Superior articular process
Inferior articular process
Spinous process

22

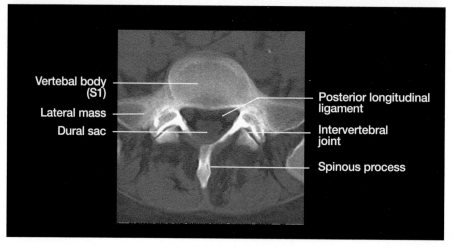

Vertebal body (S1)
Lateral mass
Dural sac

Posterior longitudinal ligament
Intervertebral joint
Spinous process

23

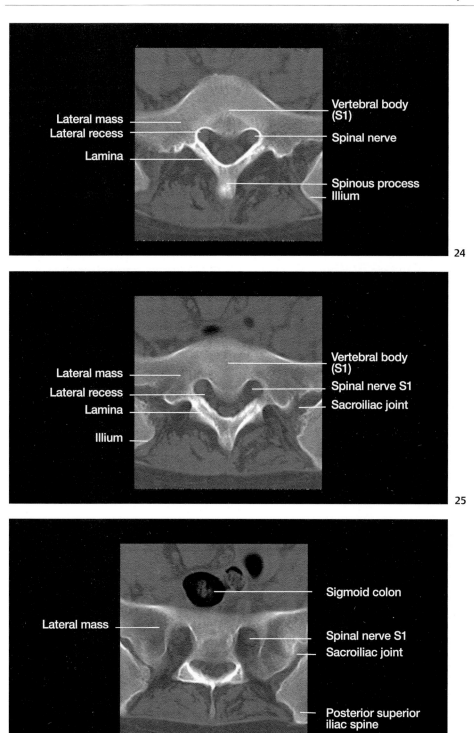

Fig. **21–26** Axial scans of the lumbar spine, parallel to vertebral endplate—bone window

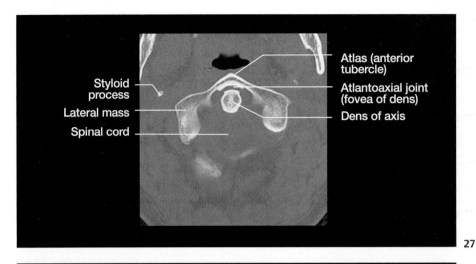

Styloid process
Lateral mass
Spinal cord

Atlas (anterior tubercle)
Atlantoaxial joint (fovea of dens)
Dens of axis

27

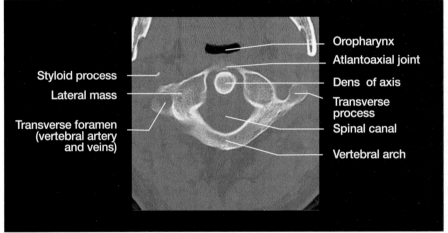

Styloid process
Lateral mass
Transverse foramen (vertebral artery and veins)

Oropharynx
Atlantoaxial joint
Dens of axis
Transverse process
Spinal canal
Vertebral arch

28

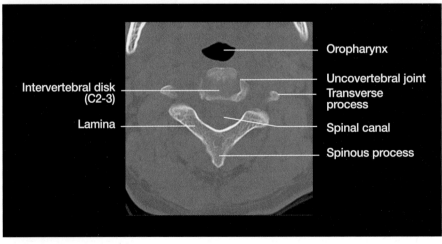

Intervertebral disk (C2-3)
Lamina

Oropharynx
Uncovertebral joint
Transverse process
Spinal canal
Spinous process

29

Fig. 27–29 Axial 5 mm scans of the cervical spine—bone window

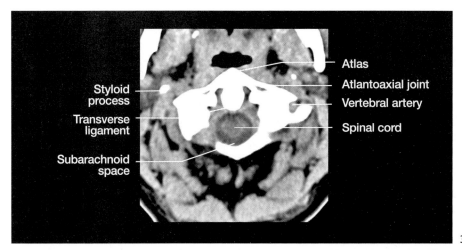

Styloid process

Transverse ligament

Subarachnoid space

Atlas

Atlantoaxial joint

Vertebral artery

Spinal cord

30

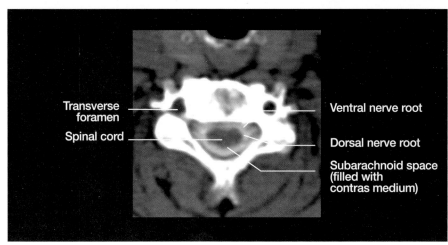

Transverse foramen

Spinal cord

Ventral nerve root

Dorsal nerve root

Subarachnoid space (filled with contras medium)

31

Fig. **30**   Single axial slice at the level of C1—soft tissue window setting

Fig. **31**   Single axial scan at the level of C 3/4, obtained after administration of contrast with subarachnoid space (post-myelography-scan)

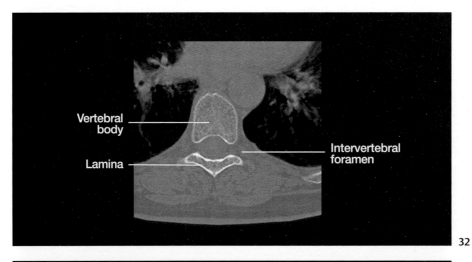

32

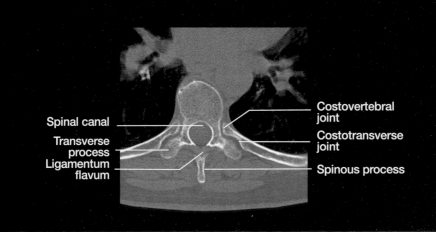

33

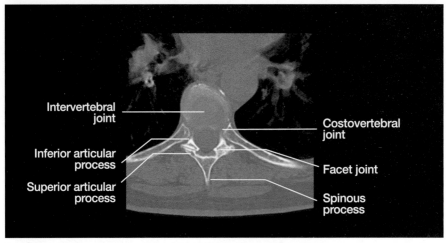

34

Fig. **32-34** Axial 5 mm scans at the thoracic level—bone window setting

10 Fundamentals

Clinical Aspects

Computed tomography (CT) is widely used in the diagnosis of spinal disorders, providing information of extremely high quality for a variety of indications. At the same time, CT is a prime example of the problems involved in examining a predominantly longitudinal organ system with a modality that is designed for imaging on axial planes. Unlike magnetic resonance imaging (MRI), CT cannot furnish a primary survey of the vertebral column with a few sagittal scans, followed by the selective evaluation of sites with apparent abnormalities. This limits the value of spinal CT in several respects:

- As a screening examination
- For imaging pathology with significant longitudinal extent
- For finding lesions located at an unknown level

Because of these limitations, the clinical findings and any additional imaging studies have a crucial role in focusing the investigation on a specific region. If there is no clinical information from the referring physician and such information cannot be easily obtained, the radiologist should try to narrow the examination based on the history, diagnostic findings, and previous imaging studies if the patient's condition permits and the situation is not an emergency.

CT should not be used to investigate nonspecific symptoms such as "unexplained back pain" unless all other diagnostic options have been exhausted.

Frequent Indications for Spinal Computed Tomography

Disk Herniation

CT is most commonly used in the spine to evaluate for an intervertebral disk protrusion or herniation encroaching on nerve roots, cauda equina fibers, or the spinal cord. This indication is much more common in the lumbar spine than in the cervical or thoracic areas.

■ Clinical Manifestations

A basic distinction is drawn between the following clinical presentations:

- Low back pain or neck pain with a nonsegmental or radicular pattern of pain projection and no neurologic deficits.
- Lumboischialgia or cervicobrachialgia, which can usually be attributed to nerve root compression during the physical examination.

Nerve root compression may be caused by a central herniation of the disk above the nerve root or by a lateral, intraforaminal disk herniation at the same level. This pattern defines a limited region for CT evaluation.

In patients with symptoms of L1–3 lumbar root compression and normal CT findings at the adjacent levels, the compression may be caused in rare cases by a lateral disk herniation at a more caudal level. The herniated disk impinges on the descending, paravertebral portion of the root after it has exited the neuroforamen. In these cases, the radiologist may have to extend the examination to the lower adjacent levels after consulting with the referring physician.

■ Examination Technique and Sources of Error

In patients examined for a herniated disk, the standard CT technique for visualizing the intervertebral disks is to acquire single slices directed parallel to the disk spaces. This requires readjusting the gantry angle for each level imaged. Because most units have a maximum gantry angle of 20–25°, the lowest level often cannot be imaged precisely parallel to the disk space. This should be taken into account when evaluating L5–S1 herniations that extend beyond the disk space. It is one reason why spiral (helical) CT scanning without gantry angulation is often recommended in patients undergoing evaluation for a herniated disk.

The need for multiple gantry angulations creates another potential source of misinterpretation: adjusting the gantry angle separately for each level causes the slices on the posterior side to overlap. In some circumstances, this may cause a herniated disk to be imaged twice, as the apparently contiguous craniocaudal images portray two ruptured disks separated by redundant, normal-appearing spinal segments. In reality, the scans merely cut the same herniated disk twice at different angles.

To evaluate the imaged structures and detect or exclude a herniated disk, it is also helpful to keep in mind the causal mechanism of beam-hardening artifacts (see p. 288).

■ Differential Diagnosis

When examining a patient with low back pain, it is important to evaluate all imaging findings critically and consider the full range of diagnostic possibilities. These include:

- A narrow spinal canal
- Bony lesions of the sacrum
- Abnormalities of bone density and trabecular structure, especially in patients with osteoporosis
- A defect in the vertebral arch (spondylolysis)
- Other potential causes of nerve root compression
- Retroperitoneal lymph nodes
- Aortic aneurysm

Fractures and Other Trauma

Another frequent indication for CT examination of the spine is a search for traumatic changes. At some trauma centers, CT is used as a primary screening study in injured patients. Spiral CT is used to evaluate the head, chest, and abdomen, depending on the pattern of the injury.

Next, the regions that have the highest statistical involvement for a particular clinical presentation or trauma mechanism are selectively reexamined.

The lesions of primary interest in spinal trauma are vertebral body fractures. These injuries are difficult to detect in whole-body examinations, however, and they cannot be reliably excluded unless selective thin CT slices are acquired.

Clinical signs such as pain and neurologic deficits, as well as secondary fracture signs such as paravertebral or retroperitoneal hematomas in spiral CT scans of the chest or abdomen, always warrant an additional bone-window examination of the adjacent vertebral bodies using thin CT slices.

Two-dimensional reformatted images are often helpful as well. Sagittal reformatting is particularly useful for mapping fracture patterns in the sagittal plane.

Whenever possible, the radiologist should correlate the CT images with conventional radiographs.

Intraspinal Masses

The primary goals in the CT diagnosis of intraspinal masses are to define the precise level of the mass and establish its identity. Intravenous contrast administration is therefore usually recommended. A dynamic contrast study can help in making a differential-diagnostic classification.

The most important criterion in the differential diagnosis of an intraspinal mass, however, is its location. Tumor masses are classified as follows:

- Extradural
- Intradural extramedullary
- Intramedullary

The most common entities within these groups are listed in Table 10.**1.**

Table 10.**1** The most common spinal tumors

Location	Entity
Extradural (55%)	<ul><li>Metastases (e.g., from breast, prostatic or bronchial carcinoma, gastrointestinal tract tumors, melanoma)</li><li>Osteogenic tumors (e.g., chordoma, osteoma, bone cyst)</li><li>Tumors that invade the spinal canal secondarily from a paravertebral location (e.g., retroperitoneal paravertebral lymphoma, pleural mesothelioma, neuroblastoma)</li><li>Rare location of predominantly intradural masses (e.g., meningioma)</li></ul>
Intradural extramedullary (40%)	Meningioma, schwannoma, epidermoid
Intramedullary (5%)	Astrocytoma, ependymoma, angioblastoma

Evaluation and Interpretation of Findings

Particularly in patients undergoing examination for degenerative disk disease, it is important to evaluate and interpret the morphologic imaging findings correctly in relation to the patient's clinical symptoms, since degenerative changes can be found in many asymptomatic patients. The detection of a disk protrusion in itself does not mean that the protrusion is causing the symptoms. Familiarity with the clinical symptoms is thus important both as a plausibility check and as a way of judging the significance of the findings.

At a time when cost efficiency greatly influences the choice of diagnostic procedures, the CT findings should not only help furnish a diagnosis, but should also influence patient management. Like other imaging modalities, CT should be part of the diagnostic algorithm and help the referring physician decide which surgical or nonsurgical options are appropriate for treating a particular set of clinical symptoms.

Technical Aspects

Since CT was introduced clinically in the early 1970s, rapid progress in hardware and software development and advances in computer technology have made the method an important tool in the basic work-up of spinal disorders. Despite the advent of MRI, the role of CT has become even more firmly established.

Like MRI, CT continues to play a large part in the investigation of difficult clinical problems using special diagnostic strategies, and it is even preferable to MRI for certain applications. While MRI quickly established its superiority for the visualization of soft-tissue structures and especially for detecting spinal cord lesions, CT is still the method of choice for detecting bony abnormalities of the spine. CT is also superior to MRI for detecting calcifications in the setting of neoplasias and other diseases.

In addition, the introduction of spiral CT scanning, with the option for improved high-resolution views, including surface reconstructions and multiplanar reformatting, has further solidified the role of CT in the diagnosis of spinal disorders.

and signal-to-noise ratio, but they lead to poorer spatial resolution along the z axis, with greater partial volume effects.

A slice thickness of 5–8 mm is recommended for an extended survey examination of the spinal canal, and it can be combined with a table feed of up to 20 mm. The search for a vertebral fracture requires contiguous scanning with a slice thickness of 1–2 mm.

Slice thicknesses of 3–5 mm are usually suitable for intervertebral disk examinations.

If two-dimensional or three-dimensional reconstructions are needed for applications such as fracture mapping or preoperative planning, thin CT slices are generally preferred to ensure a consistently high spatial resolution in all reconstructed planes (isotropism). If threshold-based three-dimensional surface-rendered views are desired, the scans should be acquired with a soft-tissue reconstruction filter to reduce image noise.

If the goal is to obtain image data sets for multiplanar reformatting, spiral CT acquisition is preferable to single-slice scanning.

Single-Slice CT Scanning

A single-slice CT examination is a "step-and-shoot" technique in which one scan is acquired by one rotation of the roentgen-ray tube, the table is incremented, the next scan is acquired, and so on. The breath is held in inspiration or expiration at each level to maintain a constant respiratory position. The slice thickness in this technique is determined by the tube collimation, and the slice increment is determined by the table feed.

It may be necessary or desirable to vary the slice thickness, depending on the nature of the study. The following principles apply:

- Thinner slices improve spatial resolution but result in a lower signal-to-noise ratio.
- Thicker slices improve contrast resolution

Spiral CT Scanning

■ **Advantages over Conventional Single-Slice Scanning**

Most of the advantages of modern spiral (helical) CT are based on the significant reduction in total examination time. Patient comfort is improved, motion artifacts are reduced, and the ability to make overlapping reconstructions increases the longitudinal resolution of the examination compared with single-slice scanning. These benefits are obtained with no increase in radiation exposure.

It has been shown that the longitudinal resolution of a thin-slice reconstruction from a spiral CT data set is equal to the resolution achieved with single slices acquired with a 50% overlap. This means that spiral CT provides the same longitudinal resolution in less time and with less radiation exposure. This is particularly important in pediatric examinations and in patients who are examined frequently.

With the ability of modern scanners to acquire images in less than one second (0.75–0.8 s), it is possible to cover a large volume in a short time, or to examine a given volume in thin slices and thus improve spatial resolution. This is particularly useful in the diagnosis of spinal disorders, many of which require the multiplanar reformatting of a data set acquired in a single, seamless volume with no registration errors. With fast spiral scanning, this can usually be accomplished even in seriously ill, traumatized, unstable, or uncooperative patients.

Multiplanar reformatting makes it possible to evaluate the scanned region not just in single axial slices but also in coronal, sagittal, or three-dimensional views, depending on requirements. The quality of the reconstructed image closely approaches that of a direct scan acquired in the corresponding orientation.

The information gained by evaluating the data from several perspectives is particularly helpful in evaluating complex anatomic structures such as the spinal column and skull base, and it can even be decisive—especially when used as a guide to surgical planning. Multiplanar reformatting helps in determining the resectability of a lesion, defining the surgical approach, and planning the internal fixation of fractures.

■ Spiral CT Examination Protocol

When selecting a spiral CT protocol, the examiner must consider a number of factors and adapt them to the requirements of the study as needed. These factors include the tube current and the increment (pitch) of the spiral scan.

- *Tube current.* If the visualization of bony structures is of primary interest, it may be best to use a lower mAs setting and a thin slice thickness (1 mm). While this increases the total scan time, it makes it possible to cover a larger volume without being limited by prolonged tube cooling times. If the primary goal is to define structures of low contrast (e.g., when examining for nerve root compression), a higher mAs should be used in conjunction with a somewhat greater slice thickness (3 mm) so that the entire region of interest can be scanned without tube cooling. With ongoing technical refinements in equipment, however, tube current is becoming a less important consideration.

- *Pitch.* Pitch is the ratio of the slice thickness per tube revolution to the table feed during the same period. A pitch greater than one increases the volume imaged per scan time but also causes widening of the slice profile. A pitch that produces overlapping slices reduces the maximum scan extent but improves the image quality, especially in multiplanar reformatting. It also improves the sensitivity of the examination for detecting smaller lesions.

A data set consisting of isotropic pixels is best for multiplanar reformatted images. This means that the spatial resolution of the reformatted slices is equally good in all planes. The pitch should therefore be set to produce an overlapping acquisition, especially when the slice thickness is 3 mm or more. As a general rule, the greater the slice thickness, the more the slices should be overlapped.

Performing the Examination

■ Examination Strategies

Two different strategies may be followed in CT examinations of the cervical, thoracic, and lumbar spine:

- For the diagnosis of intervertebral disk disease, it is best to acquire single slices 3–5 mm thick that are oriented parallel to the disk spaces. Coverage at each level should extend from the arch of the vertebra above the disk space to the arch of the vertebra below. The gantry tilt, or angle of the scan plane relative to the long axis of the body, is readjusted for each level. Often this is not possible for the L5–S1 level, because the angle of this level may exceed the maximum gantry tilt of 20–25°, depending on the scanner and the patient's constitution.

- Another strategy is to acquire contiguous single or spiral slices, usually thin, without gantry angulation. This provides seamless coverage of all structures, and the entire spinal canal can be evaluated for sites of bony stenosis or intraspinal fragments. Additionally, the data sets can be used to generate two-dimensional sagittal and coronal reformatted images or three-dimensional reconstructions that are useful or even necessary in evaluating vertebral fractures and other complex pathology.

Because the gantry usually cannot be angled exactly parallel to the disk spaces at all levels, with a potential for misinterpretation due to partial volume effects, many authors recommend spiral scanning with a narrow slice thickness (3 mm) for the diagnosis of disk disease and nerve root compression. The advantages of this technique include a significantly shorter examination time and the ability to evaluate the alignment of the vertebral bodies and the width of the neuroforamina in sagittal reformatting. A dual strategy, combining spiral CT with single slices parallel to the disk spaces, is practiced at some centers.

The tactics of the examination should be tailored to the specific indication and also depend on the availability of a modern spiral CT scanner.

■ Examination Procedure

Each examination starts with a digital survey radiograph called the scout view (synonyms: topogram, scanogram, localizer, scout image, pilot view). This is a lateral or anteroposterior projection obtained by moving the table through the roentgen beam while the tube remains stationary.

In examinations of the spinal column and especially the lumbar spine, it is standard practice to begin the examination with a lateral scout view. This view is very helpful for angling the gantry parallel to the disk spaces and for slice localization (i.e., assigning individual slices to a particular vertebral body or disk space). Except in trauma patients, an anteroposterior scout view should also be obtained. A combination of the lateral and anteroposterior scout views generally eliminates the need to perform conventional radiographs in non-trauma patients (Tress and Hare 1990). The scout view itself can demonstrate abnormalities of vertebral alignment, lordosis, kyphosis, and segmentation abnormalities, and it permits a simultaneous evaluation of the hip and sacroiliac joints. This enables the radiologist to recognize degenerative conditions that typically lead to "pseudoradicular" symptoms and incorporate them into an overall interpretation of the clinical and radiologic findings.

In some cases, structural lesions of the spine or of individual vertebral bodies may be visible on the scout view but not on single CT slices. This is particularly common when a 5-mm slice thickness has been used.

If conventional radiographs are already available, we recommend comparing the CT scans and roentgen films to define the levels of the vertebral bodies, especially in patients with lumbosacral junction anomalies where there is a variation in the number of lumbar vertebrae. It may even be necessary in such cases to image the entire thoracic spine, so that the vertebral bodies can be accurately counted in the craniocaudal direction.

Contrast Media

Two basic options are available for contrast administration in CT examinations of the spine:

- Intravenous administration
- Intrathecal administration

■ Intravenous Contrast Medium

Intravenous contrast medium can be administered through a peripheral or central venous line, preferably with the aid of an infusion pump. The amount and timing of the contrast injection depend on the specific diagnostic question and the examination technique (single slice or spiral CT). The usual contrast dose is 1–2.5 mL/kg body weight, administered at a flow rate of 0.7–4 mL/s.

For imaging inflammatory disease, a delay time of 70–120 seconds should be allowed after contrast administration before scanning is initiated. For other types of pathology such as arteriovenous malformations, the contrast medium should be injected rapidly after a delay time of only 15–25 seconds.

■ Intrathecal Contrast Medium

An intrathecal contrast medium such as iotrolan (Isovist) is usually administered by lumbar puncture for myelography, followed by CT scanning (postmyelographic CT), or may be administered directly for CT myelography (or cisternography) without prior conventional myelography. In this case, the attending physician may administer the contrast medium while the patient is still on the ward, depending on the indication. In other cases, it may be better to inject the contrast medium just before the start of the examination and document the cephalad flow of the material by CT fluoroscopy. This can serve various purposes, including the detection or exclusion of cystic masses that communicate with the subarachnoid space. As in classic cisternography, the examination should be repeated 2–6 hours after contrast administration, before most of the material has been absorbed (see below).

Intrathecal contrast administration generally provides good delineation of the spinal cord, conus medullaris, filum terminale, cauda equina, and any intradural masses that may be present. Without intrathecal contrast, these masses are very difficult to distinguish because of their similar attenuation to normal anatomic structures. CT myelography is particularly rewarding in patients with spinal stenosis or an equivocal conventional myelogram and in cases in which MRI is contraindicated.

There are circumstances in which a repeat CT examination after intrathecal contrast administration can help determine whether cystic masses communicate with the rest of the subarachnoid space. Opinions in the literature vary with regard to the ideal timing of the examinations. In our experience, it is best to perform the first examination at 1–1.5 hours and the second examination at 3–4 hours after contrast administration. Later examinations are generally unrewarding due to extensive contrast absorption and because more delayed contrast accumulation within a cystic mass may occur as a result of diffusion.

Interpreting the Examination

■ Window Setting

CT is technically capable of distinguishing approximately 4000 different degrees of intensity of x-ray attenuation (measured in Hounsfield units). The human eye can distinguish only about 15–20 shades of gray, however, and the theoretical range of CT attenuation values is therefore limited to a practical, diagnostically useful range. This process is called window selection. The window center (C) is set to the approximate attenuation of the structures of primary interest. The window width (W) is set so that all significant adjacent structures are displayed at a gray level that is easily distinguished visually from the target structures. The window settings listed in Table 10.2 have proved effective for common CT investigations of the spine.

The values shown in Table 10.2 are by no means optimal for all investigations in all patients and on all scanners, and they should be optimally adjusted for each individual case.

Table 10.2 Recommended window settings

	Window (W)	Center (C)
Disk disease	200–300	20–50
Fractures	2000 (maximal)	300–500
Postmyelographic CT	1400–2000	300–400
Tumor diagnosis (with contrast administration)	200–400	20–80

Nevertheless, one should try to maintain a constant window setting to establish an internal standard for routine examinations.

■ Artifacts

In addition to the many equipment-related artifacts that may occur, *beam-hardening artifacts* are a particularly common problem in spinal CT examinations. We shall therefore briefly review the mechanism by which these artifacts are produced.

When roentgen rays penetrate tissue with a high atomic number, such as bone, the lower-energy components of the beam are attenuated or completely absorbed. The net effect of this process is a hardening of the radiation, which is most apparent at the edges of cortical bone. Sites of predilection for beam-hardening artifact in the spine are the vertebral arches and facet joints. After being "hardened" in these areas, the radiation can no longer distinguish the inherently small attenuation differences that exist between epidural fat, spinal cord, and cerebrospinal fluid. As a result, the spinal canal sometimes appears on CT as a featureless area of low attenuation—i.e., it appears black or as a uniform shade of gray. Meanwhile, less attenuated portions of the beam that pass through the neuroforamina in the anterior part of the spinal canal may create the spurious appearance of a herniated disk when they encounter intraspinal structures. This is because the structures at that location appear considerably more dense than the posterior portions of the dural sac and epidural space.

Beam-hardening artifact is a common source of problems in cervical spinal diagnosis. Since the shoulder girdle is superimposed over the lower portion of the cervical spine, the increased attenuation and hardening of the roentgen beam often makes it impossible to evaluate the spinal canal. If the patient can tolerate it, this problem can be reduced by passing an elastic strap beneath the feet of the recumbent patient and fastening it to both wrists, drawing the arms and shoulder girdle downward.

In some cases, the artifact problem can be improved to some extent by modifying the scanning parameters, especially the slice thickness. Since the degree of beam-hardening artifact increases with slice thickness, this artifact can be reduced by using thinner slices. Another option is to acquire thin 1-mm slices by spiral scanning and use them to generate slices 3–5 mm thick.

■ References

Recommended for further study

Johnson BA, Tanenbaum LN. Contemporary spinal CT applications. Neuroimaging Clin N Am 1998; 8: 559–75.
  ● *Excellent overview.*
Tehranzadeh J, Andrews C, Wong E. Lumbar spine imaging. Normal variants, imaging pitfalls, and artifacts. Radiol Clin North Am 2000; 38(6): 1207–53, v vi. [Review]
  ● *Excellent overview.*

Recent and basic works

Fleischmann D, Rubin GD, Paik DS et al. Stair-step artifacts with single versus multiple detector-row helical CT. Radiology 2000; 216: 185–96.
  ● *Multiple detector-row CT produces fewer artifacts than single detector-row CT.*
Hopper KD, Pierantozzi D, Potok PS, et al. The quality of 3 D reconstructions from 1.0 and 1.5 pitch helical and conventional CT. J Comput Assist Tomogr 1996; 20: 841–7.
Hu H, He HD, Foley WD, Fox SH. Four multidetector-row helical CT: image quality and volume coverage speed. Radiology 2000; 215: 55–62.
Kasales CJ, Hopper KD, Ariola DN, et al. Reconstructed helical CT scans: improvement in z-axis resolution compared with overlapped and non-overlapped conventional CT scans. AJR Am J Roentgenol 1995; 164: 1281–4.
Levy RA. Three-dimensional craniocervical helical CT: is isotropic imaging possible? Radiology 1995; 197: 645–8.
  ● *The above studies illustrate the relationship of slice thickness and table feed to the quality of reconstructions and radiation exposure.*
Nawfel RD, Judy PF, Silverman SG, Hooton S, Tuncali K, Adams DF. Patient and personnel exposure during CT fluoroscopy-guided interventional procedures. Radiology 2000; 216: 180–4.
Sener RN, Ripeckyj GT, Otto PM, Rauch RA, Jinkins JR. Recognition of abnormalities on computed scout images in CT examinations of the head and spine. Neuroradiology 1993; 35: 229–31.
Tress BM, Hare WS. CT of the spine: are plain spinal radiographs necessary? Clin Radiol 1990; 41: 317–20.
  ● *Considers whether plain radiographs add significant information to that furnished by CT.*

11 Anatomy

The discussions of anatomy and embryology in this chapter are limited essentially to structures that either can be visualized with CT or are necessary for understanding a particular disorder. Specialized textbooks may be consulted for details on the ultrastructural morphology and zonal architecture of the spinal cord, which are outside the scope of the present work.

Bone

The spinal column has a segmental architecture consisting of seven cervical vertebrae, 12 thoracic vertebrae, five lumbar vertebrae, five sacral vertebral segments, and three to five coccygeal segments (Fig. 11.**1**).

While the total number of vertebral bodies is relatively constant, numerous "junctional anomalies" may be encountered, especially in the lumbosacral region. These anomalies may be associated with a variable number of separate lumbar vertebrae, ranging from four to six, due to the sacralization of a lumbar vertebra or the lumbarization of a thoracic or sacral vertebra. Especially in the preoperative diagnosis of disk herniation, these junctional anomalies can make it difficult to define the affected level accurately. To avoid misunderstandings, consultation with the referring physician is recommended whenever possible. In describing the junctional anomaly, the radiologist should use the term "lowest" or "second lowest level," as this conforms to the intraoperative assessment of vertebral level as determined by fluoroscopy.

It should be noted that the lateral scout view may appear to show six separate lumbar vertebral bodies. This is caused by "short ribs" on the T12 vertebra, which are distinguishable from transverse processes only by the presence of a joint space in the anteroposterior scout view or plain radiograph. This point should be noted in designating the intervertebral spaces (Fig. 11.**2**).

Except for the axis and atlas (C1 and C2), the basic structural anatomy of the vertebral bodies is consistent throughout the spine and varies only in its adaptation to regional functional demands. All the vertebrae except for C1 possess an anterior (ventral) vertebral body. The pedicles arise from the posterior (dorsal) side of the vertebral body, and combine with the laminae to form the vertebral arch. The anterior surface of the vertebral arch and the posterior surface of the vertebral body form the boundaries of the bony spinal canal. The costotransverse processes arise from the sides of the vertebral arch; they articulate with the ribs in the thoracic spine and serve basically as sites for muscular attachment in the cervical and lumbar spine. Each vertebral body has a superior and inferior articular process, also arising from the vertebral arch, by which it forms facet joints with the adjacent vertebrae.

The segmental differences between the cervical, thoracic, and lumbar regions of the spine include variations in the size and shape of the bony spinal canal. The shape of the canal along the cervical spine ranges from elliptical to triangular, with the apex of the triangle on the dorsal side. The transverse diameter of the cervical spinal canal is greater than its sagittal diameter. It diminishes rapidly from the craniocervical junction to the C3 level and then remains fairly constant through C7 (Figs. 11.**3**, 11.**4**).

In the thoracic region, the spinal canal has a rounded cross-section with approximately equal transverse and sagittal diameters. The posterior surface of the thoracic vertebral bodies is concave compared with the cervical and lumbar spine (Figs. 11.**3**, 11.**5**).

The lumbar portion of the spinal canal is wider than the thoracic portion and has a somewhat elliptical shape, with a greater transverse than sagittal diameter (Figs. 11.**3**, 11.**6**).

The following values are useful guidelines in CT evaluations of spinal canal width (e.g., in patients examined for spinal stenosis):

- The lumbar spinal canal should have an anteroposterior diameter of at least 15 mm.
- The cervical spinal canal below C3 should have an anteroposterior diameter of at least 12 mm.
- The craniocaudal distance between the vertebral arches should be at least 20 mm.

Based on information published in the literature, the following minimum values are useful for excluding spinal stenosis at any level:

- The anteroposterior diameter should measure at least 11.5 mm.
- The interpedicular distance should measure at least 16 mm.
- The width of the lateral recess (the area bounded laterally by the pedicle, posteriorly by the superior articular facet, and anteriorly by the posterolateral surface of the vertebral body) should be no less than 3 mm.
- The area of the spinal canal in axial cross-section should be at least 1.45 cm².
- The ligamenta flava should not exceed 4–5 mm in thickness.

The thickness of the intervertebral disk spaces (i.e., the disk height) diminishes craniocaudally along the cervical spine. The thoracic disk spaces are somewhat thinner, especially in the upper thoracic area, and become increasingly thick from above downward into the lumbar region. The thickest disk space normally occurs at the L4–5 level, and the L5–S1 disk is slightly thinner.

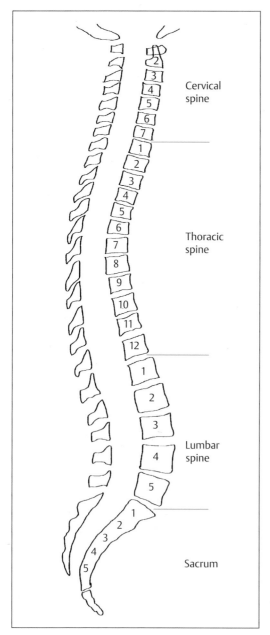

Fig. 11.**1** **Segmental architecture of the spine.**

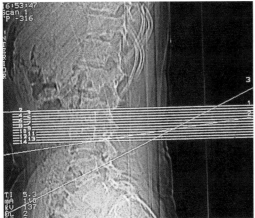

The relative orientation of the facet joints also changes in the craniocaudal direction. While the facet joints in the cervical area have an almost horizontal orientation, promoting freedom of movement in flexion and rotation, the facet joints in the thoracic and lumbar spine assume an increasingly vertical orienta-

◁ Fig. 11.**2 a–c   Junctional anomaly?**

a   The lateral scout view appears to show six separate lumbar vertebral bodies, apparently due to the lumbarization of S1.

b, c   The lateral myelogram demonstrates an L7–S1 herniated disk. The anteroposterior view shows that the presumed transverse processes of "L1" are actually short ribs. Thus, the normal segmental architecture and the segmental origin of the spinal nerves are preserved, and this must be taken into account when interpreting the images.

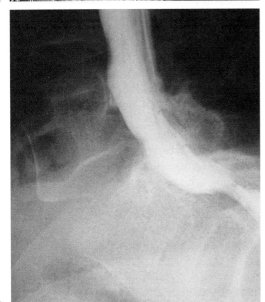

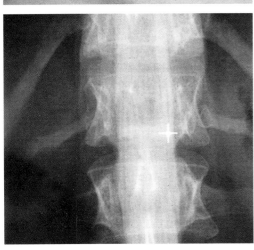

c

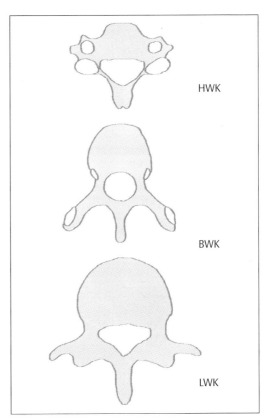

HWK

BWK

LWK

Fig. 11.**3   Varying shape of the spinal canal in the cervical, thoracic, and lumbar vertebrae.**

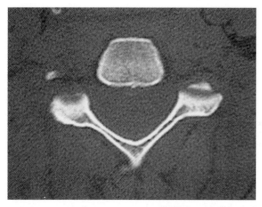

Fig. 11.**4** **Typical CT appearance of the cervical spinal canal.** Triangular cross-section.

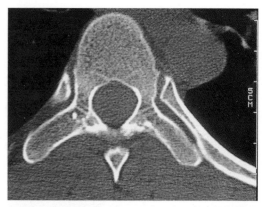

Fig. 11.**5** **Typical CT appearance of the thoracic spinal canal.** Rounded cross-section.

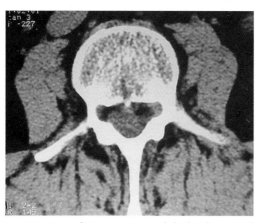

Fig. 11.**6** **Typical CT appearance of the lumbar spinal canal.** Elliptical cross-section.

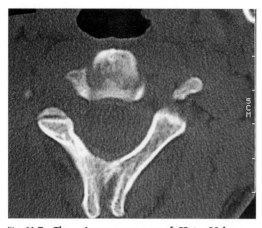

Fig. 11.**7** **The spinous processes of C2 to C6 have a variable bifid appearance.**

tion. The facet joints in the thoracic spine have a more coronal orientation, which is favorable for rotation, while the more sagittal orientation of the lumbar facet joints is favorable for movements in flexion and extension.

Segmental peculiarities of the cervical spine. The vertebral artery and a bundle of small accompanying vertebral veins runs from C6 to C1 through the transverse foramina, a series of openings in the transverse processes measuring 5–7 mm in diameter. The foramina may be congenitally open on the posterior, lateral, or anterior side. In another variant, the vertebral artery may pass through a bony "arcuate foramen" over the vertebral artery groove on the arch of the atlas before it enters the foramen magnum.

Usually, the spinous processes of C2 through C6 are bifid in varying degrees (Fig. 11.**7**).

The lateral borders of the C3 through C7 vertebral bodies each have a superiorly directed uncinate process that articulates with, and constrains the motion of, the vertebral body above it. In degenerative diseases, this process is often a nidus for appositional new bone growth, which can narrow the neuroforamina and exert pressure on the exiting spinal nerve (Figs. 11.**8**, 11.**9**).

The C7 vertebra (nuchal tubercle) is often called the "vertebra prominens" owing to the great length of its spinous process.

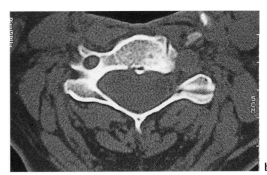

Fig. 11.**8 a, b Soft-tissue and bone-window views of a rare cause of intraforaminal nerve root compression.** The left image shows a markedly expanded vertebral artery compressing the C6 cervical nerve.

Segmental peculiarities of the thoracic spine. Each thoracic vertebra has a small facet on its superior border, just anterior to the pedicle, and on its inferior border for articulation with the heads of the ribs. Another facet on the lateral portion of the transverse processes articulates with the tubercles of the ribs.

Segmental peculiarities of the lumbar spine. In place of costal facets, the lumbar vertebrae have well-developed transverse processes, or costal processes, which represent rudimentary ribs and give attachment to muscles (Figs. 11.**6,** 11.**10**).

The atlas (C1) is the only vertebra that lacks an anterior body, consisting basically of a bony ring. This configuration allows for two essential movements at the atlas level. Each lateral mass of the atlas has a superior facet that articulates with the corresponding occipital condyle at the atlanto-occipital joint, which is responsible for nodding movements of the head. Inferiorly, the atlas transmits the load of the head and a portion of the nodding movement through the atlantoaxial joint to the second cervical vertebra (Fig. 11.**11**).

The ring-like shape of the atlas is particularly favorable for pivoting movements at the atlantoaxial joint, where the dens of the axis articulates with the dental facet on the anterior arch of the atlas (Figs. 11.**11,** 11.**12**). The trans-

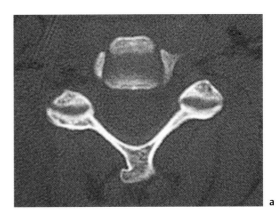

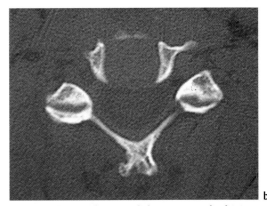

Fig. 11.**9 a, b Axial scans of the uncovertebral joint.** This joint acts like a guide rail to constrain the motion of the vertebral body above it. It is a common site of degenerative osteophytosis.

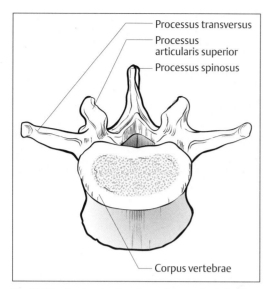

Processus transversus
Processus articularis superior
Processus spinosus
Corpus vertebrae

Fig. 11.**10** **Anatomic drawing of a typical lumbar vertebra.**

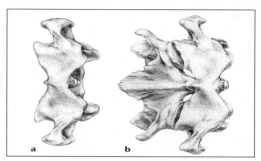

a   b

Fig. 11.**11** **Articulated view of the atlas and axis.** The form and function of C1 and C2 differ markedly from the other segments of the vertebral column.

verse ligament of the atlas retains the dens behind the anterior arch and covers it completely (see Fig. 11.**17**).

At the junction of the atlas with the foramen magnum, the average anteroposterior diameter of the spinal canal is approximately 34 mm, and its average transverse diameter is approximately 30 mm.

The axis (C2), unlike the atlas, has an anterior vertebral body from which springs the unique structure that forms a pivot for the atlas: the dens. This bony process is ossified from a separate center that fuses with the body of the axis.

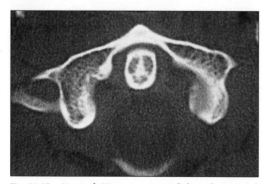

Fig. 11.**12** **Normal CT appearance of the atlantoaxial joint** between the dens and the posterior surface of the anterior arch of the atlas.

A connective tissue structure often persists at the fusion site for life and can be visualized with MRI and sometimes with CT. The presence of a separate odontoid bone in some individuals may result from a failure of fusion between the apex and body of the dens. Some authors attribute this bone to a "pinching off" of the distal portion of the dens by a congenitally short transverse ligament.

The apex of the dens generally projects 1–5 mm above the anterior arch of the atlas. Deviations from this normal range may be seen in complex anomalies such as Arnold–Chiari malformation, or may result from degenerative disease. A high position of the dens, accompanied by basilar impression, can also occur in the setting of rheumatoid arthritis. These changes can be diagnosed with conventional radiographs, however, and do not require further discussion here.

The axis, like the other cervical vertebrae through C6, has a transverse foramen for passage of the vertebral artery and the accompanying vertebral veins.

The axis is the first vertebra that bears an inferior articular process. This process forms a facet joint with the superior articular process of C3, setting the pattern for the vertebrae that follow.

Intervertebral Disks

Embryologically and phylogenetically, the intervertebral disks are viewed as fibrocartilaginous remnants of the notochord. Each disk consists of a gelatinous inner core, the nucleus pulposus, surrounded by a series of concentric fibrous rings known as the annulus fibrosus. The superior and inferior surfaces of the disk are adherent to the cartilaginous endplates of the adjacent vertebral bodies. The disks function as shock absorbers between the vertebrae, absorbing and transmitting axial body loads. They also distribute flexion, extension, and side-bending forces uniformly to the endplates of adjacent vertebral bodies. Pressures of up to 20 bar can develop within the disk space (compared with about 2 bar in an automobile tire).

The elastic resilience of the intervertebral disks depends strongly on their water content, which decreases from approximately 88 % at birth to approximately 66 % by age 70.

Altogether, the height of the intervertebral disks makes up about 25 % of the total height of the vertebral column. This accounts for the loss of body height that occurs with aging, as the disks undergo degenerative changes.

The individual height of the intervertebral disks in the cervical spine increases in the craniocaudal direction. The disks narrow again in the thoracic spine, especially the upper thoracic area, and then become thicker in the caudal direction. This pattern continues into the lumbar region, and the thickest disk space normally occurs at the L4–5 level; the L5–S1 disk is slightly narrower. The relationship of the anterior and posterior disk heights varies with the regional curvature of the spine. For example, the disk spaces in the lumbar region are higher anteriorly than posteriorly owing to the physiologic lordosis of the lumbar spine.

Until about 20 years of age, the intervertebral disks derive their blood supply from small vessels that penetrate the centers of the cartilaginous endplates. After age 20, these vessels are obliterated and the disk is supplied entirely through lymphatic channels and by the circulation of extracellular fluid. Cyclic loading and unloading of the spine creates a passive mechanism by which this fluid is exchanged.

Blood Vessels

Arteries

The spinal cord derives most of its blood supply from the anterior spinal artery, which runs anterior to the cord in the anterior sulcus. It gives rise to arteries that penetrate the spinal cord and supply its anterior portions. The posterior portions of the cord, especially the dorsal columns, are supplied by the posterior spinal arteries, which are usually paired. These vessels anastomose with the anterior spinal artery. The penetrating vessels that arise from both systems are end arteries that do not undergo further anastomosis.

The anterior spinal artery arises superiorly from the union of the spinal branches of the vertebral arteries. The posterior spinal arteries arise either from the posterior cerebellar arteries or from the vertebral arteries.

Both systems receive flow caudally from segmental arteries that enter the spinal canal through the neuroforamina and divide into an anterior and a posterior branch (Fig. 11.**13**).

The strictly metameric organization of one segmental artery for each somite in fetal life regresses during postnatal development. Most of the segmental arteries disappear, leaving only six to eight anterior and 10–20 posterior segmental arteries by adulthood. Although radicular or segmental arteries are present at the level of each vertebral segment to supply the vertebral bodies, the dura, and the segmental portions of the annulus fibrosus, facet joint, etc., these vessels are not continued as medullary arteries to supply the cord.

Table 11.1 lists the principal vessels that contribute to the blood supply of the spinal cord.

This unusual supply pattern renders the spinal cord very susceptible to ischemia, especially in the cervicothoracic region. The caudal portions of the cord have a slightly more generous provision of arterial anastomoses.

Veins

The spinal cord is drained chiefly by dorsal veins that carry blood to a posterolateral plexus in the pia mater. From there, it flows through radiculomedullary veins into the epidural venous plexus, which consists of a longitudinal system of paired anterior veins and smaller posterior veins. These vessels are interconnected by short transverse anastomoses. They also communicate with the intravertebral and basivertebral veins, which likewise drain into this plexus.

Table **11.1** Arterielle Versorgung des Myelons

Vessel	Level of entry into the spinal canal	Origin
Anterior spinal branches	C1	Vertebral arteries
Radiculomedullara artery	C2–3	Vertebral artery
Radiculomedullary artery	C5–6	Deep vervical artery, thyrocervical trunk
Radiculumedullary artery	C7-T1	Primary or secondary intercostal artery
Radiculomedullary artery	T4–5	Posterior intercostal artery
Thoracolumbar radiculomedullary artery (of Adamkiewiecz)	T9–12	Inferior intercostal artery
Lumbar arteries	L2–5	Aorta, median sacral artery

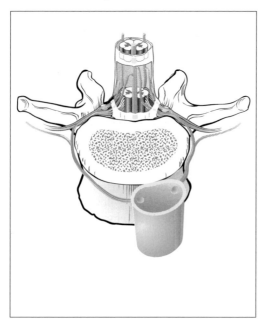

Fig. 11.**13** **The arterial blood supply of the spinal cord.**

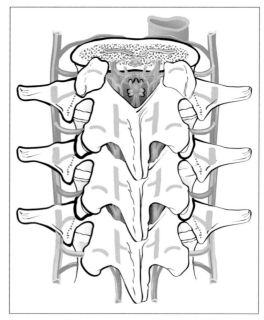

Fig. 11.**14** **The venous drainage of the spinal cord, meninges, and vertebral bodies.**

Venous blood flows from the epidural plexus into the extraspinal paravertebral veins located lateral to the pedicles. These veins carry the venous blood to the ascending lumbar veins and, at the thoracic level, to the azygos and hemiazygos veins (Fig. 11.**14**).

In some circumstances, the relationship of the intra-abdominal and intrathoracic pressures to the intraspinal pressure can cause a temporary stasis or even reversal of venous drainage from the spine. This accounts for the increased incidence of lumbar spondylodiskitis in patients with pelvic and lower extremity inflammatory disease. It also underlies the occurrence of thoracic tuberculous spondylodiskitis as a complication of pulmonary tuberculosis. When temporary flow reversal

occurs, infectious organisms that have been shed into the venous circulation may be forced into the smaller veins and venules of the vertebral bodies.

In most cases, the venous plexus cannot be clearly identified on CT scans. However, the obstruction of venous outflow (e.g., by extrinsic pressure from a mass) can markedly increase the caliber of the intraspinal veins, which then can be seen on unenhanced scans, and especially after intrathecal contrast administration. Distended intraspinal veins may be found in association with intraspinal tumors and herniated disks, and the adjacent spinal segments should always be scrutinized by CT, MRI, or myelography to detect or exclude a mass lesion (Fig. 11.**15**).

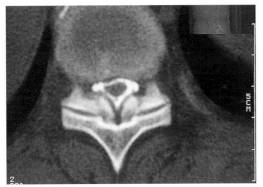 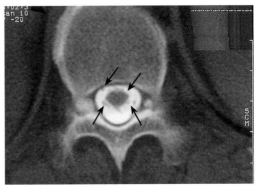

Fig. 11.**15 a, b** **Spinal stenosis.** Circumscribed thoracic spinal stenosis developed in this patient following trauma to the thoracic spine at the T10 level. Postmyelographic CT shows marked narrowing of the sub-

arachnoid space at the T10 level. The circumscribed filling defects in the opacified subarachnoid space below the stenosis *(arrows)* represent congested intradural veins.

Ligaments

The bony spinal column is stabilized by the following ligaments (Fig. 11.**17**).

Anterior longitudinal ligament. The anterior longitudinal ligament extends over the anterior surfaces of the vertebral bodies, passing from the anterolateral border of the foramen magnum, where it forms the anterior atlanto-occipital membrane, to the sacrum. It forms part of the anterior column in Denis's three-

column model, which is useful in assessing the stability of spinal fractures.

Posterior longitudinal ligament. The posterior longitudinal ligament extends from the anteromedial aspect of the foramen magnum over the posterior surface of the vertebral bodies to the sacrum. It bounds the spinal canal anteriorly and forms part of the middle column. It also forms the last barrier against

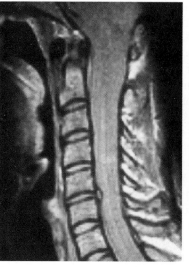 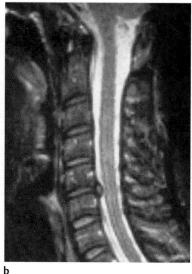

a   b

Fig. 11.16 a, b   T1-weighted and T2-weighted sagittal magnetic resonance images of the cervical spine. The posterior longitudinal ligament is clearly visualized in both sequences along with numerous other ligaments. Circumscribed elevation of the ligament is caused by a small subligamentous disk herniation.

Tectorial membrane
Apical ligament of dens
Cruciform ligament of atlas
Posterior longitudinal ligament
Posterior atlanto-occipital membrane

Nuchal ligament
Interspinous ligament
Supraspinous ligament

Ligamentum flavum
Posterior longitudinal ligament
Anterior longitudinal ligament

Fig. 11.17   **The ligaments of the cervical spine.**

the protrusion of herniated disk material into the spinal canal. Sagittal CT reformatted images often demonstrate elevation of the posterior longitudinal ligament by a subligamentous disk herniation (Fig. 11.**16**).

Ligamentum flavum. The ligamentum flavum forms an elastic ligamentous attachment between adjacent vertebral arches. It combines with the vertebral arches to form the lateral and posterior boundaries of the spinal canal. It can be identified on axial CT scans as a ligamentous structure arising from the facet joints. Between the laminae, it forms a V-shaped boundary for the spinal canal.

The ligamentum flavum is subject to involvement by degenerative disease. This leads to thickening and hypertrophy of the ligaments, with a proportionate narrowing of the spinal canal. The ligamentum flavum is one component of the posterior column.

Interspinous ligament. The interspinous ligament connects adjacent spinous processes. It is part of the posterior column.

Supraspinous ligament. This is a superficial ligament connecting the apices of the spinous processes. It is another component of the posterior column.

Cruciform ligament of the atlas. This structure is composed of the transverse ligament of the atlas, which passes from one posterior surface of the atlas to the other and holds the dens in place, and the longitudinal fascicles that pass from the body of the axis behind the dens to the anterior rim of the foramen magnum.

Apical ligament of the dens. This ligament connects the apex of the dens to the anterior rim of the foramen magnum. The bony avulsion of this ligament is presumably responsible for Anderson type I fractures of the dens.

Spinal Cord and Spinal Nerve Roots (Figs. 11.18–11.23)

The spinal cord usually appears on CT scans as a cord-like structure of uniform soft-tissue attenuation (approximately 30–40 HU). In adults, it extends caudally to the L1–2 level. There it tapers to a sharp tip, the conus medullaris, from which the filum terminale descends to the coccyx.

The two physiologic expansions of the spinal cord, known as the cervical and lumbar enlargements, result from the relatively greater amount of nerve distribution to the upper and lower extremities at those levels. They extend approximately from C3 to T1 and from T10 to L1–2.

Generally, CT cannot discriminate between the central gray matter and peripheral white matter of the spinal cord. One reason for this is

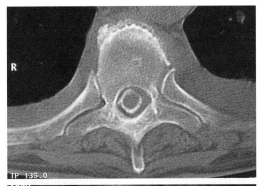

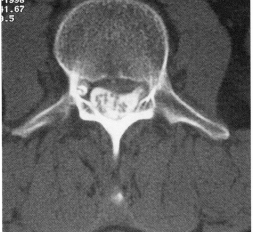

Fig. 11.**18 a, b Postmyelographic axial CT scans at the T6 and L3 levels.** While the thoracic scan demonstrates the spinal cord as a homogeneous filling defect within the subarachnoid space, the lumbar scan defines the separate filaments of the cauda equina fibers. Subligamentous portions of a left-sided disk herniation are visible on both scans. This is a common finding in the lumbar region, but is extremely rare at thoracic levels.

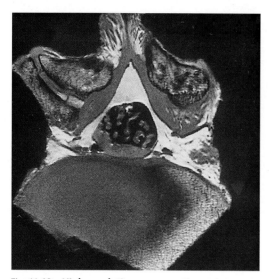

Fig. 11.**19 High-resolution magnetic resonance image of a vertebral body specimen.** As in the previous figure, the cauda equina fibers are clearly visualized.

that the cord is encased by radiographically dense compact bone, which gives rise to significant beam-hardening artifact.

The physiologic ascent of the spinal cord is associated with a relative descent of the spinal nerve roots along with the bony vertebral column. The lower the level at which a nerve root exits the spinal canal, the more pronounced this discrepancy.

The eight cervical spinal nerves each exit the neuroforamen that is located above the corresponding vertebral body. For example, the C6 root exits the spinal canal above the C6 vertebra, between C5 and C6, while the C8 root exits below C7 and above T1. At more caudal levels, all the nerve roots exit the spinal canal below the corresponding vertebral body.

This arrangement is subject to numerous variations, however—such as two conjoined roots exiting through one foramen.

In evaluating nerve root compression that does not appear to be consistent with the reported clinical findings, it should be considered that segmental innervation is also subject to variations. Thus, pain or neurologic defi-

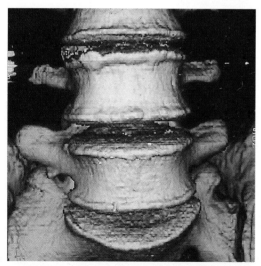

a

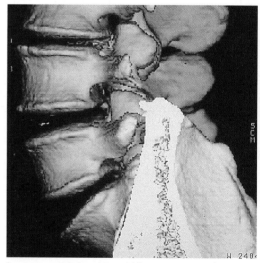

Fig. 11.**20 a–d Threshold-based shaded surface reconstructions of the lower lumbar spine.** These views were generated on the control console using the post-processing software that comes with most CT scanners. They are most commonly used to visualize complex

fractures and deformities and for preoperative planning—i.e., in situations that require a three-dimensional portrayal of spinal anatomy.
a Anterior view.
b Lateral view.

Abb. 11.**20 c** u. **d** ▷

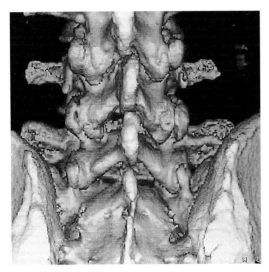

Fig. 11.**20 c**   Posterior view.

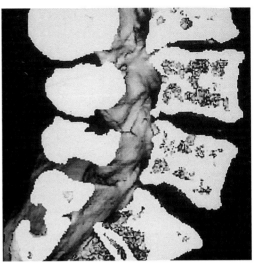

Fig. 11.**20 d**   Lateral view after computerized elimination of the near half of the vertebral bodies.

cits that follow the classic distribution of the S1 root, for example, may rarely be caused by compression of the L5 root.

There is no spinal cord below the L1–2 level in adults, only the cauda equina, composed of descending spinal nerve roots surrounding the non-neural filum terminale. The latter descends from the tip of the conus medullaris to the dorsal surface of the coccyx. The cauda equina fibers and filum terminale are clearly visualized by postmyelographic CT, which can also demonstrate the attachment site of the filum. This is particularly helpful in evaluating a tethered cord syndrome and planning the operative approach.

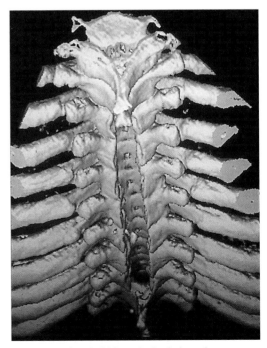

Fig. 11.**21   Threshold-based shaded surface reconstruction of the thoracic spine following an extended laminectomy from T1 to T7.** This surgery was performed for rapid decompression of an acute epidural hematoma.

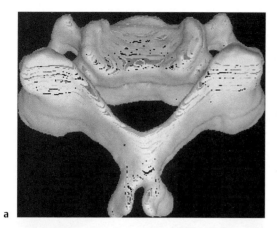

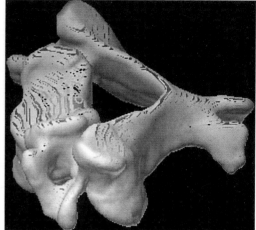

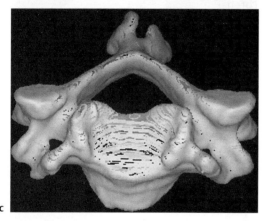

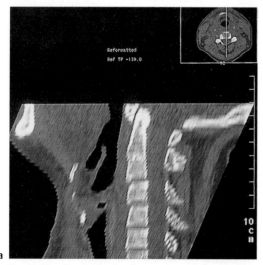

Fig. 11.**22 a–c** **Three-dimensional shaded surface reconstructions of a cervical vertebra specimen.**
a Posterior view.
b Lateral view.
c Anterior view.

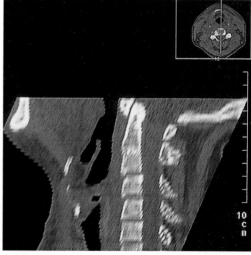

Fig. 11.**23 a, b** **Sagittal reformatting of the healthy cervical spine of a young man evaluated for a dens fracture.** The hyperdense band-like structure at the base of the dens is a commonly observed remnant of the fusion site of the separately formed portions of C2.

Spinal Meninges

The dura mater continues out through the foramen magnum from the cranial cavity to form the intraspinal dural sac. This sac extends inferiorly to the sacrum, generally to S2, where it is anchored to the dorsal surface of the coccyx as the dural terminal filament, which contains the filum terminale.

The dural sac has sheath-like extensions on each side that extend into the neuroforamina and cover the origins of the spinal nerve roots. They contain the spinal ganglion of the corresponding side. Nerve root compression caused by a herniated disk, for example, sometimes appears on postmyelographic CT as a filling defect in the affected root sheath. Because the root sheaths are directed slightly anteriorly, opacification of the sheaths can be improved by performing the CT examination in the prone position.

The dura is intimately adherent to the spinal arachnoid, a web-like tissue that completely fills the space between the dural sac and the pia mater that directly overlies the cord. This space is a continuation of the intracranial subarachnoid space and is filled with CSF. Contrast material is injected into the subarachnoid space for conventional myelography and postmyelographic CT.

The subarachnoid space on each side of the cord is traversed by the denticulate ligament, a coronal fibrous sheet with openings at the level of the spinal nerve roots. It establishes an attachment between the spinal cord and dural sac.

Epidural Space

The epidural space is a space between the dural sac and spinal canal wall that contains fat and predominantly venous vessels in the form of a plexus. It may be partly or completely occupied by pathology such as a herniated disk, tumor mass, or spinal stenosis. CT in these cases shows obliteration of the hypodense (– 80 to – 100 HU) epidural fat surrounding the dural sac. The epidural space is clinically important because of its frequent hematogenous involvement by metastatic tumors, inflammatory processes, and other disease.

■ References

Recommended for further study

Lang J. Anatomy of the craniocervical junction. In: Voth D, Glees P, editors. Diseases of the craniocervical junction. Berlin: de Gruyter, 1987: 27–61.

Wackenheim A. The pathogenesis of two distinct cervico-occipital malformations. In: Voth D, Glees P, editors. Diseases of the craniocervical junction. Berlin: de Gruyter, 1987: 63–7.

Senol U, Cubuk M, Sindel M et al. Anteroposterior diameter of the vertebral canal in cervical region: comparison of anatomical, computed tomographic, and plain film measurements. Clin Anat 2001; 14(1): 15–8.

12 Functional and Structural Abnormalities

Congenital Functional and Structural Abnormalities of the Spine

Spinal Arteriovenous Malformation

Frequency: rare; approximately 3–11% of intradural extramedullary masses.

Suggestive morphologic findings: an arteriovenous malformation (AVM) appears as a scalloped mass of very high density after bolus contrast administration. Early postinjection scans show rapid clearance of the contrast medium.

Procedure: contiguous thin slices before and after bolus contrast administration.

Other studies: magnetic resonance imaging (MRI) and spinal angiography. Myelography was the gold standard prior to MRI and spinal angiography, but today these studies are indispensable for diagnosis and treatment planning.

Checklist for scan interpretation:
▶ Extent of AVM?
▶ Significant cord compression?
▶ Evidence of prior hemorrhage?

■ Pathogenesis

The pathogenesis of arteriovenous malformations is controversial, but they are believed to result from anomalous vascular differentiation during about the sixth week of embryologic development. This leads to a persistence of thin-walled vessels with a deficient intima and media, primitive capillaries and precapillary channels, and arteriovenous shunts (Fig. 12.**1**).

Spinal AVMs are most commonly found on the dorsal aspect of the lower spinal cord. Embryologically, this has to do with the earlier differentiation of the ventral and rostral portions of the spinal vascular system. Spinal AVMs usually span a length of four or five vertebral segments, and may have one or more feeding arteries. They are classified into four types and numerous subtypes according to their location, extent, supply, and size. An AVM cannot usually be classified on the basis of the computed tomography (CT) findings, however.

The symptoms of spinal AVMs depend on their location and the associated change in intraspinal hemodynamics. Ischemic changes in the spinal cord may result from direct compression of the cord by the mass itself. They can also result from venous hypertension, with damming back of blood and outflow obstruction, or from an arterial steal effect. Hemorrhage, thrombosis, and water-hammer pulse have also been discussed as pathophysiologic factors. This explains why the location of the AVM does not always correlate with the location of the associated cord injury.

■ Frequency

Although they are rare, spinal AVMs are the most common spinal vascular anomaly. According to a study published in 1978, spinal AVMs make up approximately 3.3–11% of intradural extramedullary masses. Males predominate by a ratio of 4 : 1, and the peak occurrence is in the fourth and fifth decades.

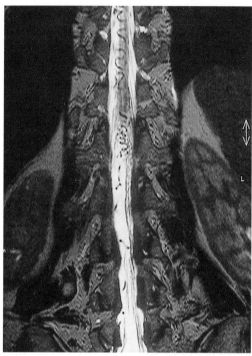
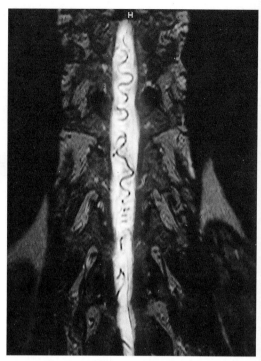

a

Fig. 12.**1 a, b T2-weighted coronal magnetic resonance images** show an intradural mass of tangled vessels extending all along the imaged region. The arteriovenous malformation (AVM) occupies the dorsal portion of the spinal canal and overlies the dorsal aspect of the cord. Most of the depicted vessels are dilated and tortuous veins, but not the AVM nidus itself, which can usually be identified only by angiography.

■ Clinical Manifestations

The initial symptoms typically appear between 35 and 40 years of age. In most cases they are indistinguishable from cord compression symptoms caused by other mass lesions. Pain is the most common initial symptom, and it often projects in a radicular pattern. Frequently the pain is worse at night and may increase after a hot bath. Approximately 65 % of patients experience a symptom complex of sensorimotor disturbances in the lower extremities and anal sphincter dysfunction.

■ CT Morphology

A spinal AVM can be difficult to identify on unenhanced CT scans, on which it appears as an elongated, isodense intradural extramedullary mass. Following intravenous contrast administration, the AVM appears as a scalloped mass of very high density, often containing tortuous blood vessels that may extend over several segments. Whenever an AVM is suspected, the contrast medium should be administered by bolus injection, and the arterial phase of enhancement should be evaluated. AVMs are characterized by intense enhancement during the arterial phase and by a rapid fading of enhancement on early postinjection scans.

AVM appears on postmyelographic CT scans as a filling defect with the features described above.

Congenital Spinal Stenosis

Frequency: relatively common; often coexists with acquired abnormalities.

Suggestive morphologic findings: narrow spinal canal, short pedicles (anteroposterior diameter < 12 mm at cervical level, < 11.5 mm at lumbar level; low interpedicular distance 20 mm), decreased epidural fat.

Procedure: contiguous CT slices with secondary reconstructions.

Other studies: myelography has several applications in spinal stenosis, such as determining whether cerebrospinal fluid (CSF) exchange is maintained past the site of the stenosis. Myelography should be combined if possible with postmyelogram CT. With cervical stenosis, MRI is useful for detecting cervical myelopathy.

Checklist for scan interpretation:
▶ Degree and craniocaudal extent of the stenosis?
▶ Other circumscribed lesions (disk protrusions, spondylophytes) that could account for clinical symptoms?
▶ Facet hypertrophy?

Pathogenesis

Despite marked individual variations in the width of the cervical, thoracic, and lumbar spinal canal, numerous studies have been published on normal values, especially in the lumbar spine. The following minimum values are a useful guide for excluding spinal stenosis, regardless of the affected segment:

- The anteroposterior diameter should be at least 11.5 mm.
- The interpedicular distance should measure at least 16 mm.
- The width of the lateral recess should be no less than 3 mm.
- The area of the spinal canal should measure at least 1.45 cm² in axial cross-section.
- The ligamenta flava should not exceed 4–5 mm in thickness.

For simplicity, it may be said that spinal stenosis is present whenever the spinal canal and lateral recess are disproportionately narrow in relation to the structures they contain.

Congenital spinal stenosis usually results from shortening of the pedicles. This may be an idiopathic condition or may result from a genetic disease such as achondroplasia. Symptoms are caused by a disproportion between the diameter of the dural sac and the width of the spinal canal or lateral recess. With achondroplasia, this disproportion typically increases in the craniocaudal direction, whereas in dysraphic syndromes and other conditions it may be circumscribed and confined to a few segments. Overall, however, congenital spinal stenosis is rare compared with acquired stenosis caused by degenerative diseases such as spondylarthrosis, facet hypertrophy, and disk protrusions. Many of these patients have a relative congenital narrowing that becomes symptomatic when a space-occupying condition supervenes. The symptoms may result from cord or nerve root compression, or from the compression of intraspinal blood vessels.

Frequency

Congenital spinal stenosis rarely occurs in isolation. Symptoms usually appear when acquired degenerative changes cause additional stenosis of a congenitally narrow spinal canal.

Clinical Manifestations

Back pain is a common early symptom. Lumbar stenosis is frequently marked by spinal claudication, with a slowly progressive decline in walking distance. Bladder dysfunction and anal sphincter dysfunction may subsequently develop. Cervical stenosis may be associated with spinal ataxia and other signs of cervical myelopathy.

The classification of spinal stenosis is discussed in connection with acquired structural abnormalities on p. 357 (Fig. 12.**2**).

CT Morphology

Scans parallel to the disk spaces demonstrate narrowing of the spinal canal. The anteroposterior canal diameter should be at least 11.5 mm in the lumbar region and 12 mm in the cervical

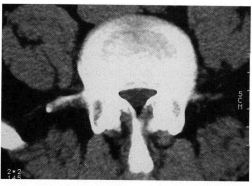 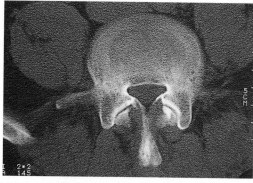

Fig. 12.**2a, b** **Congenital spinal stenosis, with short pedicles encroaching on the dural sac.** The cross-sectional area of the spinal canal is definitely less than 1.45 cm².

region. The interlaminar distance should be at least 16 mm, and the cross-sectional area at least 1.45 cm². In addition, CT often shows a reduction or obliteration of epidural fat.

Spondylosis, Spondylolysis, Spondylolisthesis (Figs. 12.2–12.7)

Frequency: common.

Suggestive morphologic findings: osteophytic spurs and facet hypertrophy, leading to stenosis of the lateral recess and neuroforamina; a cleft defect in the pedicles (spondylolysis) or a step-off due to spondylolisthesis.

Procedure: CT may consist of contiguous slices or scans parallel to the disk spaces. Suspected spondylolysis is evaluated with reformatted images or direct scans parallel to the pedicles.

Other studies: MRI and radionuclide scans are useful for detecting spondylolysis and checking for activity or sclerosis of the bone margins. Compression of the subarachnoid space is evaluated by myelography and postmyelographic CT (Fig. 12.**3a**). Conventional radiographs. Function views.

Checklist for scan interpretation:
▶ Degree of stenosis?
▶ Degree of spondylolisthesis?
▶ Spondylolysis: is there a visible defect in the pedicles? Do adjacent portions of the pedicles have sclerotic margins?

■ Pathogenesis

Spondylosis. This term is used for nonspecific degenerative spinal disease.

Spondylolisthesis. Spondylolisthesis refers to the anterior subluxation of one vertebral body over another. The most common form is displacement of L5 over S1, followed by L4 over L5.

Spondylolisthesis may result from spondylolysis, or a defect in the pedicles. Pseudospondylolisthesis can also occur due to degenerative or inflammatory changes in the facet joints (e.g., in patients with rheumatoid arthritis).

In the commonly used Meyerding classification, spondylolisthesis is divided into four grades, depending on the degree of vertebral body displacement, with each grade representing one-quarter of the longitudinal diameter of the displaced vertebral body (0–25 % = grade I, > 75 % = grade IV). This classification does not correlate with clinical manifestations, however (Fig. 12.**3**).

Complete slippage of one vertebral body over another is called spondyloptosis.

Spondylolysis. This refers to a unilateral or bilateral pars defect—i.e., a discontinuity in the part of the vertebral arch located between the superior and inferior articular processes. The defect may be congenital, but acquired forms can result from a posttraumatic nonunion or fatigue fracture of the vertebral arch (Fig. 12.**5**).

Most cases are asymptomatic or cause non-specific symptoms in the form of recurring back pain. Rarely, spondylolysis can cause nerve root compression that requires surgical stabilization of the affected site.

Pars defects most commonly occur in the L5 vertebra, followed by L4. Spondylolysis is rare in the cervical vertebrae, where C6 is the most frequent site of occurrence. The linear defect or fracture line corresponds to the "collar" of the Lachapel dog figure in conventional oblique spinal radiographs.

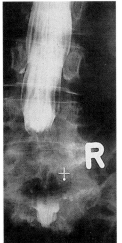
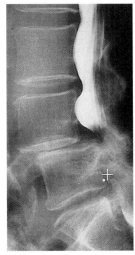

a

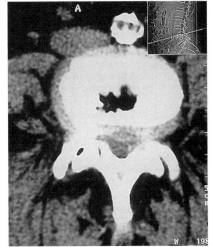

b

Fig. 12.**3 a–c Spondylolisthesis.**

a Anteroposterior and lateral lumbar myelograms of a woman with grade II spondylolisthesis at L4–5 caused by bilateral spondylolysis of the L4 pedicles. The dural sac is severely compressed at the level of the step-off. Contrast medium injected above the stenosis can pass through the compressed site, but passage of contrast is considerably delayed, and it does not reach the caudal portions of the dural sac until the end of the examination.

b Axial CT scan through the affected level shows an apparently broad-based disk protrusion or excessive prominence of a real protrusion caused by the vertebral slippage. The lateral scout view, taken in the recumbent position, shows less slippage than the standing myelogram.

c The bone-window scan clearly demonstrates the excessive load placed on the intervertebral disk and facet joints by the hypermobility at the affected level. Note the clusters of nitrogen bubbles in the disk space and right facet joint.

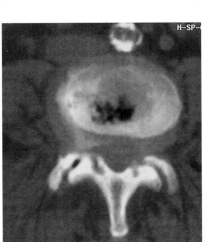

c

Retrolisthesis. Retrolisthesis is the opposite of spondylolisthesis, denoting the posterior displacement of one vertebral body over another. Generally it does not result from a vertebral arch defect but from a decrease in the height of an intervertebral disk space. As the facet joints assume an oblique anterosuperior-to-posteroinferior orientation, the height reduction can lead to varying degrees of posterior slippage (Fig. 12.**4**).

■ Frequency

Nonspecific *spondylosis* is a very common degenerative condition. CT scans or radiographs demonstrate the changes in:

- 5–10% of patients 20–30 years of age
- > 50% of patients by age 45
- > 90% of patients by age 60

Spondylolisthesis, usually of low grade, is found in up to 20% of conventional lumbar spinal radiographs, according to Frymoyer (1988).

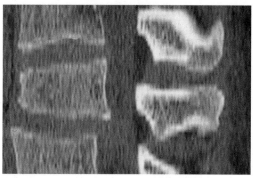

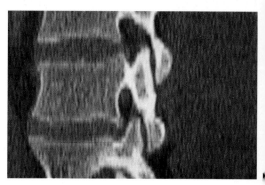

Fig. 12.**4a, b   Retrolisthesis.** An L4–5 disk herniation has caused a substantial height reduction at the affected level.
a The pronounced retrolisthesis in the sagittal reformatted image is a result of the height reduction.

b The inferior articular process of L4 slips posteriorly downward on the superior articular process of L5, as on an inclined plane.

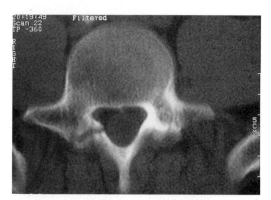

Fig. 12.**5   Spondylolysis.** Spondylolysis may be unilateral or bilateral and can result from trauma. Chronic overload can lead to a fatigue fracture, or a single traumatic event can fracture the vertebral arch, followed by the development of a nonunion. This image is a bone-window view of a right-sided spondylolysis caused by trauma.

Spondylolysis with a demonstrable pars defect is present of 4–7% of the general population and is frequently asymptomatic.

■ Clinical Manifestations

Symptoms are usually nonspecific, and include the following:

- Low back pain
- Root compression syndromes
- Compression of the conus medullaris and cauda equina

■ CT Morphology

Soft-tissue and bone-window CT scans will usually demonstrate the degenerative changes of *spondylosis* in the form of marginal bone spurs and hypertrophic facet joints. The radiologist needs to assess the extent to which these changes could produce clinically relevant central canal stenosis or lateral recess stenosis (see p. 337).

Spondylolisthesis is often apparent on CT scout views. It appears on single slices as an abrupt discontinuity between adjacent vertebral bodies. This can create the appearance of a broad-based protrusion of the intervening disk. (*Caution:* the degree of slippage may appear much greater in the standing patient and may become clinically relevant only in that position. We recommend comparing the scans with conventional standing radiographs or function views of the spine.)

Spondylolysis is best demonstrated by bone-window CT scans parallel to the pedicles, which slope slightly downward in an antero-superior-to-posteroinferior direction. The gantry angulation should be adjusted accordingly (Fig. 12.**6**).

When the scans are interpreted, it may be important for the referring physician to know whether the margins of the pars defect are sclerotic. If they are not, there is a chance that nonoperative immobilization will be beneficial. It may be helpful to add a radionuclide bone scan when addressing this question. Intense tracer uptake, signifying active bone metabolism, again suggests that fusion of the site may be accomplished without operative treatment.

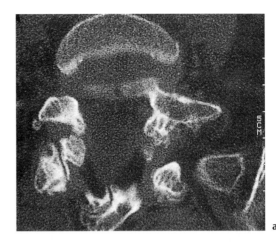

a

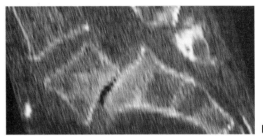

b

Fig. 12.**6 a, b** **Spondylolisthesis.** Bilateral arch defects in L5 have led to a Meyerding grade II–III spondylolisthesis at the L5–S1 level.
a Axial bone-window scan.
b Sagittal reformatting.

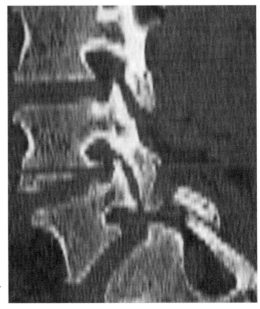

Fig. 12.**7** **Vertebral arch defects** are often clearly visu- ▷ alized on sagittal CT reformatted images.

Syringomyelia, Hydromyelia
(Figs. 12.**8**–12.**10**)

Frequency: often associated with other anomalies such as Arnold–Chiari malformation.

Suggestive morphologic findings: intramedullary area of low attenuation extending over several segments. The spinal cord may be expanded or atrophic. Postmyelographic CT may show rapid or delayed opacification of the canal by contrast medium.

Procedure: contiguous slices with secondary reconstructions. Postmyelographic CT can establish whether the syrinx communicates with the subarachnoid space.

Other studies: MRI (Figs. 12.**9**, 12.**10**), with a CSF pulsation study. Postmyelographic CT can determine the degree of CSF exchange with the subarachnoid space.

Checklist for scan interpretation:
▶ Longitudinal and lateral extent of the lesion?
▶ Does the canal enhance on postmyelographic CT? When does this occur?
▶ If CT findings are equivocal, proceed with MRI.

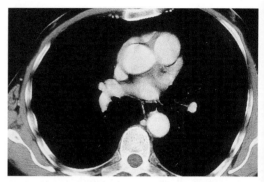

Fig. 12.**8 Central hypodensity of the spinal cord.** Thoracic CT scan in a man who sustained an L1 fracture about 10 years previously in a motor vehicle accident. For years, he had progressive lower extremity pain and weakness and bladder dysfunction. Even this survey scan, acquired for other reasons, clearly demonstrates a central hypodensity of the spinal cord. (The lesion was investigated further by magnetic resonance imaging.)

▪ Pathogenesis

Syringomyelia and hydromyelia are benign malformations of the spinal cord marked by the presence of an elongated, fluid-filled intramedullary cavity. Syringomyelia is distin-

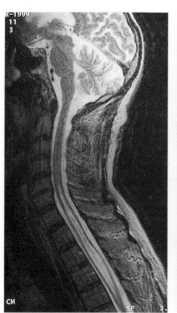

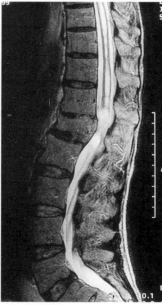

Fig. 12.**9 a, b Sagittal T2-weighted magnetic resonance imaging of the cervical spine and thoracolumbar junction area.** The central canal of the spinal cord is expanded from the cervical cord to the level of L1. The height of L1 is reduced as the result of a fracture, which has caused impairment of cerebrospinal fluid circulation.

a   b

guished by an intramedullary cavity that may be independent of the central canal, or may communicate with it but lacks an ependymal lining. Hydromyelia denotes persistence and expansion of the ependyma-lined central canal, which communicates with the fourth ventricle. The two anomalies are difficult to distinguish by CT in any given case. The central or lateral position of the expansion provides an uncertain clue to the identity of the lesion.

Both conditions can occur as a *congenital or acquired anomaly* of the spinal cord. Congenital forms usually occur in the setting of a complex syndrome. For example, from 20% to 70% of patients with Arnold–Chiari malformation have syringomyelia.

Other diseases that are frequently associated with syringomyelia or hydromyelia are as follows:

- Dysraphic disorders
- Dandy–Walker malformation
- Very severe scoliosis
- Klippel–Feil syndrome

Because the malformation is caused by altered hydrodynamics, it can develop in all diseases that lead to a congenital or acquired obstruction of CSF drainage.

The currently favored theory oɪ. the pathogenesis of syringomyelia is the *hydrodissection theory,* advanced by Williams et al. (1981). When actions occur that raise the intra-abdominal pressure, such as coughing or sneezing, and when communication between the spinal and intracranial extra-axial CSF spaces is impaired (e.g., due to herniation of the cerebellar tonsils into the foramen magnum), a check-valve mechanism is created.

The intra-abdominal pressure is transmitted through epidural veins to the intraspinal space. This leads to an upward movement of the pressure wave, allowing CSF to flow into the cranial cavity. As the intraspinal pressure subsides, the check-valve mechanism prevents a compensatory downward pulsation in the extra-axial CSF spaces. The resulting negative pressure tends to increase the CSF pulsation in the central canal of the spinal cord (hydromyelia) and also increases interstitial fluid out-

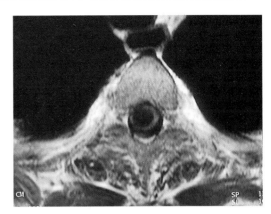

Fig. 12.**10** **Syringomyelia** documented by axial T1-weighted magnetic resonance imaging.

flow, leading to the development of syringomyelia. Histopathologic studies of the cord in such cases have found dilated perivascular spaces. In many cases, the wall of the syrinx was rich in small arteries and veins.

This led Ball and Dayan (1972) to theorize that CSF and extracellular fluid enter the cavity through the Virchow–Robin spaces of the spinal cord. Another theory, advanced by Pillay et al. in 1992 and based largely on MRI studies, assumes that approximately 30% of CSF formation is intraspinal. Thus, any type of outflow obstruction caused by trauma or arachnoiditis, for example, can lead to intramedullary cavity formation by the mechanism described above.

■ Frequency

Syringomyelia or hydromyelia is commonly found in association with other anomalies.

■ Clinical Manifestations

Many patients experience a gradual progression of the following neurologic symptoms:

- Dissociated sensory loss at the level of the affected segments
- Motor disturbances and weakness mainly affecting the upper extremity
- Very severe pain in some cases

■ CT Morphology

CT sometimes demonstrates a circumscribed, elongated region of low attenuation within the spinal cord (Fig. 12.**8**). The cord may be expanded or atrophic. The cavity may already occupy most of the cord diameter. There is frequent widening of the bony spinal canal. On postmyelographic CT, the canal may enhance rapidly through direct connections with the subarachnoid space, or it may opacify slowly over 4–8 hours due to gradual contrast permeation.

Klippel–Feil Syndrome
(Figs. 12.**11**, 12.**12**)

Frequency: rare.

Suggestive morphologic findings: the fusion of two or more vertebral bodies (Fig. 12.**11**).

Procedure: contiguous thin CT slices with secondary reconstructions.

Other studies: conventional radiographs. MRI can evaluate for cervical myelopathy.

Checklist for scan interpretation:
▶ Craniocaudal extent of the fusion?
▶ Evaluate the remaining unaffected segments, since compensatory hypermobility leads to early degenerative changes that may cause clinical symptoms.

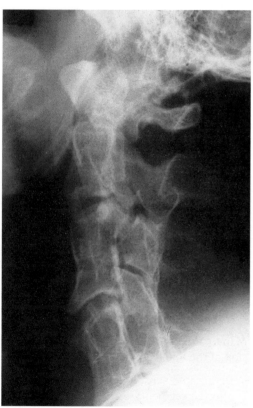

a

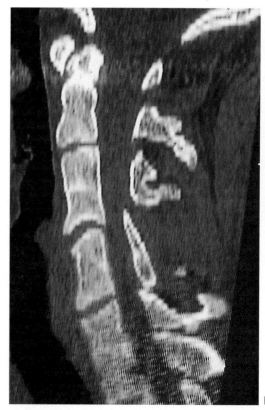

b

Fig. 12.**11 a, b Klippel–Feil syndrome** as demonstrated by a conventional radiograph and sagittal CT reformatted image of the cervical spine. The images show interbody fusion and atypical segmentation of the entire cervical spine, manifested clinically by a profound limitation of neck motion in this young patient.

◼ Pathogenesis

Klippel–Feil syndrome is based on the congenital fusion of two or more cervical vertebrae. The fusion may be limited to the vertebral bodies or may affect the entire vertebra including the posterior elements. In most cases the vertebrae are flattened, and the associated disk spaces are absent or hypoplastic. The neuroforamina are narrowed. Patients with Klippel–Feil syndrome often have coexisting clinical abnormalities.

The classic triad of the Klippel–Feil syndrome consists of:

- Short neck
- Limited motion of the cervical spine
- Low nuchal hairline

Less than 50% of patients exhibit all three of these features, however.

Other associated anomalies are listed below:

- Platybasia
- Basilar impression
- Syringomyelia
- Encephalocele
- Cranial asymmetries
- Syndactyly
- Renal anomalies
- Anal atresia
- Cardiac anomalies
- Supernumerary pulmonary lobes
- Cleft lip and palate
- Deafness due to inner ear anomalies

Another frequent anomaly, found in approximately 25–40% of cases, is a unilateral elevation of the scapula (Sprengel's deformity).

Klippel–Feil syndrome is probably based on a hereditary developmental error, with deficient segmentation of the cervical somites between the third and eighth weeks of embryonic development. Similar changes, including interbody fusion, are also found in children with alcoholic embryopathy or chromosome abnormalities (Figs. 12.**11**, 12.**12**).

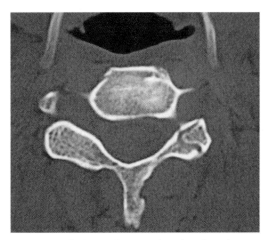

Fig. 12.**12** **Block vertebrae in Klippel–Feil syndrome.** Besides absence of the disk space, single axial CT slices show partial assimilation of the facet joints, which is typical of the partial or complete fusion of adjacent vertebral bodies.

◼ Frequency

Klippel–Feil syndrome is rare. Its true incidence is unknown, since many cases of block vertebrae are asymptomatic.

◼ Clinical Manifestations

Most cases are asymptomatic. When symptoms occur, they usually result from early osteoarthritic degeneration of the hypermobile adjacent segments. Rarely, compression syndromes of the cervical cord or nerve roots are observed.

◼ CT Morphology

CT demonstrates the fusion of two or more cervical vertebrae.

Dysraphic Disorders

Spina Bifida

Frequency: a common incidental finding.

Suggestive morphologic findings: incomplete closure of the vertebral arch with no associated meningeal anomaly.

Procedure: obtain secondary reconstructions only if the defect is clinically relevant.

Other studies: conventional radiographs. MRI may be helpful to exclude involvement of the meninges and spinal cord.

Checklist for scan interpretation:
▶ Extent of the defect?
▶ Is the defect limited to bony structures?
▶ Check for associated anomalies (lipomas, etc.).

■ Pathogenesis

Spina bifida is based on a congenital absence of the spinous processes and portions of the vertebral arch. It is not associated with meningeal or cord protrusion. In some cases, the defect can be detected by external palpation.

■ Frequency

Spina bifida is a common defect. Mild forms are detected in approximately 20–30% of the population.

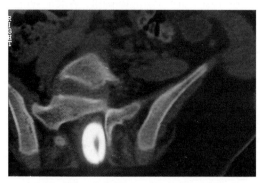

Fig. 12.**13** **Spina bifida.** A postmyelographic CT in sacral spina bifida demonstrates a meningocele plus dorsal adhesion of the filum terminale.

■ Clinical Manifestations

Spina bifida is not necessarily associated with neurologic deficits. Often the diagnosis is made incidentally or is suggested by coexisting anomalies such as diastematomyelia, lipoma, tethered cord syndrome, dermoid, or by a hairy nevus overlying the defect.

■ CT Morphology

CT shows incomplete closure of the neural arch with no accompanying anomaly of the meninges, underlying cord, or nerve roots (Fig. 12.**13**).

If spina bifida is detected incidentally, no further studies are necessary.

Myelomeningocele

Frequency: common.

Suggestive morphologic findings: herniation of leptomeninges and variable neural elements through a bony defect.

Procedure: contiguous CT slices with secondary reconstructions.

Other studies: MRI to demonstrate the entire neural axis in sagittal section (often permits better evaluation of associated anomalies).

Checklist for scan interpretation:
▶ Location and extent of the myelomeningocele?
▶ Any evidence that the lesion has ruptured?

■ Pathogenesis

Myelomeningocele is a dysraphic anomaly in which a sac covered by leptomeninges and containing CSF and variable neural elements herniates through a bony defect in the spine. If the sac does not contain neural elements, it is classified as a meningocele.

As in spina bifida, the etiology of myelomeningocele is based on a neural tube defect in the area of the caudal neuropore, which normally closes by the 28th day of embryologic development. Myelomeningocele is frequently associated with other anomalies such as Arnold–Chiari malformation, congenital scoliosis, vertebral anomalies, syringomyelia or hydromyelia, and tethered cord syndrome.

A special form is traumatic meningocele following the avulsion of nerve roots (e.g., from the brachial plexus).

■ Frequency

With an incidence of one per 1000–2000 live births, myelomeningocele is the most common congenital anomaly of the central nervous system (CNS).

■ Clinical Manifestations

The clinical symptoms depend on the size and location of the myelomeningocele. High cervical lesions can cause complete lower extremity paralysis in severe cases.

■ CT Morphology

CT demonstrates the herniation of leptomeninges and variable nerve structures through a bony defect in the spine. The defect is usually located in the dorsal lumbosacral or suboccipital area and is associated with widening of the spinal canal at that level. Special forms are anterior sacral myelomeningocele and lateral thoracic meningocele.

Tethered Cord Syndrome

Frequency: often accompanies myelomeningocele and other syndromes.

Suggestive morphologic findings: low conus medullaris, thickened filum terminale, visible fatty tissue at the site of attachment.

Procedure: postmyelographic CT is ideal for positively identifying the filum terminale and its site of attachment (Figs. 12.**13**, 12.**14**).

Other studies: sagittal MRI is useful for detecting signs of myelopathy.

Checklist for scan interpretation:
▶ Level of the conus medullaris in relation to the lumbar spine?
▶ Diameter of the filum terminale?
▶ Coexisting anomalies?

■ Pathogenesis

Tethered cord syndrome involves a low position of the conus medullaris combined with a short, thickened filum terminale. It occurs when the dural attachment of the filum terminale acts as a checkrein to the physiologic ascent of the cord. Often a lipoma is found at the broad-based site of attachment. As the vertebral column grows in length, it exerts traction on the spinal cord leading to chronic recurring ischemia.

Tethered cord syndrome is commonly associated with myelomeningocele.

■ Frequency

The majority of patients with myelomeningocele also have radiologic evidence of tethered cord syndrome.

■ Clinical Manifestations

The most common symptoms are:
– Pain
– Accompanying anomalies such as scoliosis and foot deformities

Many patients also have motor deficits such as unsteady gait, micturition difficulties, and incontinence. Skin changes such as nevi and hairy patches are often found over the defect.

Tethered cord syndrome is assumed to be present in all myelomeningocele patients who develop scoliosis, gait deterioration, progressive lower extremity spasticity, or voiding difficulties and pain. These developing symptoms usually permit a diagnosis to be made between 5 and 15 years of age.

■ CT Morphology

Even without contrast administration, CT can demonstrate a lipoma at the site where the filum is tethered. A low conus medullaris combined with a thickened filum terminale (> 2 mm in diameter) confirms the diagnosis, but postmyelographic CT is the only imaging study that can unequivocally define the tethered filum (Fig. 12.**14**).

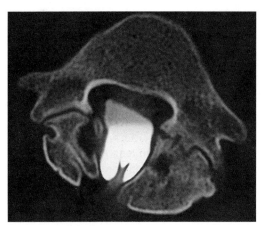

Fig. 12.**14 Tethered cord syndrome.** The dorsal attachment of the tethered filum is clearly visualized by postmyelographic CT.

Correct window and center settings (e.g., W = 2500, C = 1000) should be used to reduce partial volume effects caused by the surrounding contrast medium.

Diastematomyelia (Myeloschisis)
(Figs. 12.**15**–12.**17**)

Frequency: rare.

Suggestive morphologic findings: a bony or fibrous septum splitting the spinal cord into halves in the sagittal plane.

Procedure: contiguous thin CT slices, secondary reconstructions, bone window.

Other studies: MRI, postmyelographic CT. Unlike MRI, CT can distinguish between a bony and fibrous septum.

Checklist for scan interpretation:
▶ Height and extent of the lesion? Composition of the septum?
▶ Are there any other anomalies that could affect operative treatment (e.g., tethered cord syndrome)?

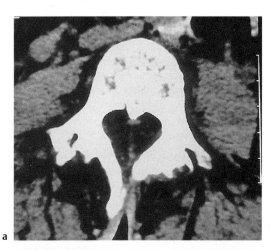

a

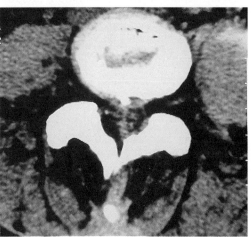

b

◁ Fig. 12.**15 a, b   Diastematomyelia.** In diastematomyelia, the affected portion of the spinal cord is split into two separate parts by a midline septum. The septum may be fibrous, as in this example, or may consist of a bony spur (see Fig. 12.**16**).

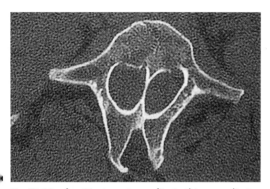

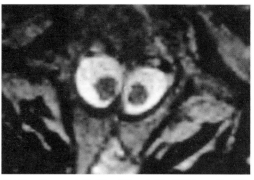

b

Fig. 12.**16 a, b   Diastematomyelia.** In this case, diastematomyelia is one feature of a complex malformation. CT is superior to magnetic resonance imaging (MRI), in that it can establish the bony nature of the septum dividing the cord. Neither T1-weighted MRI nor the T2-weighted image shown here can positively distinguish between a bony and fibrous septum.

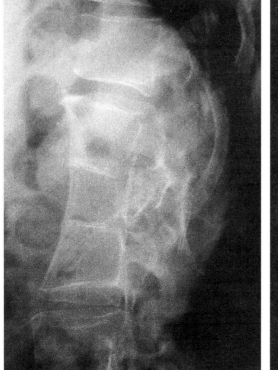

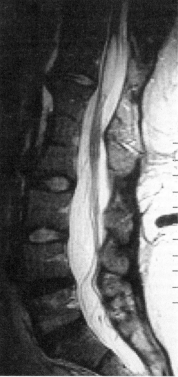

a   b

Fig. 12.**17 a–c   Diastematomyelia** (same patient as in Fig. 12.**16**). Fusion of the T12–L3 vertebral bodies is seen in a conventional radiograph (**a**), sagittal T2-weighted magnetic resonance image (**b**), and in a shaded surface display reconstructed from CT slices (**c**).

Fig. 12.**17 c** ▷

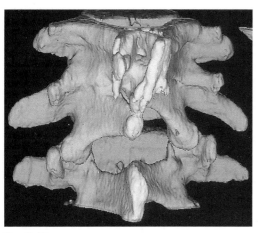

Fig. 12.**17 c**

■ Pathogenesis

Diastematomyelia is a congenital anomaly that occurs during embryologic development when the neural tube becomes folded over due to adhesions between the ectoderm and endoderm. This leads to a division of the spinal cord, conus medullaris, and filum terminale by a fibrous membrane (25%) or bony septum (75%) located in the midsagittal plane. Diastematomyelia is frequently accompanied by myelomeningocele, tethered cord syndrome, and congenital scoliosis, and is associated with clinical stigmata such as hairy patches on the back and foot deformities. The condition most commonly occurs in the lower thoracic and upper lumbar regions. It is common to find a marked decrease in vertebral height or complete absence of the disk spaces at the level of the defect. Interbody vertebral fusion is also common. A variant of diastematomyelia is diplomyelia, in which two separate hemicords occupy a common dural sac with no demonstrable fibrous or bony septum.

■ Frequency

Diastematomyelia is a rare anomaly. Females are predominantly affected, by a ratio of about 3 : 1.

■ Clinical Manifestations

The clinical symptoms are very similar to those that may occur in tethered cord syndrome.

■ CT Morphology

CT usually shows a conspicuous division of the spinal cord along the sagittal plane. The division is effected by a bony or fibrous septum and is almost always associated with other anomalies.

Lipomyeloschisis (Dural Lipoma, Lipomyelomeningocele, Fibrolipoma of the Filum Terminale)

> **Frequency:** common in the setting of complex dysraphisms.
>
> **Suggestive morphologic findings:** intramedullary, intradural or extradural mass of fat density, often in the setting of dysraphic pathology.
>
> **Procedure:** contiguous CT slices, especially in complex malformations.
>
> **Other studies:** MRI to define the extent of the anomaly in the sagittal plane.
>
> **Checklist for scan interpretation:**
> ▶ Location in relation to a lumbar or sacral vertebral body?
> ▶ Extent and degree of the anomaly?

■ Pathogenesis

The dysraphic disorders include the various forms of lipomyeloschisis:

● Intradural lipoma
● Lipomyelomeningocele
● Fibrolipoma of the filum terminale

These anomalies are typically associated with a low position of the conus medullaris, a posterior neural arch defect affecting one or more vertebral bodies, and changes in the overlying skin.

Most lipomas occur in the extradural space of the lumbosacral area, where the lesion often extends into the subcutaneous tissue. Lipomas can occur anywhere along the spine, however, and may occasionally affect the entire spinal canal. Intradural and even intramedullary occurrence has also been described.

■ Frequency

Lipomyeloschisis often occurs in the setting of a complex dysraphism. Intraspinal lipomas may also occur independently of other anomalies, and some do not become symptomatic until adulthood. Males and females are affected equally.

■ Clinical Manifestations

If a complex malformation is present, its severity determines the clinical presentation. The dominant features usually consist of motor and sensory disturbances in the lower extremity and bladder dysfunction.

■ CT Morphology

CT scans show an intramedullary, intradural, or extramedullary mass of fat attenuation (–100 HU) that does not enhance after contrast administration. Frequently these masses are found in the setting of a complex dysraphic disorder. For example, they may occur at the level of attachment of the filum terminale in a patient with tethered cord syndrome (Fig. 12.**18**).

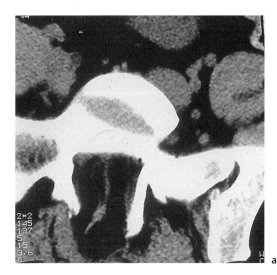

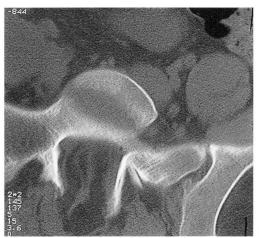

Fig. 12.**18** **Lipomyeloschisis.** CT scans at the S1 level show a congenital neural arch defect accompanied by dorsal tethering of the filum terminale and an intraspinal lipoma.
a Soft-tissue window.
b Bone window.

Spinal Meningeal Cysts (Figs. 12.**19**, 12.**20**)

■ **Frequency:** common incidental finding.

Suggestive morphologic findings: variable-size cystic mass of CSF density, which may compress the dural sac or individual nerve roots and may erode bony structures.

Procedure: postmyelographic CT is best for determining whether the cyst communicates with the rest of the subarachnoid space.

Other studies: myelography (type I and II cysts appear as contrast-filled outpouchings). MRI shows a cystic mass whose contents are isointense to CSF (Fig. 12.**20**).

Checklist for scan interpretation:
▶ Spinal meningeal cysts are usually detected incidentally.
▶ Nerve root compression?
▶ Does the cyst envelop the nerve root?

■ Pathogenesis

Spinal meningeal cyst is the term applied to cystic or diverticular, intradural and extradural outpouchings of the spinal meninges. They are known by various other names as well:

- Tarlov cyst
- Spinal arachnoid cyst
- Dural diverticulum
- Root sheath cyst

A classification proposed in 1988 is shown in Table 12.**1**.

Most spinal meningeal cysts are asymptomatic and are detected incidentally. Some are large enough, however, to produce symptoms of nerve root compression. Large cysts can have sufficient extent to compress nerve roots on both the affected side and the opposite side.

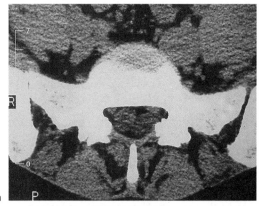
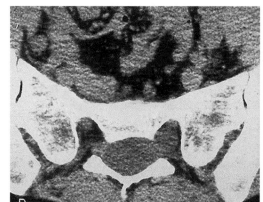

a

Fig. 12.**19a, b Spinal meningeal cyst.** CT demonstrates a sacral extradural mass displacing the dural sac and nerve roots and almost completely filling the sacral spinal canal. Note how the cyst had displaced the left S1 nerve root against the posterior surface of the neuroforamen. This classifies the lesion as a type Ia spinal meningeal cyst that does not contain a nerve root (see Table 12.**1**).

Table 12.**1** Classification of spinal meningeal cysts

Type	Description
I	Extradural meningeal cyst that does not contain a nerve root Ia Extradural meningeal cyst Ib Occult sacral meningocele
II	Extradural meningeal cyst that contains a nerve root (perineural Tarlov cyst, root-sheath cyst)
III	Intradural arachnoid cyst

■ **Frequency**

Spinal meningeal cysts are a common incidental finding, especially in postmyelographic CT.

■ **Clinical Manifestations**

Most spinal meningeal cysts are asymptomatic. If large enough, however, type I cysts in
particular can cause root compression with associated symptoms.

■ **CT Morphology**

CT demonstrates a cystic mass of variable size
that arises from the meninges and is filled with
fluid of CSF density. In postmyelographic CT
scans of type I and II cysts, the contrast distribution always confirms a communication
between the cyst and subarachnoid space.
Type III cysts most commonly occur in the dorsal subarachnoid space. Larger lesions of long
duration can cause bone erosion with
widening of the spinal canal and neuroforamina (Fig. 12.**19**).

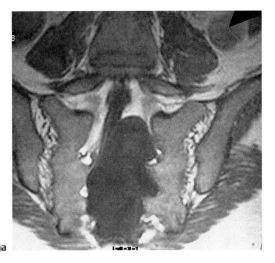

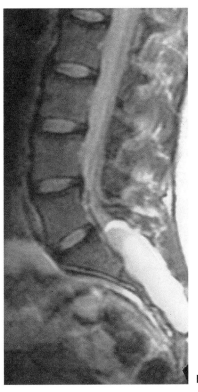

Fig. 12.**20 Spinal meningeal cyst.**
a The T1-weighted coronal magnetic resonance image
(MRI) defines the full craniocaudal extent of the cyst,
and reveals its mass effect on the dural sac and nerve
roots.
b The T2-weighted sagittal MRI reconfirms the cystic
nature of the mass. The cyst contents are isointense
to cerebrospinal fluid in both the T1-weighted and
T2-weighted images.

Acquired Functional and Structural Abnormalities of the Spine

Spinal Trauma

Fractures (Figs. 12.**21**–12.**27**)

Frequency: common.

Suggestive morphologic findings: step-off or contour irregularity; fragmentation, attenuation, irregularity, or fine linear disruption of the trabecular architecture. Associated soft-tissue injuries, paravertebral or intraspinal hematoma.

Procedure: contiguous thin CT slices, secondary reconstructions, bone window.

Other studies: compare CT findings with conventional radiographs.

Checklist for scan interpretation:
▶ Fracture type?
▶ Signs of displacement or instability?
▶ Extent of associated soft-tissue injuries?
▶ Narrowing of the spinal canal?
▶ Compression of the dural sac?
▶ Describe the fracture.
▶ Evaluate for possible instability using the three-column model.

There are various ways that CT can be used in the evaluation of spinal fractures. The choice in a given case depends mainly on the communication between the radiologist and the traumatologist at the facility where the patient has been admitted.

Frequently, conventional plain radiographs are the first step in the radiologic work-up of spinal trauma patients. Levels at which plain films show a fracture or possible structural injury are then evaluated with thin axial CT slices. If conventional radiographs are negative, CT scans are obtained at the levels that correlate with presenting neurologic deficits.

CT is the initial examination at some trauma centers, especially in multiple injury patients, in whom it can be used to screen for associated injuries to internal organs as well as bony injuries to the pelvis and spine. If the initial findings are abnormal or suspicious, the affected spinal segments can be selectively reevaluated using thin CT slices. This study may include scans acquired with parallel gantry angulation to the disk spaces.

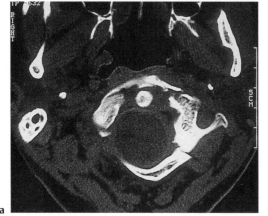 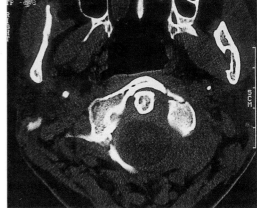

a

Fig. 12.**21 a, b** **Jefferson fracture.** The axial CT demonstrates a burst fracture of the anterior and posterior arches of the atlas caused by axial compression trauma to the spine.

If two-dimensional or three-dimensional reconstructions are desired, however, ultrathin slices should be acquired without gantry angulation, and spiral acquisition is preferred. This will eliminate respiratory artifacts and spontaneous motion-induced artifacts that could mimic step-offs in the reconstructed images.

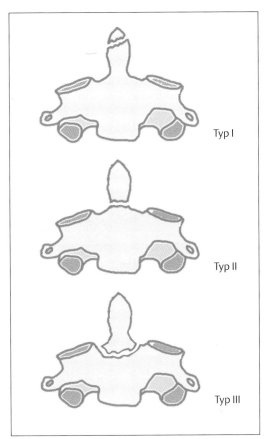

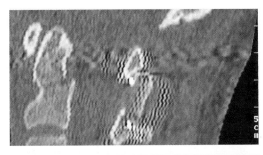

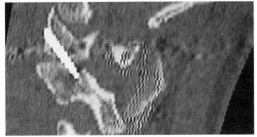

Fig. 12.**22 Anderson–D'Alonzo classification of dens fractures.** This classification is based on the level of the fracture line through the dens.

Fig. 12.**23 a, b Anderson type III fracture of the dens.** A fracture through the base of the dens has been stabilized by internal fixation with transpedicular screws. The reformatted images show slight residual displacement.

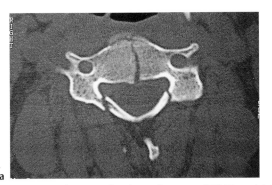

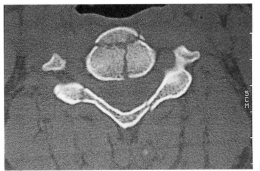

Fig. 12.**24 a, b Complete burst fracture of C4.** The axial CT demonstrates a complete sagittal fracture through the vertebral body, combined with fracture-separation of the vertebral arch.

Regardless of the sequence in which the studies are applied, it is always prudent to compare the CT images with conventional radiographs, especially if severe trauma has caused marked displacement of spinal segments or bone fragments, which can be difficult to correlate with a specific level in axial CT slices.

Spinal fractures are classified according to the affected spinal segment and the mechanism of the trauma.

■ Cervical Fractures

Atlas Fractures (C1)

Atlas fractures account for approximately 3–13 % of fractures of the cervical spine. In a series of 57 patients with atlas fractures, 56 % had an isolated fracture of C1, 44 % had combined fractures of C1 and C2, and 9 % had additional cervical vertebral fractures involving segments 3–7. Twenty-one percent of the patients also had

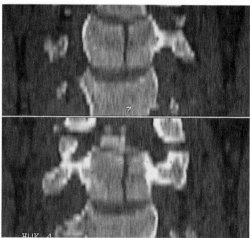
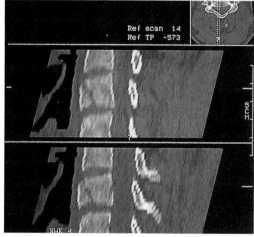

a

b

Fig. 12.**25 a, b** **Complete burst fracture of C4.** The sagittal and coronal CT reformatted images define the complex pattern of the C4 fracture. Despite posterior rim involvement, the images confirm the absence of spinal canal encroachment.

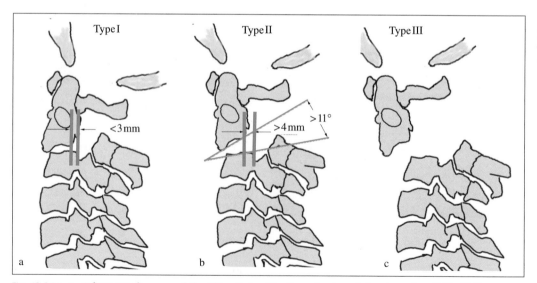

Fig. 12.**26 a–c** **Schematic diagram of the Effendi classification of axis arch fractures** (see Table 12.**3**).

significant craniocerebral injury. Of the isolated atlas fractures, 56% consisted of bilateral or multiple ring separations, 31% were unilateral ring fractures, and 13% of the fractures were confined to the lateral mass, leaving the arch intact.

Jefferson fracture. The Jefferson fracture is a burst fracture of the atlas caused by an axial compression injury (Fig. 12.**21**). The transverse ligament is ruptured, and the anterior and posterior arches are fractured and laterally displaced. Consequently, there is no encroachment on the spinal canal, and the fracture may not be associated with a neurologic deficit. Surgical treatment is still necessary, however, because the fracture is unstable.

A Jefferson fracture may occur in isolation, but in 41% of cases there is an associated fracture of C2.

On anteroposterior radiographs, the lateral mass of the atlas projects laterally past that of the axis. According to the Spence rule (Spence et al. 1970), a total lateral offset greater than 7 mm on both sides is proof that the transverse ligament is torn.

The diagnostic procedure of choice in this case is thin-slice CT scanning from C1 to C3. This will clearly define the burst fracture of the atlas arch while also detecting or excluding any small associated fractures of C2. These scans can also demonstrate spinal canal encroachment, if present, and can detect associated soft-tissue injuries or epidural hemorrhage.

Axis Fractures (C2)

Axis fractures account for approximately 20% of cervical fractures. The most common form is a type II dens fracture by the Anderson classification.

Dens fractures. Fractures of the dens constitute 10–15% of cervical fractures. Considerable force is needed to fracture the dens in a young patient, and most dens fractures are sustained in motor vehicle accidents, skiing accidents, or falls from a height. In older patients, however, dens fracture can result from a simple fall. The most common causal mechanism is hyperflex-

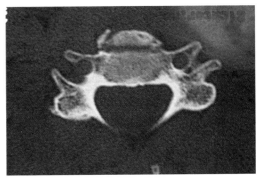

Fig. 12.**27** **Teardrop fracture** with separation of an anterior fragment from the vertebral body.

ion of the head and neck, causing C1 to displace forward relative to C2. Extension injuries are a much less frequent cause of posteriorly displaced dens fractures.

In all cases, the displacement of C1 relative to C2 narrows the spinal canal and may cause compression of the medulla oblongata. Initial death from this mechanism is estimated to occur in 25–40% of cases.

Treatment and prognosis depend mainly on the location of the fracture line, which is also the basis for the widely used Anderson classification of dens fractures (Table 12.**2**).

The question of stability is controversial, especially in *type I fractures.* We disagree with the assertion that the relatively rare type I fracture is inherently stable. The mechanism of the fracture is a bony avulsion of the dens apex, to which the apical ligament is attached. This ligament connects the apex of the dens to the anterior rim of the foramen magnum. A type I dens fracture, therefore, is the radiologic correlate of an atlanto-occipital dislocation.

Type II fractures cause significant atlantoaxial instability and require internal or external fixation to stabilize the site and prevent nonunion (pseudoarthrosis).

Type III fractures through the vertebral body of C2 are usually stable and do not require primary surgical intervention for internal stabilization. Approximately 90% will heal with 8–14 weeks of external stabilization (Fig. 12.**23**).

Table 12.**2**   Anderson classification of dens fractures (Anderson and D'Alonzo 1974)

Type	Description
I	Fracture line runs above the attachment of the transverse ligament, in the upper third of the dens
II	Fracture line runs through the neck of the dens in the lower third and below the attachment of the transverse ligament
	IIa Same as type II, plus displaced fragments at the level of the fracture line
III	Fracture line runs through the C2 vertebral body with involvement of the medullary cavity

Odontoid bone. A separate ossicle with radiographically smooth, sclerotic margins may be found (incidentally or during trauma work-up) in place of the normal dens. Often called the odontoid, this bone may create problems of differential diagnosis. The view that the odontoid is a developmental variant based on a failure of fusion between the dens and body of C2 is currently accepted only for the "terminal ossicle," or an apex that is separate from the dens body. The fact that an odontoid may be found in many patients who had a normal dens on previous radiographs suggests that at least some cases represent nonunion of an older dens fracture.

Axis arch fracture (hangman's fracture, traumatic spondylolisthesis of the axis). The term "hangman's fracture" dates from a 1965 article by Schneider et al. noting that the hyperextension–distraction mechanism of a legal hanging (the knot is placed beneath the chin of the condemned prisoner) consistently produces a bilateral fracture through the pedicles of C2. Today, the most common mechanism for this type of fracture is hyperextension or hyperflexion combined with violent axial compression sustained in a motor vehicle accident or sports injury (e.g., diving head-first into shallow water). The fracture line runs through each pars interarticularis of the axis arch.

Three fracture types are distinguished according to the degree of displacement of C2 in relation to C3 (Table 12.**3**; Figs. 12.**26**, 12.**38**).

Subaxial Cervical Fractures (C3–7)

CT has a much less important role between C3 and C7 than in the area of the craniocervical junction. Most fractures and dislocations that occur between C3 and C7 are clearly visible on conventional radiographs, and ligamentous injuries in that region are well demonstrated by MRI. Nevertheless, CT is used in this region to evaluate combined injuries of the cervical spine, and when a fracture is suspected from plain films, CT can reliably detect or exclude bony injuries and spinal canal compromise as part of the initial work-up (Fig. 12.**25**).

Interfacet Dislocation

Strong flexion of the cervical spine can cause a dislocation of the facet joints, in which the posterior part of the inferior articular process of the upper vertebral body slips in front of the anterior part of the superior articular process of the lower vertebral body. Pure flexion usually leads to a bilateral interfacet dislocation (BID), while flexion plus rotation tends to cause a unilateral interfacet dislocation (UID).

A UID can occur without significant associated ligament injury and without a neurologic deficit. The clinical manifestations consist

Table 12.**3** Effendi classification of axis arch fractures (Effendi et al. 1981)

Type	Description
I	Axis (C2) shows < 3 mm subluxation relative to C3. The fracture is usually stable, and the patient has no neurologic deficits. The causal mechanism is usually axial compression and extension
II	Disruption of the posterior longitudinal ligament and C2–3 disk, with subluxation of 4 mm or more and more than 11° angulation of the C2 and C3 endplates. The usual causal mechanism is axial compression, extension, and subsequent rebound flexion
	Type IIa is like type II, but shows pronounced angulation and little subluxation
III	The causal mechanism of flexion plus axial compression leads initially to rupture of the C2–3 facet joint capsules and an isthmus fracture, followed by extensive dislocation and subluxation, with rupture of the posterior and anterior longitudinal ligaments or separation of the anterior longitudinal ligament from the ventral surface of C3.

of pain and a characteristic tilted, rotated position of the head ("robin's head" position).

A BID requires considerably greater force, which generally ruptures the juxtafacet ligaments, the ligamentum flavum, the anterior and posterior longitudinal ligaments, the interspinous ligament, and the annulus fibrosus. BID is usually associated with injuries of the cervical cord and/or spinal nerve roots.

Teardrop Fracture (Fig. 12.**27**)

This is an unstable fracture caused by strong hyperflexion of the cervical spine. It is usually associated with extensive combined bony and ligamentous injuries. It consists of a combination of the following structural injuries:

- Avulsion of a small fragment from the anterior inferior vertebral body (the "teardrop").
- Frequently there is a midsagittal fracture through the affected vertebral body (often not visible on conventional radiographs).
- Posterior displacement of the fractured vertebra (retrolisthesis).
- Compression of the vertebral body, with anterior wedging and resultant kyphosis.
- Dislocation of the facet joints.
- Extensive prevertebral soft-tissue swelling due to internal bleeding (reflects the severity of the trauma).
- Narrowing of the disk space caudal to the fracture.

This type of injury has a much poorer prognosis than other cervical fractures below C1 and C2. Many patients sustain a complete cord lesion at the affected level.

CT is often the only imaging modality that can distinguish a teardrop fracture from a simple bony avulsion of the anterior longitudinal ligament. CT can also detect associated soft-tissue injuries, prevertebral hemorrhage, sagittal plane fractures, and any accompanying cord compression.

Other Fractures

Other isolated fractures that are not caused by severe trauma and do not produce neurologic deficits (e.g., a fracture of the spinous process) generally are not an indication for CT examination.

■ Frequency

Atlas fractures account for approximately 3–13% of cervical fractures. Axis fractures account for 20%, with dens fractures making up about 10%. The most common dens fracture is the type II fracture through the base. Type I fractures are very rare. Teardrop fractures have been found in approximately 5% of patients with cervical spine injuries using conventional radiographs.

■ Clinical Manifestations

The most common symptom of a C1 and C2 fracture is pain in the upper cervical spine. The pain may radiate to the occipital region due to irritation of the greater occipital nerve, which arises from the C2 segment. Other common symptoms are limitation of neck motion and muscle spasms and paresthesias of the upper extremity. A typical clinical feature is a tendency for the patient to support the head manually while moving the trunk. Subaxial fractures, especially of the teardrop type, require considerable force and are usually associated with severe cervical cord injury or even a complete cord lesion.

If patients with an odontoid bone or nonunion develop clinical symptoms or show signs of significant atlantoaxial instability, surgical fusion should be performed in the same way as for an acute, displaced fracture of the dens. Nonoperative immobilization will not be sufficient to achieve fusion in these cases.

■ CT Morphology

CT is the method of choice for detecting or excluding the fracture of a cervical vertebra, especially a dens fracture. As on conventional radiographs, a fracture may appear on CT as a step-off, contour irregularity, displaced fragment, or as a fine lucency, linear discontinuity, or irregularity in the trabecular structure.

Sagittal CT reformatted images are almost indispensable for determining the fracture type and assessing its relationship to the spinal canal. Three-dimensional surface reconstructions are particularly helpful for planning surgical intervention and reconstructing the spinal column.

Thoracolumbar Spinal Fractures
(Figs. 12.**28**–12.**39**)

The three-column model proposed by Denis (1983) is a helpful tool for the clinical and radiologic classification of thoracolumbar fractures. It is particularly useful for evaluating the stability of a fracture (Fig. 12.**28**):

- The *anterior column* in this model consists of the anterior half of the vertebral body and intervertebral disk and the anterior longitudinal ligament.
- The *middle column* consists of the posterior part of the vertebral body and intervertebral disk and the posterior longitudinal ligament.
- The *posterior column* includes the entire vertebral arch along with the interspinous ligament, supraspinous ligament, ligamentum flavum, and facet joint capsule.

A basic distinction is made between mild and severe thoracolumbar injuries.

Mild Injuries

These include injuries that involve only part of one supporting column, leaving the rest of the column intact. Examples are fractures of a transverse process or an articular process, or a pars fracture involving a portion of the vertebral arch. This category also includes isolated fractures of a spinous process. These injuries are considered stable, and in the absence of significant associated injuries they do not require special treatment.

Severe Injuries

- *Compression fracture of the anterior column.* The middle column is intact in these cases, and the posterior column may be intact or distracted, depending on the severity of the trauma. The spinal canal is not narrowed or compressed, and there are no neurologic deficits. This type of injury most commonly affects the region from T6 to T8 and from T12 to L3 (Figs. 12.**29**, 12.**30**).
- *Vertebral body burst fracture.* This is an axial compression injury caused, for example, by jumping from a height and landing on the feet. The fracture involves the entire vertebral body and thus affects both the anterior and middle columns. CT shows a discontinuity in the posterior rim of the vertebral body, and may demonstrate a bone fragment protruding into the spinal canal (Fig. 12.**39**). This fracture mechanism can cause narrowing of the spinal canal, with compression of the spinal cord or cauda equina.

- *Flexion fractures.* Flexion fractures of the middle and posterior columns ("seatbelt fractures") can be classified into several groups, depending on the fracture pattern:
  - Horizontal vertebral fractures involving all the bony elements, known also as a Chance fracture (Fig. 12.**34**).
  - Fractures that involve only ligamentous structures within one level.
  - Fractures that involve the bony elements of the middle column along with anterior and posterior ligamentous structures, affecting two levels. These are distinguished from fractures that involve only the ligamentous structures of two adjacent levels.
- *Fracture-dislocations.* Fracture-dislocations affect all three columns, and are caused by the addition of a rotary or translational component. Complete spinal cord lesions are common, due to the shearing effect on the cord.

■ Frequency

Sixty-four percent of vertebral body fractures occur at the thoracolumbar junction, most commonly in the T12–L1 segment.

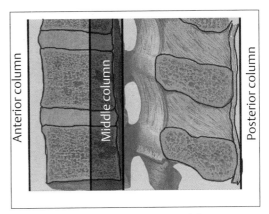

Fig. 12.**28**   **Denis's three-column model.**

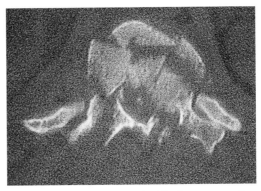

Fig. 12.**29 Thoracic vertebral-body compression fracture involving all three columns.** Bone fragments protrude into the vertebral canal, compressing the spinal cord.

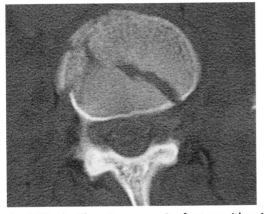

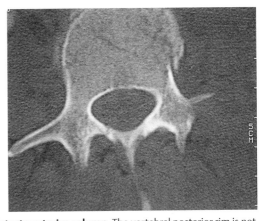

a   b

Fig. 12.**30 a, b   Thoracic compression fracture with an intact posterior column.** The vertebral posterior rim is not involved, and consequently there is no cord impingement.

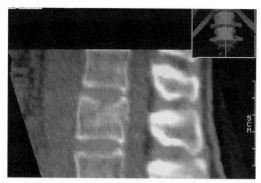

a

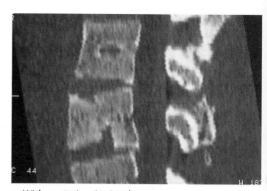

Fig. 12.**31 Sagittal reformatted images of thoracic compression fractures.**

a With posterior rim involvement.
b Without posterior rim involvement.

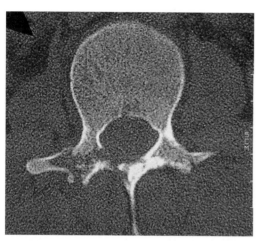

Fig. 12.**32 Fracture sustained in a motor vehicle accident.** This patient was involved in a head-on collision with another vehicle. The axial CT scan at the L1 level shows a fracture line in the posterior column, predominantly involving the right pedicles in this plane of section. The overall fracture pattern was difficult to appreciate in single slices.

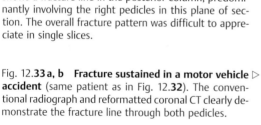

Fig. 12.**33 a, b Fracture sustained in a motor vehicle** ▷
accident (same patient as in Fig. 12.**32**). The conventional radiograph and reformatted coronal CT clearly demonstrate the fracture line through both pedicles.

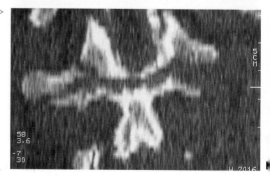

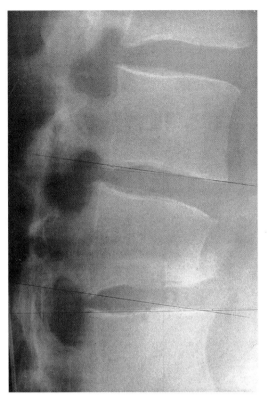

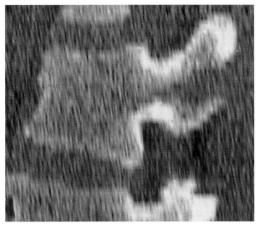

Fig. 12.**34a, b** **Chance fracture.** Both the lateral plain radiograph and the sagittal CT reformatted image show a fracture extending through the pedicles and the whole vertebral body. Separation of the pedicles has occurred posteriorly due to the fracture mechanism, and a vertebral body compression fracture is visible anteriorly.

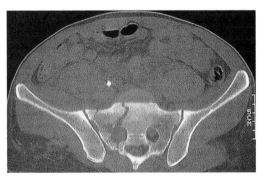

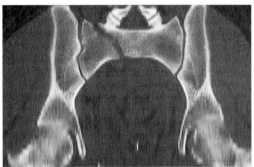

Fig. 12.**35a, b** **Sacral fracture.** Axial loading (e.g., jumping or falling from a height) is the most common mechanism producing a unilateral or bilateral trans-foraminal fracture of the sacrum. The case shown is a unilateral transforaminal sacral fracture, which is best appreciated in the reformatted coronal image.

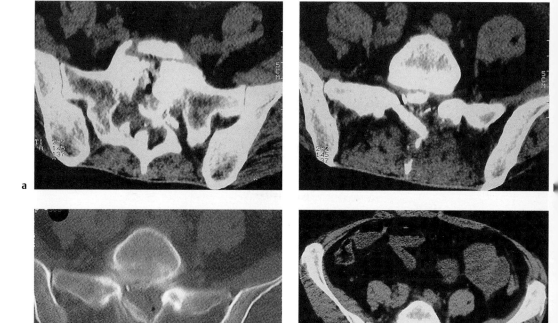

Fig. 12.**36 a–d** **Complex sacral fracture caused by a gunshot injury.** The missile track in this case runs through the sacrum and through the spinal canal. The bone-window view in particular demonstrates intraspinal air and bone fragments. The crescent-shaped collection just above the missile track is a right-sided epidural hematoma.

■ Clinical Manifestations

The neurologic deficit can be quite severe, depending on the degree of cord compression.

■ CT Morphology

A particular difficulty in the CT evaluation of flexion fractures is the horizontal course of the fracture, which runs parallel to the axial scan plane. As with cervical fractures, sagittal reformatted images should be obtained so that the fracture can be surveyed in one view and does not need to be traced through multiple axial sections. The sagittal reformatted image is also better for assessing the degree of height reduction caused by compression of the affected vertebral body.

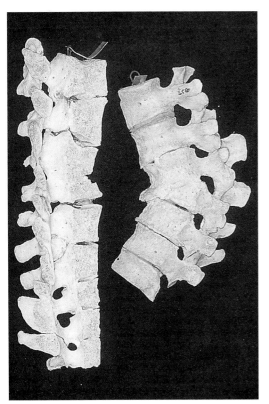

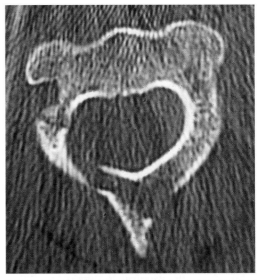

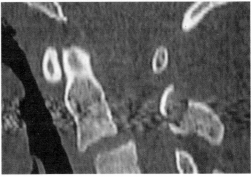

Fig. 12.**37** **Vertebral-body compression fracture.** The impaction or even fusion of two adjacent vertebral bodies can occur, especially after a predominantly anterior compression fracture. The resulting kyphosis depends on the degree of vertebral body compression.

Fig. 12.**38 a, b** **Effendi type II fracture of the axis arch.** The base of the dens is displaced 4 mm anteriorly.

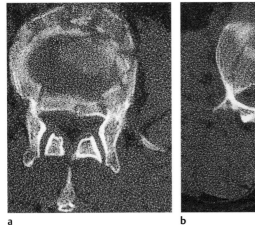

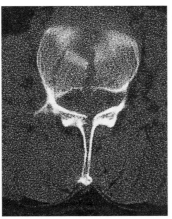

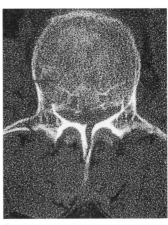

a   b   c

Fig. 12.**39 a–c** **Burst fracture of a lumbar vertebra** with depression of the endplates, retropulsion of a fragment into the spinal canal, and fracture-separation of the vertebral arch.

Traumatic Disk Herniation

Frequency: rare.

Suggestive morphologic findings: often located in the thoracic spine, usually coexists with fractures or ligamentous injuries.

Procedure: contiguous slices or scans parallel to the disk spaces.

Other studies: correlate with conventional radiographs. MRI can detect ligamentous injuries.

Checklist for scan interpretation:
▶ Degree of cord or dural sac compression?
▶ Associated injuries?

■ Pathogenesis

A traumatic disk herniation is a disk protrusion that occurs in response to adequate trauma, with no evidence of degenerative disease. It is reasonable to assume, however, that most traumatic disk herniations that are not associated with vertebral body fractures or tears of the posterior longitudinal ligament are secondary to degenerative changes that have developed in the nucleus pulposus and annulus fibrosus. This particularly applies to disk herniations in the lumbar and cervical regions.

■ Frequency

Approximately 25% of thoracic disk herniations have a traumatic etiology.

Hemorrhage

Frequency: epidural hematomas are more common than subdural hematomas, although both are rare.

Suggestive morphologic findings: a mass extending over several segments, usually posterior to the thoracic cord, and often showing a crescent shape on axial scans. The mass is hyperdense in the acute stage.

Procedure: contiguous spiral scans with secondary reconstructions.

Other studies: sagittal MRI. The epidural or subdural location of the hemorrhage is easier to define with MRI than CT.

Checklist for scan interpretation:
▶ Location and extent of the hemorrhage?
▶ Degree of cord compression?
▶ *Caution:* due to the risk of a transverse cord lesion, notify the referring physician at once if cord compression is observed.

■ Pathogenesis

The CT density of a hemorrhagic collection depends on its age. Fresh blood from 30 min to 2–3 weeks old appears hyperdense to surrounding tissues, owing to its high hemoglobin content. As the blood is reabsorbed, it initially becomes isodense and difficult to identify. Finally it appears hypodense to surrounding structures. The duration of these stages depends on the size and location of the hemorrhage, because iron removal from the hemoglobin is a key factor in the gradual decrease in attenuation.

With a peracute hemorrhage, the density of the extravasated blood may closely approximate that of the blood within the vascular system.

Epidural Hematoma

Spinal epidural hematoma most frequently occurs in the thoracic spinal canal, usually appearing as an elongated mass of high density (up to 100 HU) on the dorsal aspect of the dural sac. It may be caused by a vertebral body fracture or dislocation, vascular injury (e.g., during lumbar puncture), hypertension, arteriovenous malformation, vertebral body hemangioma, or especially a coagulation disorder due to hemophilia or treatment with heparin or anti-coagulant medication. A significant factor in the pathogenesis of epidural hemorrhage is the fact that the thin-walled, valveless veins of the epidural space are loosely embedded in fatty tissue and are therefore very sensitive to sudden increases in intra-abdominal or in-trathoracic pressure. There have been numerous reports of epidural hematomas brought on acutely by coughing or sneezing. In approximately 50% of cases, a definite cause of the hematoma cannot be ascertained.

Subdural Hematoma

As this type of intraspinal hemorrhage is much rarer than epidural hematoma and has basically the same clinical symptoms, little information has been published on its causes and imaging features. An electron-microscopic study by Haines et al. (1993) on the structure of the meninges supplied a possible explanation for the mechanism by which intracranial subdural hematomas can be transmitted to the spinal canal. The authors claim that the two-layer structure of the dura is responsible for the spread of subdural hematomas. The outer dural layer contains numerous fibroblasts and extracellular collagen, while the inner layer consists only of a loose aggregation of fibroblasts, making it vulnerable to traumatic disruption. This suggests that the term "subdural space" is a misnomer, since it is not a true anatomic space, but a space that is artificially created when the boundary cell layer of the dura is mechanically disrupted. Despite this discovery, the term "subdural space" remains in general use.

■ Frequency

Epidural hematomas are more common than subdural hematomas, but both entities are rare. To date, several hundred cases with varying etiologies have been described in the literature. Most of these cases were secondary to a coagulation disorder.

■ Clinical Manifestations

Patients usually complain of very severe back pain of acute onset, often located between the shoulder blades and sometimes showing a radicular distribution. Neurologic deficits may develop over a period of several hours and may progress to a complete cord lesion; other cases show a more insidious clinical progression. When neurologic symptoms progress slowly, motor deficits may be overlooked in a patient who is bedridden due to pain.

■ CT Morphology

Epidural hematoma typically appears on CT as an elongated, sometimes crescent-shaped mass of high attenuation usually located post-erolateral to the dural sac in the thoracic spine. The collection may cause compression of the dural sac. Subdural hematomas, being similarly confined, may also appear as a circumscribed crescentic mass of high attenuation (Figs. 12.**40**, 12.**41**).

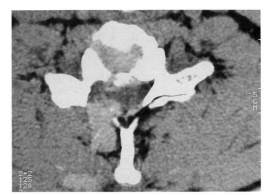

Fig. 12.**40 Epidural hematoma in the cervical spine**, caused by bleeding after surgery for a herniated disk. Axial CT shows that the hemorrhage has spread beyond the epidural space to the paravertebral soft tissues.

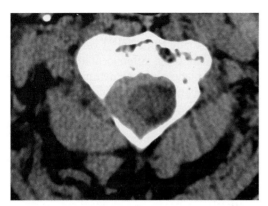

Fig. 12.**41** **Epidural hemorrhage** in a woman receiving anticoagulant medication who denied a history of trauma. The patient presented clinically with acute right-sided hemiparesis.

■ Spinal Subarachnoid Hemorrhage

Frequency: rare.

Suggestive morphologic findings: CT may show diffusely increased density in the subarachnoid space or circumscribed areas of hyperdense coagulated blood.

Procedure: contiguous spiral scans are acquired before and during intravenous contrast administration to locate the source of the hemorrhage (e.g., a spinal arteriovenous malformation).

Other studies: MRI, angiography.

Checklist for scan interpretation:
▶ Locate the source of the hemorrhage.
▶ Report the findings without delay.

Spinal subarachnoid hemorrhage is rare. It may be caused by trauma, interventional procedures, or a ruptured blood vessel (e.g., in a spinal arteriovenous malformation). Because the hemorrhage can spread more or less freely within the CSF-filled subarachnoid space, it often appears on CT only as a diffuse, faint hyperdensity surrounding the lower-density spinal cord or cauda equina filaments. The main goal of diagnostic studies is to locate and identify the source of the hemorrhage. MRI, with its capacity for sagittal plane imaging, is much better for this purpose than CT. MRI is also more sensitive in detecting small amounts of blood.

Degenerative Diseases of the Spine

Degenerative Disk Disease (Disk Protrusion, Disk Herniation, Sequestered Disk)

Frequency: very common.

Suggestive morphologic findings: tissue of disk attenuation protruding into the spinal canal or neuroforamen.

Procedure: contiguous spiral scans permit secondary reconstructions for better evaluation of the neuroforamina. Standard CT work-up consists of scans parallel to the disk spaces.

Other studies: MRI (coronal and sagittal), myelography, and postmyelographic CT are better for evaluating compression of the subarachnoid space.

Checklist for scan interpretation:
▶ Location (level) of the herniated disk and affected side?
▶ Subligamentous or transligamentous herniation?
▶ Osteophytic reaction?
▶ Predominantly bony narrowing?

■ Pathogenesis

As noted in Chapter 11, degenerative changes start to develop in the intervertebral disks at about 20 years of age. In some cases these changes are demonstrable by MRI at an early stage, appearing as a reduction of T2-weighted signal intensity in the nucleus pulposus. This reflects a decrease in the water content of the nucleus.

CT cannot demonstrate these early changes, and typically is used only when degenerative disk disease in the form of a disk protrusion or herniation has already led to back pain or symptoms of nerve root compression.

Degenerative disk disease almost always affects the entire motion segment between two adjacent vertebral bodies in varying degrees. A motion segment consists of the nucleus pulposus, the annulus fibrosus, and the surrounding ligaments, most notably the posterior longitudinal ligament and ligamentum flavum. The facet joints create a true articular connection between the adjacent vertebral bodies. With the progression of degenerative changes, all of these structures usually show a significant degree of involvement. The pathophysiology of degenerative disk diseases is briefly reviewed below.

Degeneration of the intervertebral disk tissue, especially the nucleus pulposus, begins at approximately 20 years of age. As the nucleus pulposus undergoes progressive dehydration, it becomes less resilient and less able to absorb mechanical forces efficiently. Another effect of this fluid loss is a reduction in disk height, leading to laxness of the motion segment composed of the intervertebral disk, ligament apparatus, and facet joints. In turn, the altered mechanical properties of the motion segment promote more rapid degeneration and hypertrophy of the facet joints, facet osteoarthrosis, or even spondylarthrosis.

The intervertebral disk may calcify, as an expression of further degeneration.

As the intervertebral disk loses its resiliency, physiologic loads on the affected segment can cause an alternation of increased pressure and intermittent negative pressure within the disk space. This creates a *vacuum phenomenon* in which nitrogen gas is aspirated from the tissue. The free nitrogen remains trapped in the disk space, appearing as a lucent collection on CT scans (Figs. 12.**42**, 12.**43**). Sometimes a disk herniation can cause the gas bubbles to leave the disk space and enter the spinal canal.

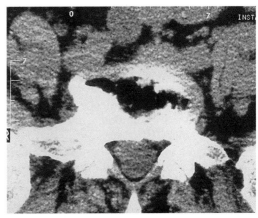

Fig. 12.**42** **Vacuum phenomenon.** Degenerative disk changes give rise to intermittent negative pressures within the disk space. Nitrogen aspirated from the tissue by this mechanism appears as a lucent collection on CT.

As degenerative changes progress, the annulus fibrosus becomes friable and fissured, compromising its ability to constrain the nucleus pulposus. A discontinuity in the annular fibers allows protrusion (Fig. 12.**44**) and eventual herniation (Fig. 12.**45**) of the degenerated nuclear tissue.

Herniated nuclear material that has become detached from the parent disk is called a free fragment or *sequestered disk* (Fig. 12.**46**).

This free fragment may migrate from the site of rupture. With a posterolateral lumbar disk herniation, the fragment usually migrates

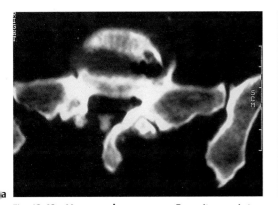

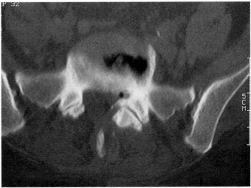

Fig. 12.**43** **Vacuum phenomenon.** Free nitrogen is trapped in the disk space, and may enter the spinal canal along with protruding disk tissue or in isolation, as shown in this case of a lateral disk herniation.

cephalad into the ipsilateral lateral recess (Fig. 12.**47**).

Approximately 20% of sequestered disks migrate cephalad. An *axillary sequestrum* comes to lie between the nerve root and the dural sac, caudal to the root sleeve (Fig. 12.**48**).

Multiple separate fragments at various locations are a common finding with sequestered disks.

In addition to acute disk herniation (sometimes called a "soft" herniation), degeneration of the nucleus pulposus can lead to bulging and stretching of the annulus fibrosus. These stresses are transmitted via the Sharpey fibers of the annulus (Fig. 12.**49**) to the posterior margins of the vertebral endplates, creating a stimulus for appositional bone growth.

This osteophytic counterpart of the soft herniation is sometimes called a "hard" herniation or *buttress reaction.* It is a common accompanying feature of degenerative disk disease, especially in the cervical region (Fig. 12.**50**).

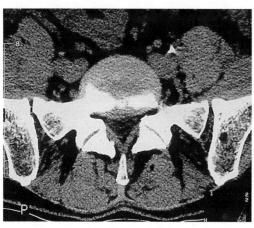

Fig. 12.**44** **Broad-based, convex disk protrusion.** The annulus fibrosus and posterior longitudinal ligament are stretched, but still intact.

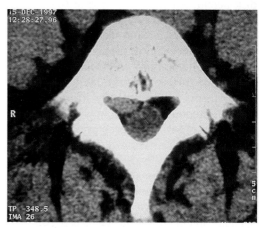

Fig. 12.**45** **Lateral lumbar disk herniation.** The disk material in the spinal canal is markedly hyperdense to the dural sac.

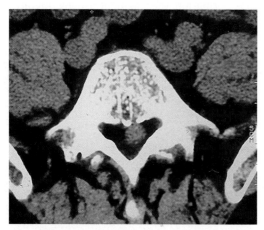

Fig. 12.**46** **Free sequestered disk fragment.** The hyperdense nuclear material within the spinal canal has separated completely from the parent disk.

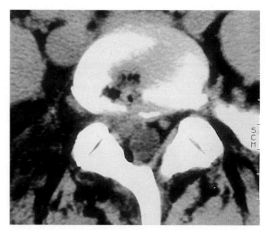

Fig. 12.**47** **Sequestered disk with a vacuum phenomenon at the level of the herniation.** The free disk fragment is lodged in the ipsilateral recess, where it compresses the spinal nerve root.

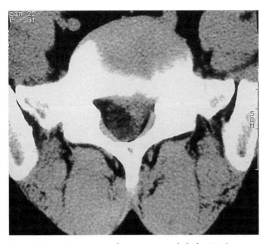

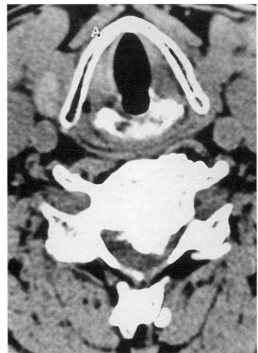

Fig. 12.**48** **Fragmented sequestered disk.** CT demonstrates a subligamentous fragment under the posterior longitudinal ligament and an intraspinal axillary sequestrum between the dural sac and spinal nerve root.

The bulging disk tissue eventually stretches the outer portions of the annulus fibrosus and the posterior longitudinal ligament. These structures have a relatively rich nerve supply, and mechanical disruption of them leads to back pain. It should be noted that these structures derive their sensory innervation from the sinuvertebral nerve (of von Luschka), which anastomoses with the dorsal root of the corresponding spinal nerve at the affected level, with the two segments of the spinal nerves above it, and with the sympathetic trunk.

The nerve supply to the outer portion of the annulus fibrosus, similar to its vascular supply, appears to depend partly on degenerative processes within the disk. It has been shown, for example, that healthy disks can withstand considerable pressure and manipulation (e.g., during diskography) without causing pain.

A normal motion segment is painless even under very heavy loading, whereas a diseased segment can cause severe pain even when subjected to ordinary loads.

When the nucleus finally ruptures through a complete tear in the annulus and also

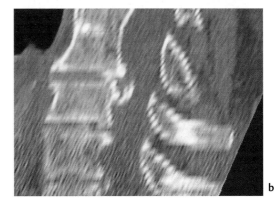

Fig. 12.**49 a, b** **Disk bulge.** A long-standing disk bulge causes stretching of the Sharpey fibers, creating a stimulus for appositional bone growth. Sometimes called a "buttress reaction," osteophytic spurs on the posterior margins of the vertebral bodies are commonly seen with a long-standing disk bulge.

through the posterior longitudinal ligament, the patient often perceives the release of annular fiber tension as a sudden shifting of pain from the back to a lower extremity. This is a consequence of the resulting nerve root compression, which causes pain that radiates in a

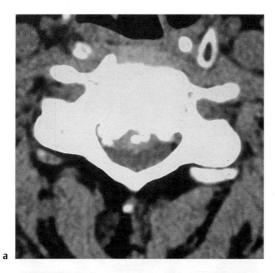
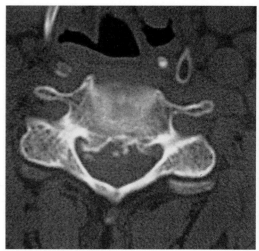

a

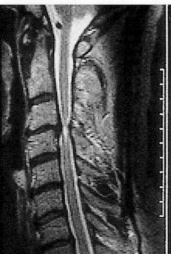
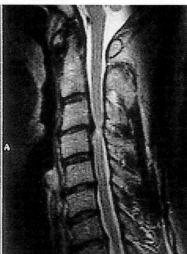

c

Fig. 12.**50 a–c Bony spinal stenosis.** A result of prolonged disk herniation, this osteophytic narrowing of the spinal canal is frequently responsible for the clinical manifestations of cervical myelopathy. Its imaging correlate is a prominent, circumscribed hyperintense area in sagittal T2-weighted magnetic resonance imaging.

radicular distribution. In extreme cases, a massive disk herniation can cause compression of the spinal cord, conus medullaris, or cauda equina with transverse cord symptoms or a cauda equina syndrome (Fig. 12.**51**).

Lumbar disk herniation. The posterior longitudinal ligament, which interconnects the posterior aspects of the vertebral bodies within the spinal canal and forms part of the middle supporting column of the spine, is less well developed in the lumbar region than at higher levels because of the physiologic lumbar lordosis. Meanwhile, the lower lumbar spine carries the highest gravitational load, and the lower segments of the lumbar spine are connected to the sacrum, which has very little craniocaudal mobility. These factors explain why the great majority of disk herniations occur at the L4–5 and L5–S1 levels. According to reports from different authors, these levels account for 65–95% of lumbar disk herniations.

Table 12.**4** shows the frequency distribution of lumbar herniations by levels.

The most common intraspinal disk herniation, regardless of the affected level, is the *posterolateral herniation* in the area of the lateral recess. This form accounts for approximately 50% of disk herniations. Disks tend to herniate posterolaterally because of an anatomic weak point in the annulus fibrosus: while the medial portion of the ring is firmly blended with the posterior longitudinal ligament, the lateral portion receives little or no ligamentous reinforcement (Fig. 12.**52**).

Table 12.**4** Frequency distribution of lumbar disk herniation by levels

Level	%
L4–5	35
L5–S1	27
L3–4	19
L2–3	14
L1–2	5

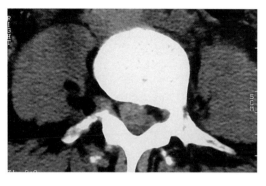
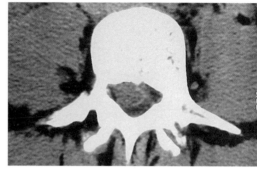

b

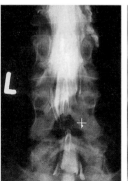
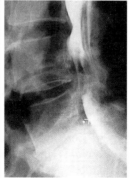

d

Fig. 12.51 Massive disk herniation at L4–5.

a CT demonstrates a massive L4–5 disk herniation, with marked dural sac compression and clinical symptoms of compression of the conus medullaris and cauda equina. Initially it was unclear whether the lesion was a massive disk herniation or a spinal tumor, and additional scans were therefore obtained after intravenous contrast administration.

b The mass itself does not enhance, but the postcontrast scan clearly shows a displaced intraspinal vein located between the herniated disk and the displaced dural sac.

c Myelography documents the degree of dural sac compression.

d The T2-weighted sagittal magnetic resonance image localizes the mass to the L4–5 level. The L4–5 disk space is hypointense, as it has become dehydrated due to degeneration.

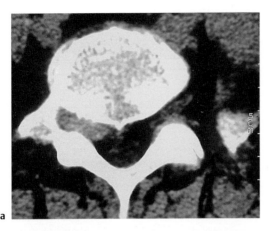

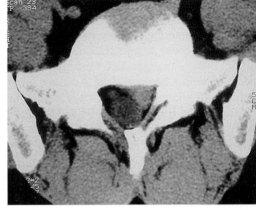

Fig. 12.**52 a–c** **Posterolateral disk herniation.**
a Right posterolateral disk herniation at L4–5.
b Left posterolateral disk herniation at L5–S1.
c Left posterolateral disk herniation with an axillary free fragment.

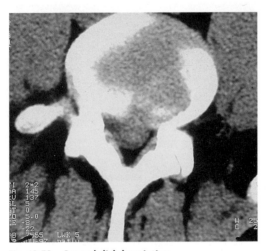

Fig. 12.**53** **Central disk herniation.**

A posterolateral herniated disk can compress multiple nerve roots in some cases, and rare cases at the thoracic level can compress the spinal cord in addition to one or more nerve roots.

Central disk herniations account for approximately 8% of herniations. They can exert direct pressure on the spinal cord or cauda equina from the anterior side (Fig. 12.**53**).

Lateral (Fig. 12.**54**) and *intraforaminal herniations* (Fig. 12.**55**) together make up about 10% of herniated disks. They typically cause compression of only one nerve root.

Extraforaminal and anterior disk herniations (Figs. 12.**56**, 12.**58**) together make up about 29% of cases and are often missed on sectional imaging studies. Extraforaminal herniations, when extensive, can compress the spinal nerve descending from the level above.

Special forms include bilateral disk herniation (on both sides of the posterior longitudinal

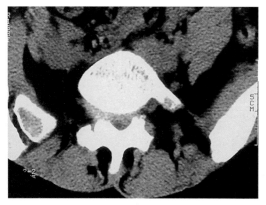

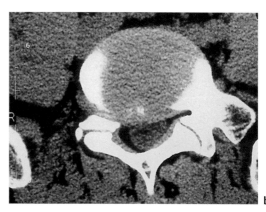

b

Fig. 12.**54** **Lateral disk herniation.**

a Right lateral L5–S1 disk herniation with an intraforaminal and extraforaminal component. The L5 root is elevated and compressed against the roof of the neuroforamen.

b Broad-based right lateral disk herniation at L5–S1, with an intraforaminal and extraforaminal component.

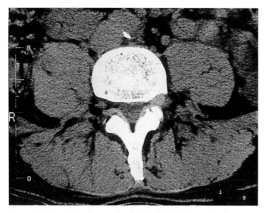

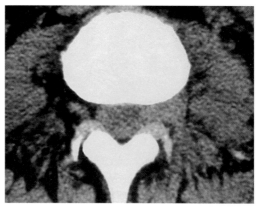

Fig. 12.**55** **Intraforaminal L4–5 disk herniation** on the left side.

Fig. 12.**56** **Extraforaminal L3–4 disk herniation** on the left side.

ligament) and intraosseous herniation, known also as a Schmorl nodule (Fig. 12.**57**).

Intraosseous herniations account for approximately 14% of herniated disks, but most are asymptomatic and represent an incidental finding or a manifestation of disk degeneration.

An extremely rare variant is the *intradural disk herniation,* in which a free disk fragment erodes through dura that is adherent to the posterior longitudinal ligament or annulus fibrosus. This is extremely difficult to detect on standard CT scans, but most cases can be detected by postmyelographic CT.

Cervical disk herniation. The cervical intervertebral disks, unlike the lumbar disks, are subject less to axial body loads than to loads resulting from the segmental mobility of the cervical spine—flexion, extension, rotation, and their combinations.

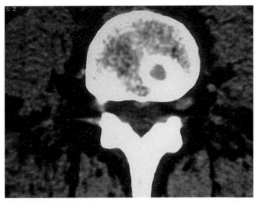
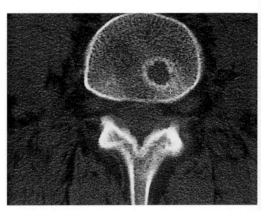

a

Fig. 12.**57** **Schmorl nodule.** CT shows an intraosseous disk herniation with marginal sclerosis. The eccentric location of the lesion and its sclerotic margins distinguish it from congenital abnormalities, such as remnants of the notochord.

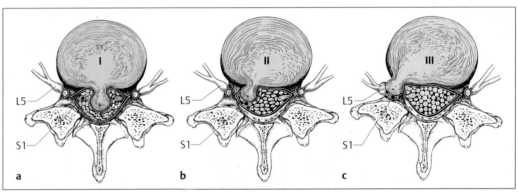

Fig. 12.**58** **Central, posterolateral, and lateral disk herniation.**

a A central disk herniation exerts pressure on the dural sac (cauda equina).

b A posterolateral herniation presses on the dural sac and on the nerve root from the segment below the affected disk.

c A lateral herniation compresses the nerve root from the segment above the disk. A large herniation can also compress the root exiting at the level of the affected disk.

As in the lumbar spine, the posterior longitudinal ligament in the neck is stronger centrally than laterally. Consequently, a herniated disk tends to protrude laterally in the area of the uncinate process, where it compresses the nerve root as it leaves the spinal canal. Because the cervical canal is narrower than the lumbar canal, even very small fragments in the lateral recess that are barely perceptible on CT scans can cause significant symptoms (Fig. 12.**59**).

Segments C5–6 and C6–7 are most commonly affected, presumably because most flexion and extension occur at those levels. Herniations at the C5–6 and C6–7 levels together make up approximately 90% of cervical herniated disks.

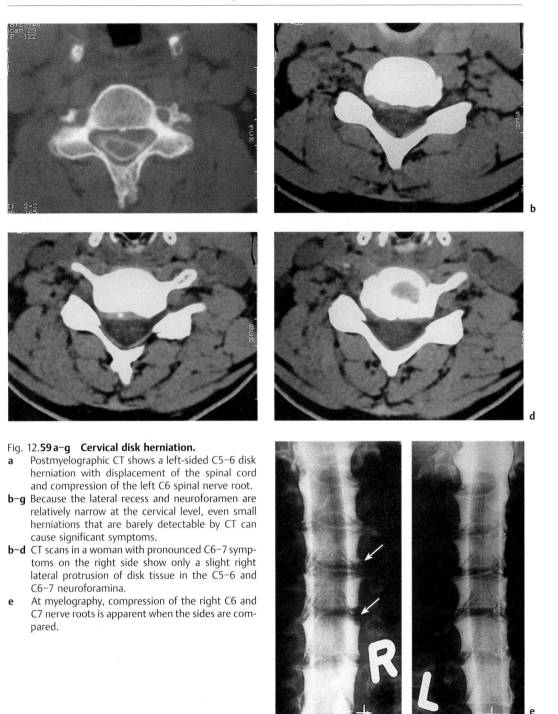

Fig. 12.**59 a–g   Cervical disk herniation.**

a   Postmyelographic CT shows a left-sided C5–6 disk herniation with displacement of the spinal cord and compression of the left C6 spinal nerve root.

b–g   Because the lateral recess and neuroforamen are relatively narrow at the cervical level, even small herniations that are barely detectable by CT can cause significant symptoms.

b–d   CT scans in a woman with pronounced C6–7 symptoms on the right side show only a slight right lateral protrusion of disk tissue in the C5–6 and C6–7 neuroforamina.

e   At myelography, compression of the right C6 and C7 nerve roots is apparent when the sides are compared.

Fig. 12.**59 f** u. **g** ▷

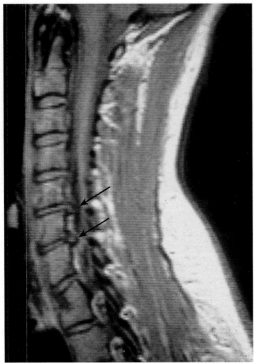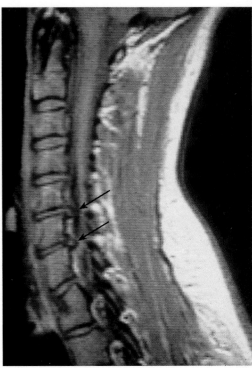

f

Fig. 12.**59 f, g** One advantage of magnetic resonance imaging over CT is its ability to display direct sagittal sections. The herniated disk tissue at C5–6 and C6–7 is clearly visualized *(arrows)*.

The frequency distribution by levels is shown in Table 12.**5**.

Thoracic disk herniation. Herniated disks are far less common in the thoracic spine than in the cervical and lumbar regions, accounting for just 0.25–0.75 % of cases, depending on the source. Only about three thoracic herniations are treated surgically for every 1000 lumbar herniations that come to operation.

Table 12.**5** Frequency distribution of cervical disk herniation by levels

Level	%
C6–7	70
C5–6	20
C7–T1	10
C4–5	2

There are several reasons for this. First, the thoracic spine is subject to less axial loading than the lumbar spine. Second, the range of motion of any given thoracic segment is relatively small. The orientation of the thoracic facet joints mainly permits movements in rotation while allowing very little forward or backward bending. This also explains why some 25 % of thoracic disk herniations have a traumatic etiology and why the peak age incidence, at 20–50 years, is lower than with lumbar herniations.

Thoracic disk herniation is often a difficult surgical problem. The relative tightness of the thoracic spinal canal compared with the lumbar canal and the high sensitivity of the cord blood supply to manipulations make it difficult to reach the thoracic disks through a posterior approach, which requires displacement of the dural sac.

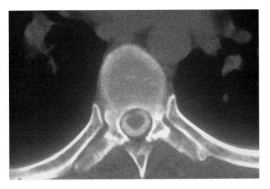

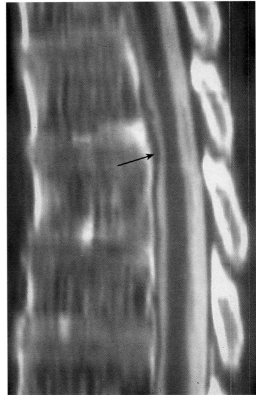

Fig. 12.**60 a, b Postmyelographic CT scan of a T9–10 disk herniation.** This small protrusion *(arrow)* did not cause neurologic deficits, and the only clinical symptom was low back pain.

An anterior approach can also be quite challenging, depending on the level of the affected segment. It is often necessary to resort to a lateral approach using a costotransversectomy.

At some centers, endoscopic surgical procedures are successfully used in the treatment of thoracic disk herniations.

Approximately 75% of thoracic disk herniations are located below T8. The T11–12 level is most commonly affected (Figs. 12.**60**, 12.**61**).

■ Frequency

Disk herniation is one of the most common indications for CT examination of the spine. Approximately 70% of the male population have at least one episode of low back pain that is investigated by sectional imaging.

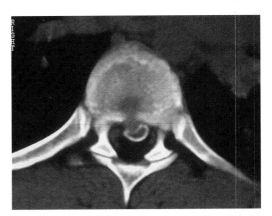

Fig. 12.**61 Postmyelographic CT scan of a T11–12 disk herniation.** Severe pain in this patient was accompanied by fluctuating deficits and especially weakness of the right lower extremity.

■ Clinical Manifestations

The symptoms frequently progress over time. They often start with back pain or nuchal pain and stiffness. Compression of a nerve root is marked by radicular pain radiating to the dermatome of the compressed root. Pain symptoms may be followed by a reduction or loss of reflexes, sensorimotor deficits with muscle weakness, hypalgesia, hypesthesia, and paresthesias. A large herniation toward the cauda equina can cause a complete or partial cauda equina syndrome (Fig. 12.**62**), the features of which include rectal dysfunction and incomplete emptying of the bladder.

If there is preexisting spinal stenosis, or if the herniation is large, the radiculopathy from a herniated cervical disk may be accompanied by lesions of the long spinal tracts, a Brown–Séquard complex, or compression of the anterior spinal artery (Fig. 12.**63**). This combined pattern of nerve-root and cord involvement is termed radiculomyelopathy.

■ CT Morphology

The sensitivity of CT in the diagnosis of lumbar disk herniation is 80–95%, and its specificity is approximately 68–88%. The efficacy of CT in this setting is based largely on its ability to detect even subtle differences in the radiographic density of different tissues.

Intervertebral disk material is hyperdense to all physiologic intraspinal structures on CT scans. Even a novice can recognize the protrusion of this material into the spinal canal at the level of the disk space, regardless of whether the protrusion is broad-based and concentric or narrow and eccentric with irregular margins.

A broad-based, concentric protrusion usually represents a nucleus that is bulging against an intact annulus fibrosus (Figs. 12.**64**–12.**66**). A narrow, eccentric protrusion usually signifies a subligamentous herniation through a rupture in the annulus fibrosus (Fig. 12.**67**). Finally, an eccentric protrusion with irregular margins usually represents a transligamentous herniation or a sequestered disk (Fig. 12.**68**).

Two main difficulties, each fairly common, may be encountered in the CT diagnosis of herniated disks:

- An intraspinal free fragment, whether large or small, may be approximately isodense to the dural sac and cauda equina due to degeneration and rarefaction of the nuclear material. In this case, even extensive lesions are easily missed or misinterpreted as artifacts (Fig. 12.**69**). Any doubts can be resolved

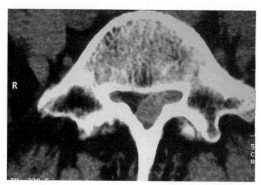

Fig. 12.**62 Massive right lateral disk herniation at L5–S1.** This herniation produced the clinical manifestations of a partial cauda equina syndrome.

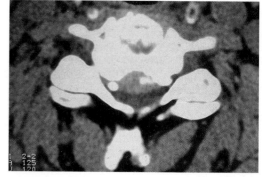

Fig. 12.**63 Cervical spinal stenosis with marked cord compression by a long-standing broad-based disk herniation.** Note the associated osteophytic reaction. The patient had marked clinical and electrophysiologic signs of cervical myelopathy.

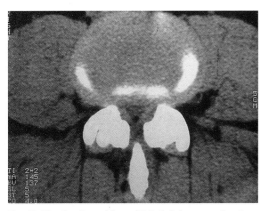 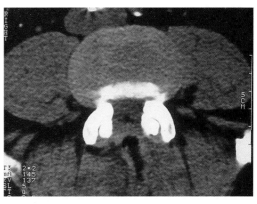

b

Fig. 12.**64 a, b** **Broad-based L4–5 disk protrusion in a constitutionally narrow spinal canal.** Note that the disk protrusion and hypertrophy of the facet joints and ligamentum flavum aggravate the preexisting spinal stenosis, causing symptoms to appear. The residual cross-sectional area of the spinal canal is well below the minimum value of 1.45 cm². The protrusion in this case leads to absolute spinal stenosis. Treatment consisted of laminectomy to decompress the dural sac.

by performing myelography and postmyelographic CT.

- If surgery has already been performed at one disk level, it is necessary to differentiate a recurrent disk herniation from postoperative scar tissue, which is also hyperdense.

The recommended action in both cases is to adjust the window setting interactively on the instrument console—IE, evaluate the finding at various window center settings. If uncertainty persists, the site should be investigated further by MRI, myelography, or other techniques.

A number of authors have recommended prolonged, high-dose contrast administration to differentiate postoperative scarring from a recurrent disk herniation. This is based on the notion that scar tissue and granulation tissue are vascularized and therefore enhance with contrast medium, whereas the nucleus pulposus is avascular and forms a circumscribed hypodensity that is easily distinguished from scar tissue.

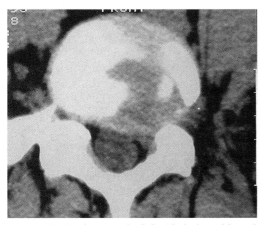 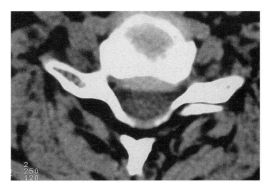

Fig. 12.**65** **Predominantly left-sided, broad-based disk protrusion** causing symptomatic compression of the L4 nerve root.

Fig. 12.**66** **Broad-based cervical disk protrusion** with smooth margins.

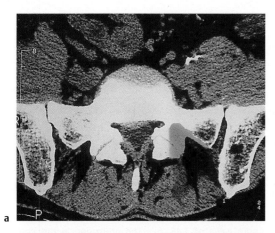

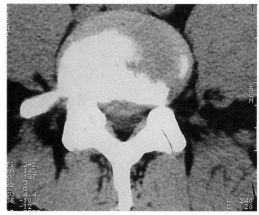

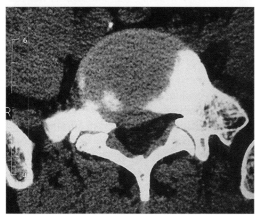

Fig. 12.**67 Subligamentous sequestered disk fragments at the L5–S1 level.**
a, b The fragment extends below the level of the disk
space (**a**) and above it (**b**).
c This fragment is located at the level of the disk
space.
As noted in the text, the posterior longitudinal ligament
is strongly developed at the midline, and is thinner laterally. This explains why lateral subligamentous sequestra-
tions are less common.

In practice, we have found that this technique is often of little help. One problem is that
nuclear material contained within the scar is
difficult to distinguish from the nerve root,
which is also hypodense (Fig. 12.**70**). Another
problem is that regressive changes within
postoperative changes can create a nonhomogeneous enhancement pattern, leading to a
false-positive study.

Another potential difficulty is that
sequestered disk tissue may eventually acquire
a blood supply through vascular ingrowth, resulting in contrast enhancement and a false-
negative study.

Ultimately, the question of whether to perform a scar resection or repair a recurrent disk
herniation will depend mainly on the degree of
root compression and thus on the clinical presentation.

It was thought for many years that
herniated disks do not enhance. This is reasonable when we consider that, by 15–20 years
of age, the nucleus pulposus is a bradytrophic,
avascular tissue. It is possible, however, for
herniated disk tissue and especially intraspinal
sequestered disks to acquire a blood supply
through vascular invasion and thus enhance
after intravenous contrast administration.
There are even reports of lateral herniations
being mistaken preoperatively for schwannomas because of their intense enhancement
and their expansion of the neuroforamen (Fig.
12.**71**).

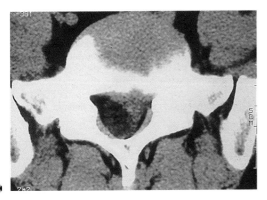

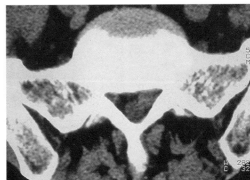

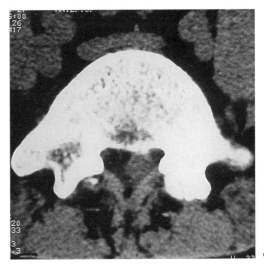

Fig. 12.68 Sequestered disks.

a Classic appearance of a transligamentous lumbar sequestered disk. The fragment has caused a broad-based, concentric elevation of the posterior longitudinal ligament. The hyperdense, eccentric fragment protrudes into the spinal canal on the left side, and is already compressing the left L1 nerve root.

b An eccentric sequestered disk at L5–S1. The nuclear fragment is more isodense to the dural sac than in **a**.

c This free fragment has partially compressed the dural sac and displaced it to the right. The dural sac is poorly defined in this scan due to the relatively hard (narrow) window setting, and a less experienced examiner might misinterpret the fragment as part of the dural sac. It is always wise to compare the density of the questionable finding with the density of the dural sac at the upper or lower adjacent level.

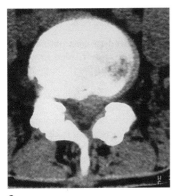

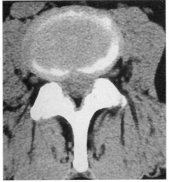

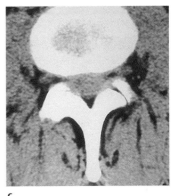

a   **b**   **c**

Fig. 12.69 a–f Sequestered disks.

a A fresh sequestered fragment from a left posterolateral disk herniation. The density of the fragment contrasts markedly with that of the compressed, displaced dural sac.

b, c In these scans from a patient with marked symptoms of conus medullaris–cauda equina compression, a massive disk herniation is difficult to recognize because of the subtotal compression and because its density almost matches that of the dural sac. Fig. 12.69 d–f ▷

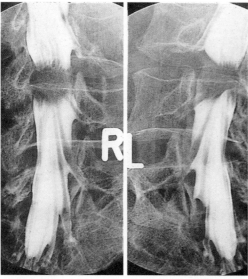

d

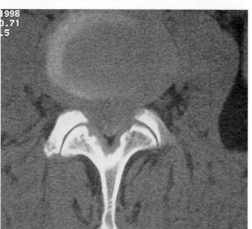

e

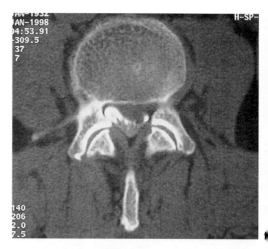

f

Fig. 12.**69**
d Myelography shows bilateral compression of all roots caudal to L3 by a massive disk herniation.
e, f Postmyelographic CT shows subtotal compression of the subarachnoid space at the level of the disk. The contrast medium passes through the narrow point, however, and the cauda equina fibers just below that level are again clearly defined.

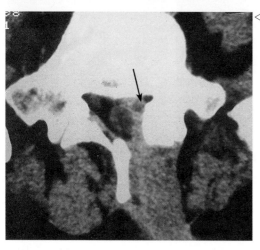

◁ Fig. 12.**70** **Contrast-enhanced CT in a patient who presented with a recurrence of left-sided low back pain 12 weeks after disk surgery** (interlaminar fenestration and nucleotomy). A tract of enhancing granulation and scar tissue is clearly visible extending from the disk space to the subcutaneous level. Embedded in this tissue in the left lateral recess is a nodular-appearing structure (arrow) that is identified as a spinal nerve root only by its continuity in adjacent slices.

Synovial Cyst, Facet Ganglion

Frequency: relatively rare.

Suggestive morphologic findings: cystic mass arising from the facet joint. The mass may contain hemorrhagic areas or gas and may enhance after contrast administration.

Procedure: contiguous slices or scans parallel to the disk spaces, bone window.

Other studies: MRI (T2-weighted) can demonstrate the cystic nature of the lesion.

Checklist for scan interpretation:
▶ Juxtafacet cyst? (Differentiate from a sequestered free fragment.)
▶ Location and size of the lesion?

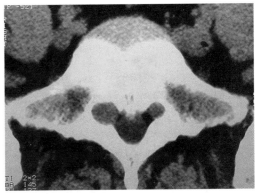

Fig. 12.**71 The right neuroforamen at S1 is expanded by an intraforaminal free fragment.**

■ Pathogenesis

Synovial cysts and ganglia arising from the facet joints are important entities that require clinical and CT differentiation from intervertebral disk disease. They can be particularly difficult to distinguish from an intraspinal sequestered disk fragment lodged in the lateral recess.

Synovial cysts and facet ganglia, which cannot be confidently distinguished by their imaging features, were first described by Kao et al. (1974), who called them *juxtafacet cysts.* The pathogenesis of these cystic lesions is not fully understood, but presumably results from degenerative processes—due, for example, to myxoid degeneration and synovial protrusion associated with hypermobile facet joints. This is supported by clinical series showing that the average patient age was between 58 and 63 years and that most patients had significant degeneration of the intervertebral joints or degenerative spondylolisthesis.

In purely morphologic terms, each type of juxtafacet cyst represents a mass arising from the facet joint that may produce clinical symptoms of nerve root compression.

■ Frequency

Juxtafacet cysts are relatively rare, though precise data are lacking. In one series of 1500 consecutive CT examinations of the lumbar spine,

only three cases were observed. The systematic analysis of clinical series indicates an average patient age of 58–63 years, with a slight female predominance. The most common site of occurrence is the L4–5 level. Bilateral occurrence has also been described.

■ Clinical Manifestations

The main clinical features are root compression symptoms similar to those caused by a herniated disk. Since the pressure is mostly from the dorsal side, predominant compression of the dorsal root may lead only to pain and sensory deficits without necessarily causing a motor deficit. Intracystic hemorrhage can cause an acute exacerbation of symptoms.

■ CT Morphology

CT demonstrates a mass that arises from the facet joint and may display cystic features (Figs. 12.**72**, 12.**73**).

The cystic mass often extends toward the intervertebral foramen and compresses the nerve root from the dorsal side. The cyst wall may enhance after contrast administration. The wall may also calcify, appearing hyperdense on unenhanced scans. Intracystic hemorrhage sometimes occurs. Transient negative pressure in the joint can create a vacuum phenomenon leading to gas inclusions in the cyst.

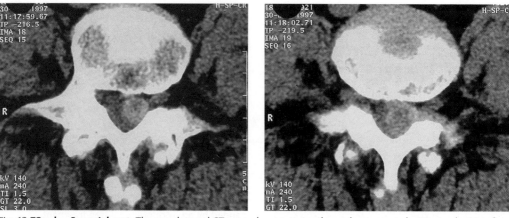

Fig. 12.**72 a, b** **Synovial cyst.** The unenhanced CT scans demonstrate a hyperdense mass abutting and arising from the intervertebral joint.

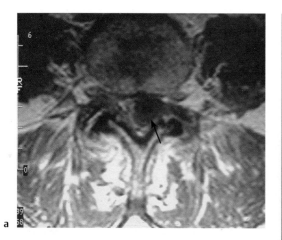

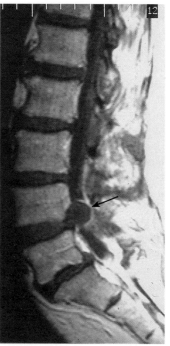

Fig. 12.**73 a–c** **Synovial cyst on magnetic resonance imaging** (MRI). T1-weighted MRIs in all three planes demonstrate the relationship between the cystic mass and the facet joint *(arrow)*.

Fig. 12.**73 c** ▷

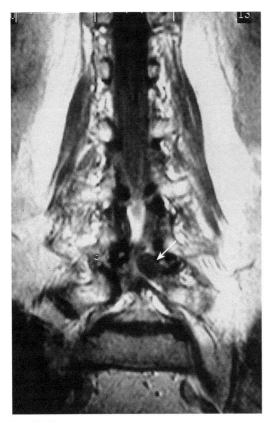

Fig. 12.**73 c**

Spinal Stenosis (Figs. 12.**74**–12.**78**)

Frequency: common.

Suggestive morphologic findings: narrowing of the spinal canal, which may be caused by appositional new bone growth or hypertrophy of the facet joints or ligamentum flavum. May complicate congenital stenosis. "Steerhorn-shaped" spinal canal, displacement of epidural fat.

Procedure: scans may be contiguous or directed parallel to the disk spaces. Secondary reconstructions provide better visualization of the neuroforamina.

Other studies: myelography combined with post-myelographic CT can document the degree of compression of the subarachnoid space and root sleeves (Fig. 12.80). MRI can detect myelopathy (circumscribed hyperintensity in T2-weighted image).

Checklist for scan interpretation:
▶ Degree of stenosis?
▶ Relative or absolute spinal stenosis?
▶ What segments are involved?
▶ Where is the site of maximal stenosis?
▶ Osteophytic spurs, degenerative changes in facet joints, uncovertebral osteoarthritis?

■ Pathogenesis

Spinal stenosis may have a congenital cause such as short pedicles (see p. 307) as well as a variety of acquired causes. The most frequent

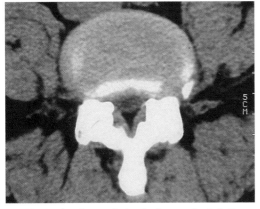

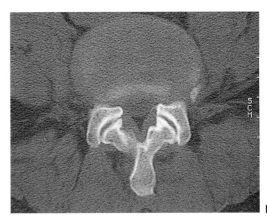

Fig. 12.**74 a, b** **Congenital spinal stenosis.** Soft-tissue and bone-window CT scans demonstrate congenital spinal stenosis based on short, symmetrical pedicles and symmetrical hypertrophy of the facet joints and ligamenta flava.

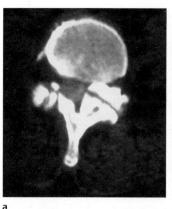
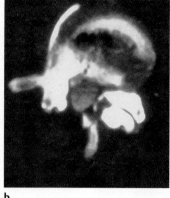

a b

Fig. 12.**75 a, b Rotational scoliosis.** With severe vertebral body deformity, as seen here in a patient with severe rotational scoliosis, unilateral loads on the facet joints promote an asymmetric degeneration that can lead to unilateral narrowing of the spinal canal, neuroforamina, and lateral recess.

Caution: there may also be significant disk degeneration, with anterior and posterior bulging and a vacuum phenomenon.

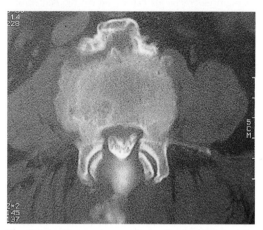
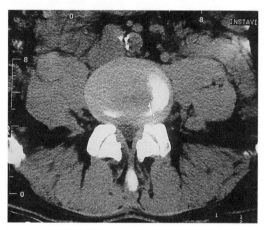

Fig. 12.**76 CT scan in a patient who had previously undergone laminectomy for cauda equina decompression.** Note the conspicuous osteophytes on the anterior margins of the vertebral body.

Fig. 12.**77 Relative spinal stenosis.** This case illustrates the way in which a preexisting relative spinal stenosis can become symptomatic, due to symmetrical hypertrophy of the facet joints and soft-tissue changes, such as a broad-based disk protrusion caused by degeneration of the annulus fibrosus.

Fig. 12.**78 Jones–Thomson ratio.** The ratio of A × B: C × D is normally less than 1:4.5.

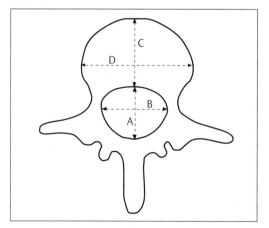

acquired causes are degenerative changes such as spondylarthrosis, which leads to hypertrophy of the facet joints and ligamenta flava.

Other degenerative changes that can produce clinically significant narrowing of the spinal canal are listed below:

- Intraspinal marginal osteophytes
- Calcification of the posterior longitudinal ligament
- Spondylolisthesis
- Disk degeneration and protrusion

In addition, systemic diseases that are associated with structural bone changes (e.g., Paget disease) as well as surgical procedures and trauma are other potential causes of spinal stenosis.

Regardless of the specific cause, a disproportion is created between the width of the remaining cervical, thoracic, or lumbar spinal canal and the diameter of the dural sac and nerve roots.

Lumbar Spinal Stenosis

The literature contains a variety of normal values for the width of the spinal canal, some dating from the pre-CT era. The values listed in Table 12.**6** are considered valid guidelines.

The *Jones–Thomson ratio* (Fig. 12.**78**) is a quantitative index of spinal stenosis that is of somewhat limited practical use. It represents the ratio of the anteroposterior diameter of the spinal canal (A) multiplied by the interpedicular distance (B) to the transverse diameter (C) of the vertebral body multiplied by its transverse diameter (D). Normally, this ratio should range between 1: 2 and 1: 4.5. If the ratio is greater than 1: 4.5, stenosis is present.

Jones–Thomson ratio: $(A \times B): (C \times D) \leq 4.5$

To simplify matters, *relative stenosis* is said to be present when the anteroposterior diameter of the spinal canal is less than 15 mm, and *absolute stenosis* is present when this diameter is 10 mm or less.

Stenosis of the lateral recess can also cause root compression symptoms, regardless of whether there is accompanying central canal

Table 12.**6** Normal dimensions of the spinal canal (from Ulrich et al., *Radiology* 1980; 134: 137–43)

Anteroposterior diameter	At least 11.5 mm
Interpedicular distance	At least 16 mm
Width of lateral recess	At least 3 mm
Axial cross-sectional area	At least 1.45 cm²
Thickness of ligamenta flava	No more than 4–5 mm

stenosis. The most frequent cause of lateral recess stenosis is hypertrophy of the superior articular process, which may be combined with a slight disk bulge. The L4–5 level is the most common site of occurrence.

The lateral recess should measure at least 4 mm on CT to exclude stenosis. A value less than 2 mm confirms lateral recess stenosis.

Other potential causes of circumscribed stenosis are neoplastic and metabolic disorders of the vertebral bodies.

■ Frequency

Lumbar spinal stenosis is particularly common. Most patients are between 35 and 50 years old when symptoms first appear. Stenosis due purely to degenerative changes is most common between the ages of 50 and 60.

■ Clinical Manifestations

The typical symptoms of lumbar spinal stenosis range from low back pain and spinal claudication with decreased walking distance to paraparesis of the lower extremity.

■ CT Morphology

CT slices parallel to the disk spaces demonstrate narrowing of the spinal canal. In severe cases, this can lead to obliteration of the epidural fat plane. It is very common to find hypertrophy of the facet joints and ligamenta flava. This may be associated with short pedicles, giving the spinal canal a "steerhorn" shape in axial section.

Cervical Spinal Stenosis (Figs. 12.79, 12.80)

■ Pathogenesis

Cervical spinal stenosis is rarely congenital, and most cases result from degenerative changes. These include *soft* and *hard disk herniations*, the latter consisting mainly of an osteophytic "buttress reaction" to a soft disk protrusion.

Other changes that can lead to cervical spinal stenosis are as follows:

- Hypertrophy of the laminae
- Hypertrophy of the dura
- Hypertrophy of the posterior longitudinal ligament

Hypertrophy of the posterior longitudinal ligament may be confined to a focal area or may be more extensive and diffuse. The anteroposterior diameter of the cervical spinal canal should measure at least 12 mm.

■ Frequency

Cervical spinal stenosis is a common disease that usually becomes symptomatic after 45–50 years of age.

■ Clinical Manifestations

The following symptoms are typical of cervical myelopathy due to spinal stenosis:

- Motor and sensory deficits in the upper extremities
- Paresis chiefly affecting the proximal portion of the lower extremities
- Spasticity of the lower extremities
- Sphincter dysfunction
- Ataxic gait

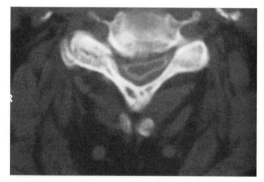

Fig. 12.**79 Cervical spinal stenosis.** Cervical postmyelographic CT in a patient with symptomatic nerve root compression and clinical signs of long-tract compression secondary to cervical spinal stenosis.

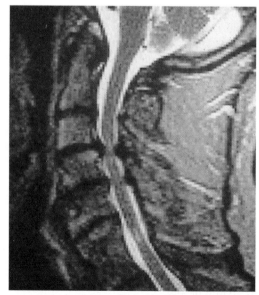

Fig. 12.**80 Cervical spinal stenosis.** The sagittal T2-weighted magnetic resonance image shows conspicuous areas of increased signal intensity in a patient with clinical manifestations of cervical myelopathy.

■ CT Morphology

As with lumbar spinal stenosis, narrowing of the spinal canal is the primary feature that suggests the diagnosis on CT scans. Obliteration of the epidural fat is seen in advanced cases. The most common demonstrable causes are marginal osteophytes, spondylophytic changes in the uncovertebral joint, and hypertrophy of the facet joints and posterior longitudinal ligament. Soft or hard disk herniations are also causative in many cases (diskogenic stenosis, Fig. 12.**79**).

Osteoporosis (Fig. 12.**81**)

Frequency: common.

Suggestive morphologic findings: rarefaction of trabeculae, cortical thinning, accentuation of vertical trabeculae (hypertrophic atrophy), decrease in vertebral body height with biconcave deformity of the endplates (fish vertebrae).

Procedure: thin slices parallel to the disk spaces, bone window setting. Bone mineral content can be determined by dual-energy scanning or comparison with a reference standard.

Other studies: acoustic impedance measurement at the heel, dual-photon absorptiometry (DPX). Conventional radiographs, T2 relaxometry.

Checklist for scan interpretation:
▶ If a fracture is present, does it involve the posterior rim of the vertebral body? Is it causing nerve compression?
(The fracture risk can be evaluated by assessing the degree of cancellous bone rarefaction and by the quantitative determination of bone mineral content.)

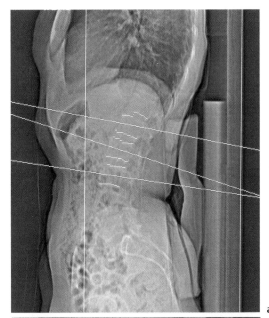

a

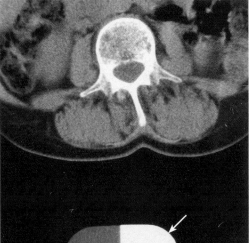

b

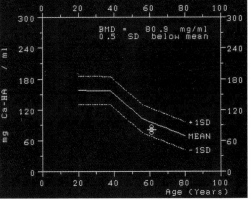

c

Fig. 12.**81 a–c CT determination of bone density.** The measured bone density is compared with a phantom *(arrow)* to determine the mineral salt content of the bone. The measured values are within one standard deviation of average compared with an age-adjusted standard population. Conclusion: CT does not show evidence of osteoporosis.

■ Pathogenesis

Osteoporosis refers to any loss of bone substance exceeding that which is normal for age. It is based on an imbalance between the removal of old bone and the formation of new bone. This may result from a decrease in new bone formation or an acceleration of bone resorption. An etiologic distinction is drawn between the more common *primary* forms of osteoporosis (95%) and the much less common *secondary* forms (5%).

Primary osteoporosis has several forms based on the age of onset:

- Juvenile form
- Presenile form
- Postmenopausal form
- Senile form

Secondary osteoporosis may be focal or generalized, depending on the cause. It is common in patients with hormonal changes and may result from the following disorders:

- Abnormalities of calcium and phosphate metabolism due to renal disease (disturbance of vitamin D metabolism leads to osteomalacia)
- Hyperthyroidism
- Hypogonadism
- Diabetes mellitus
- Corticosteroid therapy

Secondary osteoporosis can also result from:

- Immobilization
- Nicotine abuse
- Alcohol abuse
- Malabsorption

The local and generalized forms of osteoporosis have basically the same radiographic appearance.

The causes of primary osteoporosis are not fully understood. In addition to the fact that women have an inherently smaller bone mass than men, the fall in estrogen levels after menopause appears to play a central role. Some authors believe that the postmenopausal estrogen decline leads to bone loss by reducing the stimulation of osteoblast activity. Others attribute the bone loss to a lack of osteoclast inhibition.

Even in its early stage, osteoporosis is manifested on radiographs by a rarefaction of cancellous bone, with a relative sparing of trabeculae that are distributed along longitudinal stress lines. This accounts for the streak-like structure of affected vertebral bodies on conventional radiographs, but this does not appear until the bone mass has been reduced by approximately one-third.

As the disease progresses, the cortical bone becomes thinned due to resorption of the endosteal surfaces. The streak-like appearance of the vertebral bodies increases with progression of the osteoporosis, even if a balance is reestablished between bone formation and resorption. This is because bony trabeculae that have been lost cannot be replaced. As a result, there can be no complete resolution of osteoporosis, only a reinforcement of the trabecular framework that still remains. This process is often referred to as "hypertrophic atrophy."

■ Frequency

Osteoporosis is the most common skeletal disease, with an incidence of approximately 15%. It is usually manifested in the second half of life and is much more common in women than men, especially after menopause.

■ Clinical Manifestations

As the vertebral bodies lose density and become brittle and more unstable, fractures can occur. They may take the form of recurring *microfractures,* which are manifested by chronic back pain and a progressive loss of vertebral body height. Microfractures can also lead to anterior wedging of the vertebral bodies, especially in the middle and lower thoracic spine, and to concavity of the superior and inferior endplates ("fish vertebrae"), which is most common in the lower thoracic and lumbar areas. Pathologic fractures, with retropulsion of bone fragments into the spinal canal, can occur spontaneously or after trivial trauma, and may produce transverse cord symptoms that require surgical treatment.

■ CT Morphology

CT has two main tasks in the evaluation of osteoporosis:

- It is used to investigate back pain and fractures resulting from osteoporosis.
- It can help determine bone mineral content to screen for osteoporosis or document response to treatment.

Conventional radiographs in advanced stages of osteoporosis typically show picture-frame vertebra, wedged vertebrae, and possible accentuation of vertical trabeculae in lateral views. Thin axial CT slices show rarefaction of the cancellous trabecular structure, accentuated vertical trabeculae, and possible thinning of the cortices. Axial scans also commonly show fissuring of the endplates with protrusion of the nucleus pulposus into the vertebral body.

Use of CT to determine bone mineral content. CT can be used in several ways for the quantitative or semiquantitative determination of bone mineral content:

- In *densitometry,* the mineral content of the bone within a certain volume element is calculated or estimated from its roentgen-ray attenuation. This method assumes that density differences between volume elements that contain water or soft tissue and calcium are based entirely on differences in calcium content. While this assumption is correct in principle, it only allows semiquantitative measurement, as the variable fat content of the bone marrow in vertebral bodies introduces a "fat error" that can distort measurements by up to 30%. Beam-hardening artifacts and calibration errors can further limit the accuracy of the measurement, although calibration errors can be eliminated by using a reference standard of known density.
- *Dual-energy scanning* is based on the fact that different materials have different mass attenuation coefficients for roentgen rays emitted at various energy levels. Materials with a low atomic number, such as fat and water, attenuate roentgen rays at diagnostic energy levels chiefly by scattering, while materials with a higher atomic number, such as calcium, also attenuate roentgen rays by absorption. This absorption, in turn, depends strongly on the energy spectrum of the roentgen ray beam. Thus, irradiating the tissue at different kilovoltage levels (e.g., 85 and 125 kV) yields two attenuation profiles, and these can be used to generate an image that accurately reflects the calcium content of different tissues. This method is more precise than densitometry, but it is also more costly and involves greater radiation exposure.

From a clinical standpoint, the absolute accuracy of the determination of bone mineral content is not crucial in the diagnosis of osteoporosis. Given the large interindividual variations in normal bone mineral content, we cannot accurately classify measurements as normal or abnormal. A more important concern is the reproducibility of the measurements. Reproducible measurement of bone mineral content enables us to identify patients who have rapidly progressive bone loss and refer them for appropriate therapy.

Bone mineral analysis is also useful for assessing the risk of fracture in osteoporosis patients. This is done by comparing the attenuation values of the cancellous bone in several lumbar vertebral bodies with the values in a reference population. Large-scale studies have shown that the fracture risk is significantly increased when the density is more than two standard deviations below the age-normal value.

It should be added, however, that the role of diagnostic procedures in osteoporosis screening has decreased markedly in recent years as hormone replacement therapy has become more widely used. Today, the primary role of CT is in detecting fractures and evaluating the risk of fractures in patients who are known to have the disease.

■ References

Recommended for further study

Spinal arteriovenous malformation

Anson JA, Spetzler RF. Classification of spinal arteriovenous malformations and implications for treatment. Barrow Neurol Inst Q 1992; 8: 2–8.
- *Describes current criteria for classifying spinal AVMs.*

Koenig E, Thron A, Schrader V, Dichgans J. Spinal arteriovenous malformation and fistulae: clinical, neuroradiological and neurophysiological findings. J Neurol 1989; 236: 260–6.

Congenital spinal stenosis

Ulrich CG, Binet EF, Sanecki MG, et al. Quantitative assessment of the lumbar spinal canal by CT. Radiology 1980; 134: 137–43.
- *Presents the minimum values cited here for excluding spinal stenosis.*

Spondylosis, spondylolysis, spondylolisthesis

Harvey CJ, Richenberg JL, Saifuddin A, Wolman RL. The radiological investigation of lumbar spondylosis. Clin Radiol 1998; 53: 723–8.

Syringomyelia, hydromyelia

Ball MJ, Dayan AD. Pathogenesis of syringomyelia. Lancet 1972; ii: 799–801.

Pillay PK, Issam AA, Hahn JF. Gardner's hydrodynamic theory of syringomyelia revisited. Cleve Clin J Med 1992; 9: 373–80.

Williams B, Terry AF, Jones F, et al. Syringomyelia as a sequel to traumatic paraplegia. Paraplegia 1981; 19: 67–80.

Klippel–Feil syndrome

Ulmer JL, Elster AD, Ginsberg LE, Williams DW. Klippel–Feil syndrome: CT and MR of acquired and congenital abnormalities of the cervical spine and cord. J Comput Assist Tomogr 1993; 17: 215–24.
- *Compares the modalities and demonstrates the principal features of the syndrome.*

Spina bifida occulta and myelomeningocele

Barson AJ. The vertebral level of termination of the spinal cord during normal and abnormal development. J Anat 1970; 106: 489–97.

Tethered cord syndrome

Bruhl K, Schwarz M, Schumacher R, et al. Congenital diastematomyelia in the upper thoracic spine: diagnostic comparison of CT, CT myelography, MRI and US. Neurosurg Rev 1990; 13: 77–82.

Diastematomyelia (myeloschisis)

Pang D, Dias MS, Abab-Barmado M. Split cord malformation, 1: a unified theory of embryogenesis for double spinal cord malformation. Neurosurgery 1992; 31: 451–80.
- *Presents a theory on the embryogenesis of diastematomyelia.*

Lipomyeloschisis

Heinz ER, Rosenbaum AE, Scarff TB, et al. Tethered spinal cord following meningomyelocele repair. Radiology 1979; 131: 153–69.

Spinal meningeal cysts

Nabors MW, Pait TG, Byrd EB, et al. Updated assessment and current classification of spinal meningeal cysts. J Neurosurg 1988; 68: 366–77.
- *Describes the classification of spinal meningeal cysts.*

Interfacet dislocation

Leite CC, Escobar BE, Bazan C III, Jinkins JR. MRI of cervical facet dislocation. Neuroradiology 1997; 39: 583–8.

Fracture classification of Anderson and D'Alonzo

Anderson LD, D'Alonzo RT. Fractures of the odontoid process of the axis. J Bone Joint Surg Am 1974; 56: 1663–74.
- *Historical work, forms the basis for the current classification of dens fractures.*

Denis's three-column model

Denis F. The three-column spine and its significance in the classification of acute thoracolumbar spinal injuries. Spine 1983; 8: 817–31.
- *Helpful concept for assessing the stability of thoracolumbar vertebral body fractures.*

Epidural and subdural hematoma

Felber S, Langmaier J, Judmaier W, et al. [Magnetic resonance imaging of epidural and subdural spinal hematomas; in German]. Radiologe 1994; 34: 656–61.
- *Splendid illustration of the MRI features of intraspinal hemorrhages.*

Packer NP, Cummins BH. Spontaneous epidural hemorrhage: a surgical emergency. Lancet 1978; i: 356–8.

Degenerative disk diseases

Hardy RW Jr. Lumbar disc disease. New York: Raven Press, 1993.

Wesolowski DP, Wang AM. Radiologic evaluation. In: Rothman RH, Simeone FH, editors. The spine, vol. 1. Philadelphia: Saunders, 1992: 570–91.

Synovial cyst, facet ganglion

Silbergleit R, Gebarski SS, Brunberg JA, et al. Lumbar synovial cysts: correlation of myelographic, CT, MR, and pathologic findings. AJNR Am J Neuroradiol 1990; 11: 777–9.
- *Compares the modalities and provides pathologic–radiologic correlation based on good-quality images.*

Lumbar spinal stenosis

Ciric I, Mikhael MA, Tarkington JA, et al. The lateral recess syndrome. J Neurosurg 1980; 81: 699–706.

Ulrich CG, Binet EF, Sanecki MG, et al. Quantitative assessment of the lumbar spinal canal by CT. Radiology 1980; 134: 137–43.
- *Presents the minimum values cited here for excluding spinal stenosis.*

Cervical spinal stenosis

Yu YL, du Boulay GH, Stevens JM, et al. Computed tomography in cervical spondylotic myelopathy and radiculopathy: visualization of structures, myelographic comparison, cord measurements and clinical utility. Neuroradiology 1986; 28: 221–36.

Osteoporosis

Kalender WA, Klotz E, Süss C. Vertebral bone mineral analysis: an integrated approach with CT. Radiology 1987; 164: 419–23.
- *Focus on the technical principles of CT densitometry.*

Recent and basic works

Spinal arteriovenous malformation

Kohno M, Takahashi H, Yagishita A. Postmyelographic computerized tomographic scan in the differential diagnosis of radiculomeningeal arteriovenous malformation: technical note. Surg Neurol 1997; 47: 68–71.
- *Evaluates the role of postmyelographic CT in the diagnosis of spinal AVM.*

Lasjaunias P, Berenstein A. Surgical neuroangiography, part 3: vascular anatomy of brain, spinal cord and spine. Berlin: Springer, 1990: 15–87.
- *Part of an important four-volume standard reference work.*

Congenital spinal stenosis

Hinck VC, Clark WM, Hopkins CE. Normal interpeduncular distances (minimum and maximum) in children and adults. AJR Am J Roentgenol 1966; 97: 141–53.
- *Historical work on evaluating the width of the spinal stenosis in conventional radiographs.*

Spondylosis, spondylolysis, spondylolisthesis

Frymoyer JW. Back pain and sciatica. N Engl J Med 1988; 318: 291–300.
- *Review article that includes a look at the socioeconomic aspects of low back pain.*

Syringomyelia, hydromyelia

Williams B. Syringomyelia. Neurosurg Clin N Am 1990; 1: 653–85.
- *Excellent review on the causes of syringomyelia and syringobulbia, and treatment options.*

Tethered cord syndrome and diastematomyelia (myeloschisis)

Barson AJ. The vertebral level of termination of the spinal cord during normal and abnormal development. J Anat 1970; 106: 489–97.

Lipomyeloschisis

Naidich TP, McLone DG, Mutluer S. A new understanding of dorsal dysraphism with lipoma (lipomyeloschisis): radiologic evaluation and surgical correction. AJNR Am J Neuroradiol 1983; 4: 103–16.
- *Describes the various presentations of spinal dysraphisms, presents an animal model, and emphasizes the use of postmyelographic CT for determining extent and planning surgery.*

Spinal meningeal cysts

Langenbach M, Kuhne D, Brenner A, von Wickede R, Leopold HC. The value of different neuroimaging methods in the diagnosis of a congenital, spinal, epidural meningeal cyst. Neurosurg Rev 1989; 12: 245–9.
- *Describes one case of thoracic epidural cyst with myelographic, CT and MRI findings.*

Rimmelin A, Clouet PL, Salatino S, et al. Imaging of thoracic and lumbar spinal extradural arachnoid cyst: report of two cases. Neuroradiology 1997; 39: 203–6.
- *Describes several cases at different sites, presents myelographic, CT and MRI findings while assessing the communication of the cyst with the subarachnoid space.*

Fractures

Beggs I, Addison J. Posterior vertebral rim fractures. Br J Radiol 1998; 71: 567–72
- *Illustrates the MRI and CT features of posterior rim fractures.*

Blackmore CC, Mann FA, Wilson AJ. Helical CT in the primary trauma evaluation of the cervical spine: an evidence-based approach. Skeletal Radiol 2000; 29(11): 632–9.

Blackmore CC, Ramsey SD, Mann FA, Deyo RA. Cervical spine screening with CT in trauma patients: a cost-effectiveness analysis. Radiology 1999; 212: 117–25.

Effendi B, Roy D, Cornish D, et al. Fractures of the ring of the axis: a classification based on the analysis of 131 cases. J Bone Joint Surg Br 1981; 63: 319–27.

Harris JH. The cervicocranium: its radiographic assessment. Radiology 2001; 218(2): 337–51.

Keats TE, Dalinka MK, Alazraki N et al. Cervical spine trauma. American College of Radiology. ACR Appropriateness criteria. Radiology 2000; 215 (Suppl): 243–6.

Samaha C, Lazennec JY, Laporte C, Saillant G. Hangman's fracture: the relationship between asymmetry and instability. Bone Joint Surg [Br] 2000; 82(7): 1046–52.

Nunez DB Jr, Quencer RM. The role of helical CT in the assessment of cervical spine injuries. AJR Am J Roentgenol 1998; 171: 951–7.

Spence KF, Decker S, Sell KW. Bursting atlantal fracture associated with rupture of the transverse ligament. J Bone Joint Surg Am 1970; 52: 543–9.

Van Hise ML, Primack SL, Israel RS, Muller NL. CT in blunt chest trauma: indications and limitations. RadioGraphics 1998; 18: 1071–84.
- *Describes the use of contrast-enhanced spiral CT in patients with trauma and multiple trauma, stressing the value of secondary reconstructions to evaluate thoracolumbar vertebral fractures.*

Epidural and subdural hematoma

Haines DE, Harkey HL, Al-Mefty O. The "subdural" space: a new look at an outdated concept. Neurosurgery 1993; 32: 111–20.
- *Electron-microscopic study; questions the concept of a subdural space.*

Post MJD, Becerra JL, Madsen PW, et al. Acute spinal subdural hematoma: MR and CT finding with pathologic correlates. AJNR Am J Neuroradiol 1994; 15: 1895–1905.
- *Good quality images, with emphasis on MRI; describes the complementary roles of CT and MRI in the diagnosis of acute subdural hematoma.*

Degenerative disk diseases

Ashkenazi E, Pomeranz S, Floman Y. Foraminal herniation of a lumbar disc mimicking neurinoma on CT and MR imaging. J Spinal Disord 1997; 10: 448–50.
- *Case report of a sequestered disk with expansion of the neuroforamen and marked contrast enhancement, mimicking a schwannoma.*

Brant-Zawadzki MN, Dennis SC, Gade GF, Weinstein MP. Low back pain. Radiology 2000; 217(2): 321–30.

Jarvik JG, Deyo RA. Imaging og lumbar intervertebral disk degeneration and aging, excluding disk herniations. Radiol Clin North Am 2000; 38(6): 1255–66. [Review]
- *Excellent overview*

McCall IW. Lumbar herniated disks. Radiol Clin North Am 2000; 38(6): 1293–309.
- *Excellent overview*

Milette PC. Classification, diagnostic imaging, and imaging characterization of a lumbar herniated disk. Radiol Clin North Am 2000; 38(6): 1267–92. [Review]
- *Excellent overview*

Synovial cyst, facet ganglion

Deinsberger W, Schindler C, Boker DK. [Juxtafacet cysts: pathogenesis, clinical symptoms, and therapy; in German]. Nervenarzt 1997; 68: 825–30.
- *Describes this entity, which includes synovial cysts and facet ganglia, based on findings in 16 cases (mainly MRI).*

Hemminghytt S, Daniels DL, Williams NL, et al. Intraspinal synovial cysts: natural history and diagnosis by CT. Radiology 1982; 145: 375–6.

Kao CC, Winkler SS, Turner JH. Synovial cyst of spinal facet: case report. J Neurosurg 1974; 41: 372–6.

Lumbar spinal stenosis

Hahnel S, Forsting M, Dorfler A, Sartor K. [Radiologic findings in lumbar spinal stenosis; in German]. Aktuelle Radiol 1996; 6: 165–70.
- *Detailed description of pathophysiology, symptomatology, and imaging features of lumbar spinal stenosis in conventional and sectional modalities.*

Hasegawa K, Homma T. morphologic evaluation and surgical simulation of ossification of the posterior longitudinal ligament using helical computed tomography with three-dimensional and multiplanar reconstruction. Spine 1997; 22: 537–43.
- *Describes the use of spiral CT in surgical planning and simulating the surgical approach to ossifications of the posterior longitudinal ligament (in nine cases).*

Hamburger C, Buttner A, Uhl E. The cross-sectional area of the cervical spinal canal in patients with cervical spondylotic myelopathy: correlation of preoperative and postoperative area with clinical symptoms. Spine 1997; 22: 1990–5.
- *Neurosurgical work dealing with patient selection and postoperative outcomes in cervical spinal stenosis based on cross-sectional area in CT.*

Hinck VC, Clark WM, Hopkins CE. Normal interpeduncular distances (minimum and maximum) in children and adults. AJR Am J Roentgenol 1966; 97: 141–53.

Senel A, Tanik A, Akan H. Quantitative assessment of the normal adult spinal canal at the fourth lumbar vertebra by computed tomography. Neuroradiology 1994; 36: 54–5.
- *Study in 105 patients, uses the Jones–Thomson ratio to define lumbar spinal stenosis.*

Wybier M. Imaging of lumbar degenerative changes involving structures other than disk space. Radiol Clin North Am 2001; 39(1): 101–14.
- *Excellent overview*

Cervical spinal stenosis

Blease Graham C, Wippold FJ. Comparison of CT myelography performed in the prone and supine positions in the detection of cervical spinal stenosis. Clin Radiol 2001; 56(1): 35–9.

Epstein NE. Identification of ossification of the posterior longitudinal ligament extending through the dura on preoperative computed tomographic examinations of the cervical spine. Spine 2001; 26(2): 182–6.

Reul J, Gievers B, Weis J, Thron A. Assessment of the narrow cervical spinal canal: a prospective comparison of MRI, myelography and CT-myelography. Neuroradiology 1995; 37: 187–91.
- *Comparative evaluation of cervical spinal stenosis with MRI, myelography, and postmyelographic CT, which tends to overestimate moderate and higher-grade stenoses.*

Osteoporosis

Andresen R, Radmer S, Banzer D. [Development of a CT-based index for predicting fracture risk in osteoporosis patients; in German]. Aktuelle Radiol 1997; 7: 264–9

Cherian RA, Haddaway MJ, Davie MW, McCall IW, Cassar-Pullicino VN. Effect of Paget's disease of bone on areal lumbar spine bone mineral density measured by DXA, and density of cortical and trabecular bone measured by quantitative CT. Br J Radiol 2000; 73(871): 720–6.

Hopper KD, Wang MP, Kunselman AR. The use of clinical CT for baseline bone density assessment. J Comput Assist Tomogr 2000; 24(6): 896–9.

Weishaupt D, Schweitzer ME, DiCuccio MN, Whitley PE. Relationships of cervical, thoracic, and lumbar bone mineral density by quantitative CT. J Comput Assist Tomogr 2001; 25(1): 146–50.

13 Intraspinal Masses

Approximately 15% of primary central nervous system (CNS) tumors are intraspinal. The ratio of intracerebral to intraspinal sites of occurrence for primary CNS tumors is approximately 10:1 for astrocytic tumors and about 3–20:1 for ependymomas, depending on the source.

As a general rule, the majority of intraspinal CNS tumors differ from most intracerebral CNS tumors in that they are benign and become symptomatic by compressing neural tissues, rather than by invading or destroying tissues.

Classification of Intraspinal Masses

Intraspinal masses can be divided into three groups according to the compartment that they occupy. This classification also provides a guide to differential diagnosis, based on the frequency of occurrence of particular tumor entities in different spinal compartments.

Intraspinal masses are classified by location into the following groups (Fig. 13.**1**):

- Extradural spinal masses
- Intradural extramedullary spinal masses
- Intramedullary spinal masses

Extradural masses. Extradural masses are the largest group, accounting for approximately 55% of spinal tumors. They may arise from the vertebral bodies or epidural structures, or they may invade the spinal canal secondarily from nearby structures (Fig. 13.**2**).

The largest group of extradural masses consists of metastases from the primary tumors listed below.

Bone tumors that arise from the vertebral bodies are among the most important primary extradural spinal tumors. They include:

- Chordoma
- Osteoid osteoma
- Osteoblastoma
- Aneurysmal bone cyst
- Vertebral hemangioma

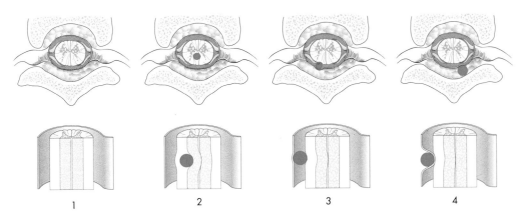

Fig. 13.**1 Sites of occurrence of intraspinal masses.**
1 Normal anatomy
2 Intramedullary mass
3 Intradural extramedullary mass
4 Extradural mass

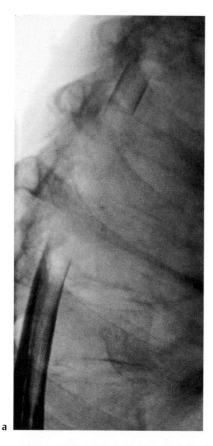

a

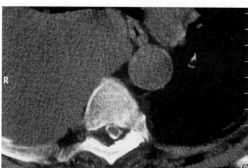

b

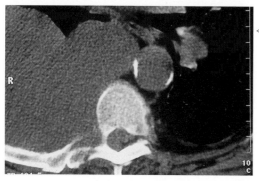

c

Neurofibromas can also occur as primary extradural lesions.

Some tumors that are predominantly intradural can occur in the extradural compartment as well. For example, approximately 15% of spinal meningiomas present as extradural masses.

Intradural extramedullary mass. These masses make up approximately 40% of spinal tumors. They arise chiefly from the leptomeninges and nerve roots. The most important are:

- Meningioma
- Schwannoma
- Lipoma
- Neurofibroma

Approximately 4% of spinal metastases occur in the intradural–extramedullary compartment.

Intramedullary masses. Intramedullary neoplasms arise directly from the spinal cord, and make up approximately 5% of spinal tumors. Astrocytomas and ependymomas each account for approximately one-third of intramedullary tumors (up to 50%, according to some sources). The remaining third consists of various tumor entities that are rare individually, or occur infrequently as spinal neoplasms. They include:

- Glioblastoma
- Dermoid
- Epidermoid
- Teratoma
- Lipoma
- Hemangioma
- Hemangioblastoma
- Lymphoma
- Oligodendroglioma

Only about 2% of spinal metastases are intramedullary.

◁ Fig. 13.2 a–c **Example of a paravertebral tumor invading the spinal canal secondarily.** A right-sided pleural mesothelioma has invaded the spinal canal at multiple levels by contiguous spread through the neuroforamina. Compression of the dural sac and nerve roots appears as an elongated filling defect on myelography and postmyelographic CT.
a Myelogram.
b, c The postmyelographic CTs above (**b**) and below (**c**) the level of dural sac compression.

Extradural Masses

Metastases (Figs. 13.**3**–13.**10**)

■ **Frequency:** spinal metastases are the most common extradural mass, occurring in approximately 10% of cancer patients.

Suggestive morphologic findings: more than 90% of spinal metastases are extradural. Bone destruction is common. Lesions are usually multiple, and enhance after intravenous contrast administration.

Procedure: if metastasis is suspected, obtain primary contrast-enhanced computed tomography (CT) scans with a bone-window setting.

Other studies: Magnetic resonance imaging (MRI) can screen the entire spinal column for metastases. Compare with conventional radiography. Watch for contrast block in postmyelographic CT.

Checklist for scan interpretation:
▶ Number, location, and extent of lesions?
▶ Signs of resulting instability?
▶ Cord compression?

■ Pathogenesis

Metastases are distinguished from other spinal masses by their propensity to occur in all three compartments. Most occur in the extradural compartment, however, and they most commonly involve the vertebral bodies (only 2–4% of metastases are intradural, 1–2% intramedullary).

The most common primary tumors that metastasize to the epidural spinal compartment are listed below:

● Lymphoma (usually due to systemic spread)
● Bronchial carcinoma
● Breast carcinoma
● Prostatic carcinoma
● Gastrointestinal tract neoplasms
● Melanoma

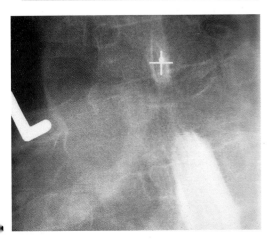

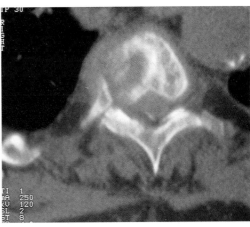

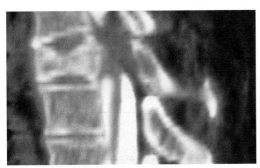

Fig. 13.**3 a–e** **Spinal metastases from bronchial carcinoma** in a patient with clinical manifestations of a partial cord lesion at the T6–7 level.

a Myelography reveals a compression fracture of the T4 vertebral body, with dural sac compression and a partial block of the contrast column.

b A sagittal reformatted image of postmyelographic CT scans clearly demonstrates spinal canal encroachment by the T4 fracture, with soft-tissue components contributing to compression of the dural sac.

c The bone-window view of the affected vertebral body (postmyelographic CT) shows an extensive mass with an intraspinal component and associated bone destruction.   Fig. 13.**3 d, e**

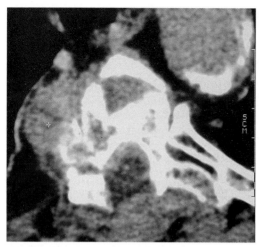

Fig. 13.**3 d**   A bone-window scan at the same level after surgical decompression of the spinal cord by laminectomy.

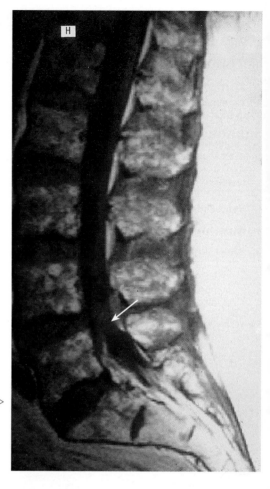

Fig. 13.**3 e**   A sagittal T2-weighted magnetic resonance ▷ image (MRI) of the lumbar spine in the same patient illustrates the higher sensitivity of MRI for detecting vertebral body metastases without an associated pathologic fracture. An additional intraspinal metastasis is also seen *(arrow)*.

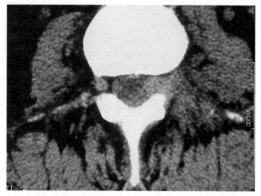

a

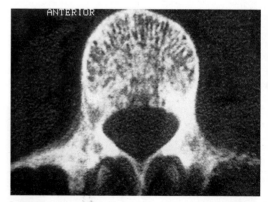

Fig. 13.**4 a, b**   **Spinal metastases from breast cancer.**
a CT scan with a soft-tissue window in a woman with known breast cancer and a radicular compression syndrome of the left L3 nerve root. An intraspinal–extradural metastasis was found at surgery.

b The bone-window view in the same patient shows diffuse, patchy sclerosis of the vertebral bodies reflecting diffuse involvement by osteoplastic metastases. Therapy-induced sclerosis should also be considered in breast cancer patients, however.

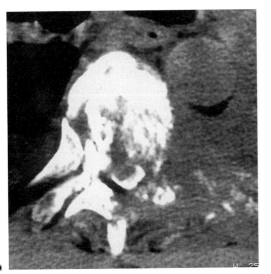
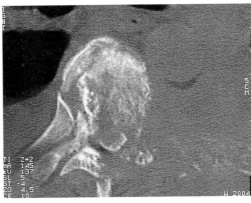

Fig. 13.**5 a, b   Soft-tissue and bone-window views of metastatic tumor in a thoracic vertebra.** The scans demonstrate an extensive soft-tissue mass with intraspinal and paravertebral components.

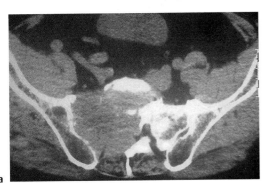
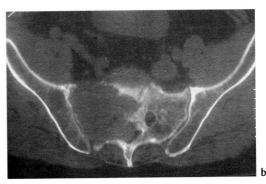

Fig. 13.**6 a, b   A large metastatic tumor in the right lateral mass of the sacrum.** The tumor has caused compression symptoms involving multiple sacral nerve roots.

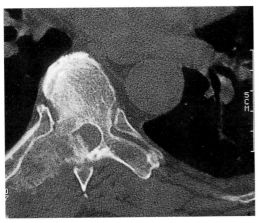
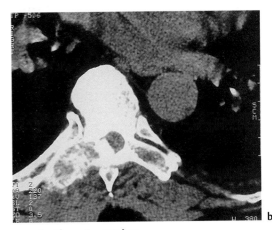

Fig. 13.**7 a, b   A metastatic tumor in the transverse process of a thoracic vertebra.**

Together, these tumors make up approximately 80% of primary tumors that metastasize to the epidural compartment of the spine.

The most common mode of spread is by hematogenous metastasis via the segmental arteries or epidural venous plexus (Batson's plexus, Fig. 13.**9**).

The distribution of metastatic lesions in the cervical, thoracic, and lumbar regions is roughly proportional to the anatomic length of region. Thoracic metastases are the most common, therefore, accounting for 50–60% of lesions.

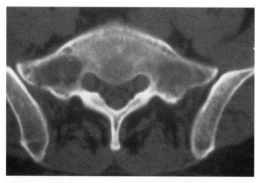

Fig. 13.**8 Metastasis in the right lateral mass of the sacrum.** So far, the tumor has caused only spinal cord displacement and trabecular destruction. The cortical bone is still intact.

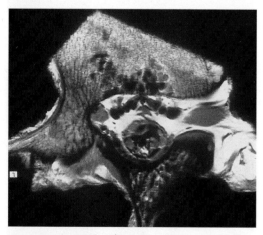

Fig. 13.**9 Communication of veins.** This high-resolution magnetic resonance image of a lumbar vertebra preparation clearly demonstrates the prominent epidural veins and the vertebral body veins that anastomose with them.

■ Frequency

Metastases are the most common extradural spinal masses, occurring in approximately 10% of cancer patients. Some 5–10% of malignant tumors present initially with clinical symptoms due to cord compression.

■ Clinical Manifestations

Pain is the initial symptom in 95% of cases. It may be focal or radicular in nature, and is generally aggravated by movement or acts that raise the intra-abdominal and epidural pressures (coughing, sneezing, bearing down).

As the mass effect of the lesion increases, it can produce a variety of cord or conus compression symptoms ranging to complete cord paralysis. Progression may be insidious as the lesion grows and exerts more pressure on the cord, or symptoms may occur acutely due, for example, to progressive vertebral body destruction that culminates in a pathologic fracture.

The most serious potential complications of spinal metastases are instability of the spinal column caused by the destruction of one or more vertebral bodies and cord compression by a space-occupying lesion within the spinal canal.

■ CT Morphology

Multifocal occurrence is common, and most metastases enhance after intravenous contrast administration. Vertebral body destruction most frequently involves the pedicles. Osteoplastic lesions that are hyperdense on CT scans are typical of metastases from prostatic and breast carcinoma. They are particularly common after treatment initiation in breast cancer patients. Dense vertebral sclerosis (ivory vertebra) may develop in Hodgkin disease (Fig. 13.**10**). The treatment of bony metastases with bisphosphonates such as pamidronate (Aredia) can induce a generalized hyperdensity throughout the skeleton.

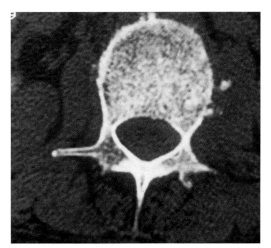

Fig. 13.**10** **Hodgkin disease.** Bone-window CT scan of an ivory vertebra in Hodgkin disease.

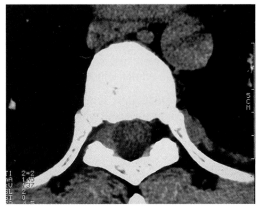

Fig. 13.**11** **Epidural involvement of the thoracic spine by non-Hodgkin lymphoma.** There is material of soft-tissue density filling the epidural space to the right of the dural sac, displacing the epidural fat in that area.

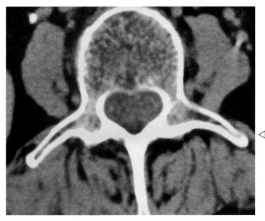

Lymphoma (Figs. 13.**11**–13.**14**)

■ **Frequency:** 0.1–10% of patients with non-Hodgkin lymphoma, depending on the source.

Suggestive morphologic findings: highly variable. All three compartments may be involved, including the bone. Contiguous invasion by paraspinal tumor is common. Some tumors are hyperdense on plain CT scans and enhance after intravenous contrast administration.

Procedure: plain and postcontrast scans, including bone window.

Other studies: MRI can demonstrate the entire spinal column and is the most sensitive study for detecting medullary involvement (Fig. 13.**13**).

Checklist for scan interpretation:
▶ Craniocaudal extent?
▶ Degree of cord compression?
▶ Bone destruction or impending instability?

■ **Pathogenesis**

Like metastases from a solid primary tumor, lymphoma can occur in all spinal compartments. Spinal involvement may be primary or metastatic. Lymphoma is sometimes difficult to distinguish from other circumscribed masses or diffusely infiltrating processes, depending on the affected compartment. The most common pattern is infiltration of the bone and invasion of the spinal canal through the intervertebral foramina by a retroperitoneal or paravertebral lesion. After entering the spinal canal, lymphoma can lead to cord ischemia through vascular compression or may compress the cord directly. Cord compression can also result from vertebral body destruction by lymphoma. Involvement of the vertebral bodies is often associated with extensive bone destruction and sclerotic changes.

◁ Fig. 13.**12** **Intradural spinal involvement by non-Hodgkin lymphoma.** This unenhanced CT scan of the lumbar spine is difficult to interpret. When the diagnosis is known, however, it can be seen that the intradural space, which normally contains only cerebrospinal fluid and cauda equina fibers at this level, shows an almost uniform hyperdensity.

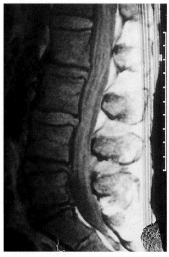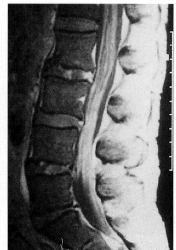

Fig. 13.**13 a, b Diffuse subarachnoid spread of lymphoma.** The sagittal T1-weighted two-dimensional fast low-angle shot (FLASH) sequences before and after contrast administration show that the spinal subarachnoid space is almost completely filled with lymphomatous tissue. This tissue is seen more clearly on the contrast-enhanced image.

a   b

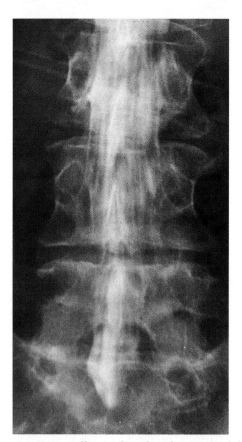

Fig. 13.**14 Diffuse subarachnoid spread of lymphoma.** Lumbar myelography (same patient as in Fig. 13.**13**) also shows diffuse lymphomatous involvement of the subarachnoid space.

Other patterns of lymphomatous involvement are:

- Leptomeningeal spread from a primary CNS lymphoma (usually diffuse, rarely focal)
- Primary intramedullary lymphoma

Primary intramedullary lymphoma is extremely rare, however, and only a few cases have been described in the world literature.

■ Frequency

Spinal involvement is present in 0.1–10% of patients with non-Hodgkin lymphoma, depending on the source. As the population infected with human immunodeficiency virus (HIV) and immunosuppressed transplant recipients have become more numerous in the past 10–15 years, there has been a marked rise in the frequency of CNS involvement by lymphoma and especially of primary CNS lymphomas. At the same time, the peak age incidence has declined from 40–70 years to the current 30–40 years.

■ Clinical Manifestations

Clinical manifestations depend on the degree of cord compression and the effects of vascular compression. A complete cord lesion may develop in severe cases.

■ CT Morphology

As noted earlier, lymphoma is often difficult to distinguish from other diseases, depending on its location and pattern of spread. Purely osseous involvement can resemble metastases from other tumors, but may feature sclerotic areas in addition to extensive bone destruction. Especially in Hodgkin disease, dense sclerosis already visible on plain films can lead to the development of an "ivory vertebra" (Fig. 13.**10**).

A lymphoma that has invaded the spinal canal from the retroperitoneum has a less ambiguous CT appearance, and is usually accompanied by signs of retroperitoneal lymphadenopathy.

Leptomeningeal spread typically appears as a diffuse sheet-like area or disseminated micronodular region of contrast enhancement.

Primary intramedullary lymphoma is extremely rare and is virtually indistinguishable from glioma. The fact that primary CNS lymphomas are often hyperdense on plain CT scans owing to their high cellular density is less helpful in the spine than in the cranium, due to the narrow confines of the spinal canal, as well as partial-volume and beam-hardening artifacts.

Lymphomas in all locations usually show intense contrast enhancement, especially on delayed images.

Osteogenic Extradural Masses

Chordoma (Figs. 13.**15**, 13.**16**)

Frequency: rare.

Suggestive morphologic findings: destruction of one or more vertebral bodies or the sacrum, associated soft-tissue mass, contrast enhancement.

Procedure: thin postcontrast CT slices, bone-window views.

Other studies: MRI or radionuclide bone scanning can exclude other lesions and differentiate chordoma from metastases. Compare with conventional radiographs.

Checklist for scan interpretation:
▶ Tumor extent and segmental location?
▶ Instability?
▶ Cord compression?

■ Pathogenesis

Chordomas are rare tumors that arise from remnants of the embryonic notochord (develops in week 4–7). Normally, the notochord differentiates into the nucleus pulposus of the intervertebral disk.

If a chordoma develops, it is usually located at one end of the notochord. This can result in a clivus chordoma, cervical chordoma, or sacrococcygeal chordoma.

There is still disagreement regarding the biologic behavior of chordomas. While many authors note that the tumor is locally invasive and causes bone destruction, they still charac-

Fig. 13.**15 Clivus chordoma.** The tumor has completely destroyed the clivus, and is causing an extensive mass effect.

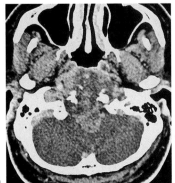 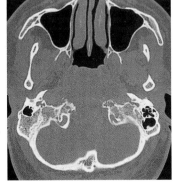

a   b

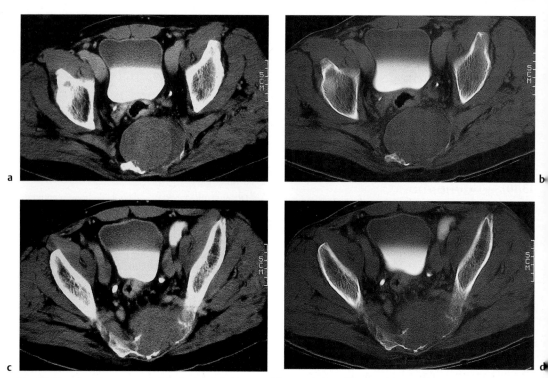

Fig. 13.**16 a–d**   **A large sacral chordoma.** Soft-tissue and bone-window CT scans demonstrate extensive erosion of the left lateral mass of the sacrum.

terize it as benign. The tumor has a high recurrence rate after excision. Distant metastases to the lung, bone, liver, and lymph nodes have also been described.

■ Frequency

Chordomas are relatively rare. They make up approximately 1–4% of "malignant" bone tumors, and their incidence is one in 2 million. While spheno-occipital chordomas affect both sexes equally, sacrococcygeal and vertebral chordomas are about twice as common in men than women. The peak age incidence is in the fifth decade.

Vertebral chordomas make up 15–20% of chordomas. The most common site of occurrence is the cervical spine, followed by the lumbar spine.

■ Clinical Manifestations

Pain is a common but nonspecific symptom. It may be local or may radiate in a radicular distribution. Compression of the spinal cord, conus medullaris, or cauda equina frequently develops over time. Even large sacrococcygeal chordomas may cause few symptoms, however.

■ CT Morphology

CT often shows extensive destruction of one or more vertebral bodies or portions of the sacrum (Fig. 13.**16**). The destruction extends beyond the disk space, and is often associated with an adjacent soft-tissue mass, which may be quite large. An intraspinal tumor component can lead to cord or nerve root compression.

The tumor often appears hyperdense on unenhanced CT scans, which show complete destruction of the trabecular structure of the affected vertebral bodies. Most chordomas enhance after intravenous contrast administration.

Eosinophilic Granuloma

Frequency: rare; almost never seen after age 30.

Suggestive morphologic findings: nonsclerotic osteolytic area with sharply defined margins and a hyperdense center (sequestrum); little or no soft-tissue or periosteal reaction; vertebral body collapse (vertebra plana).

Procedure: thin CT slices, bone window views.

Other studies: obtain conventional radiographs of other skeletal regions, especially the skull, to check for multiple lesions.

Checklist for scan interpretation:
▶ Location and extent of the lesion?
▶ Signs of instability?

■ Pathogenesis

Eosinophilic granuloma is one of a group of granulomatous disorders (Abt–Letterer–Siwe disease, Hand–Schüller–Christian disease) that are known collectively as histiocytosis X. Eosinophilic granuloma is the mildest form.

Histopathologically, eosinophilic granuloma involves a local infiltration of the bone with mononuclear and eosinophilic granulocytes that form a soft-tissue mass. As the disease progresses, the mass causes lysis of the bone.

Some tumors show a propensity for spontaneous remission.

One treatment option is resection of solitary lesions. Multiple lesions are better managed by chemotherapy or low-dose radiotherapy if the affected vertebral bodies show signs of impending instability.

■ Frequency

Eosinophilic granuloma is the most common and mildest variant of histiocytosis X. It affects children and young adults almost exclusively. A useful rule of thumb is that eosinophilic granuloma can be eliminated as a differential diagnosis in patients over 30 years of age. The peak age incidence is approximately 5–10 years, and males predominate by a ratio of about 3 : 2. Involvement is monostotic in 50–75 % of patients. The spine is the third most common site of occurrence after the calvarium and mandible, accounting for 20–25 % of cases.

■ Clinical Manifestations

The cardinal symptom in most cases is local pain.

■ CT Morphology

Eosinophilic granuloma appears as an osteolytic lesion on CT scans, often causing a dramatic decrease in vertebral body height. Generally the vertebral arches are spared. As it continues to lose height, the vertebral body assumes the shape of a thin disk (vertebra plana), which is typically seen in the thoracic region. Often, there is a central hyperdensity caused by the sequestration of bone material within the soft-tissue mass. The margins of the osteolytic lesion are well defined, but are not sclerotic. Usually, there is little or no evidence of an associated soft-tissue or periosteal reaction.

Giant-Cell Tumor (Osteoclastoma)

Frequency: rare; the spine is the primary location in only 5 % of cases.

Suggestive morphologic findings: expansile, destructive mass with associated cortical destruction and nonsclerotic margins. Shows nonhomogeneous enhancement after contrast administration.

Procedure: thin CT slices, intravenous contrast administration, bone-window views.

Other studies: conventional radiographs, radionuclide bone scan.

Checklist for scan interpretation:
▶ Location and extent (may be marked on the skin if desired).
▶ Associated intraspinal soft-tissue mass?
▶ Instability or risk of fracture?

■ Pathogenesis

Giant-cell tumor is a locally aggressive primary bone tumor that arises from osteoclasts (synonym: osteoclastoma). Spinal involvement is described in about 5 % of cases. Approximately

15% of giant-cell tumors are classified as malignant, but the radiologic, clinical, and even histologic findings may be insufficient for confident benign–malignant differentiation. Both benign and malignant forms have a high recurrence rate, even after radical excision.

The tumor most commonly affects women 20–30 years of age.

Morphologically, giant-cell tumor is an osteolytic lesion associated with a reddish-gray soft-tissue mass that may contain cysts, hemorrhagic areas, and necrosis. The cortex is usually thinned from the inside, and the zone of bone destruction does not develop sclerotic margins. A periosteal reaction may be present.

An important differentiating criterion is that giant-cell tumors always arise from epiphyseal plates that have already closed. This means that they occur only after the cessation of skeletal growth.

The most common sites of occurrence of giant-cell tumors are the epiphyses of the long tubular bones. In the spinal column, the sacrum is commonly affected. Generally the vertebral body is involved first, with subsequent extension to the vertebral arches. Associated soft-tissue masses have been described.

Treatment is geared toward the histologic tumor grade, and ranges from meticulous curettage of a benign giant-cell tumor to radical excision of a malignant form.

■ Frequency

Giant-cell tumor is a rare neoplasm, and only about 5% affect the spinal column primarily. The peak age of occurrence is between 20 and 40 years, and women are affected about twice as often as men.

■ Clinical Manifestations

Common nonspecific symptoms are local pain, limitation of motion, and occasional pathologic compression fractures. An intraspinal or paravertebral soft-tissue mass may cause symptoms of cord or nerve root compression as it enlarges.

■ CT Morphology

Giant-cell tumor appears on CT as an expansile, destructive tumor that is frequently associated with cortical destruction. Generally there is no detectable sclerotic margin. An associated soft-tissue mass may be visible. The tumor usually shows nonhomogeneous enhancement after contrast administration. It cannot be classified as benign or malignant based on its imaging appearance alone.

Osteoid Osteoma, Osteoblastoma

Frequency: relatively common, accounting for approximately 40% of benign spinal tumors and 1.4% of spinal tumors.

Suggestive morphologic findings: expansile tumor with a central, very vascular enhancing nidus and sclerotic margins.

Procedure: thin CT slices, intravenous contrast administration, bone-window views.

Other studies: the central nidus is often visible on plain radiographs. Bone scans show marked radiotracer uptake.

Checklist for scan interpretation:
▶ Location (may be marked on the skin if desired).
▶ Instability?
▶ Impending cord or root compression?
▶ Additional studies to exclude multiple lesions (e.g., radionuclide scan).

■ Pathogenesis

Osteoid osteoma is a benign tumor that arises from osteoblasts. The classic radiographic appearance is that of a small, hyperdense tumor with a central lucency called the nidus. Only the nidus presents the histologic features of osteoid osteoma: a rounded focus in cancellous bone surrounded by a sclerotic zone of cortical thickening.

The tumor is composed of numerous osteoid trabeculae, mostly uncalcified, surrounded by osteoblasts and osteoclasts in a capillary-rich stroma.

Osteoblastoma differs histologically from osteoid osteoma mainly by its richer vascular supply. Generally, a tumor that is 15–20 mm or larger is classified as an osteoblastoma. Because of its size, osteoblastoma is particularly likely to cause cord or nerve root compression.

In one study, 22% of patients with spinal osteoid osteomas had neurologic deficits while 28% of patients with spinal osteoblastomas showed signs of myelopathy.

With both forms, adolescents are predominantly affected. Lesions in vertebral bodies are most commonly located in the vertebral arch. Although both entities are benign bone tumors, complete surgical excision is indicated because of the potentially severe bone pain, which worsens at night.

■ Frequency

Primary spinal involvement occurs with approximately 40% of osteoblastomas and 25% of osteoid osteomas. Together, these tumors make up approximately 40% of benign spinal bone tumors and 1.4% of vertebragenic tumors in general. Males predominate by a 2:1 ratio. The peak age incidence is about 20–30 years.

■ Clinical Manifestations

The classic clinical symptom is local pain that worsens at night and is relieved by aspirin. This is not a consistent feature, however, as it occurs in only 40% of patients with spinal osteoid osteoma and only 25% of patients with osteoblastoma. The second most common symptom after pain is scoliosis, which may be painful or antalgic. The convexity is usually toward the contralateral side. Radicular pain and/or neurologic deficits also occur in 50% of patients.

■ CT Morphology

Osteoid osteoma and osteoblastoma typically present on CT as an expansile tumor that often affects the vertebral arches primarily. The tumor has a very vascular central nidus that is surrounded by a sclerotic zone and enhances after intravenous contrast administration.

Aneurysmal Bone Cyst

Frequency: the second most common benign spinal tumor; predominantly affects women under 30 years of age.

Suggestive morphologic findings: an expansile, predominantly cystic mass that is hypodense on plain CT scans, and has a nonhomogeneous internal structure. Shows intense, nonhomogeneous enhancement after contrast administration. May show a clam-shell pattern of periosteal calcification.

Procedure: thin CT slices before and after contrast administration (may use bolus injection), bone-window views.

Other studies: MRI can detect intracystic hemorrhage and fluid levels. Conventional radiographs.

Checklist for scan interpretation:
▶ Extent and location (may be marked on the skin if desired).
▶ Intraspinal mass?
▶ Risk of fracture?

■ Pathogenesis

Aneurysmal bone cyst is a benign osteolytic bone lesion. Unlike a juvenile bone cyst, however, it is not a primary lesion but develops in response to previous bone injury. It may also accompany a giant-cell tumor or fibrous dysplasia. Some authors disagree with this view of the pathogenesis—noting, for example, that it does not explain why 90% or more of patients are younger than age 30.

Aneurysmal bone cysts occur most frequently in the spine (approximately 30%), the long bones, and the pelvis. They usually consist of an eccentric osteolytic lesion, often expansile, bordered by a hernia-like outpouching of periosteum that breaks through the cortex and extends along adjacent vertebra, forming a beehive-like expansion that mimics the internal involvement of multiple vertebrae. The posterior elements are more commonly affected.

Frequency

Aneurysmal bone cyst is the second most common benign spinal tumor. Approximately 20–30% of aneurysmal bone cysts occur in the spine. Sites of predilection are the posterior vertebral elements of the lower thoracic and upper lumbar spine. Most patients are under age 30. Females from age 10–20 are most commonly affected.

Clinical Manifestations

Most patients have a painful swelling or merely local hyperesthesia or hyperalgesia. Up to 5% of patients sustain a pathologic fracture.

CT Morphology

Aneurysmal bone cyst typically appears as a hypodense, expansile, cyst-like mass with a nonhomogeneous internal structure. It shows intense, nonhomogeneous enhancement after contrast administration, especially when a bolus injection is used (Fig. 13.**17**).

Vertebral Hemangioma (Figs. 13.**18**, 13.**19**)

Frequency: the most common benign spinal tumor, present in approximately 9–12% of the general population. A common incidental finding.

Suggestive morphologic findings: punctate accentuation of hypertrophic trabeculae in an axial CT scan. May or may not enhance after contrast administration.

Procedure: thin CT slices, bone-window views.

Other studies: vertebral hemangioma is visible on conventional radiographs if it involves at least one-third of the vertebral body. On MRI, hemangiomas with lipomatous changes are hyperintense on T1- and T2-weighted images; expansile hemangiomas are isointense on T1-weighted images and hyperintense on T2-weighted images. Radionuclide scan can detect existing compression fractures.

Checklist for scan interpretation:
▶ Does CT confirm or exclude a suspected vertebral hemangioma?
▶ Compression fracture or risk of fracture?
▶ Expansile mass causing cord or root compression?

Pathogenesis

Cavernous hemangiomas are benign bone lesions. They are often multifocal, and become more numerous with aging. In approximately one-third of cases, up to five noncontiguous levels are affected. The most common sites of occurrence are the lower thoracic and upper

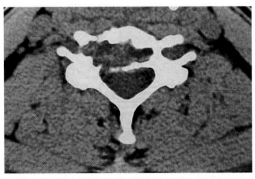

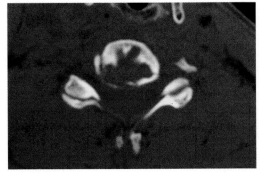

a

Fig. 13.**17 a, b Aneurysmal bone cyst.** CT typically shows a large, expansile, osteolytic intraosseous mass without sclerotic margins. This lesion has penetrated the cortex, but has not yet formed an intraspinal mass. The postcontrast scan usually shows an intense, nonhomogeneous pattern of enhancement.

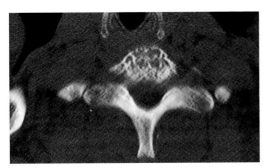

Fig. 13.**18** **Cervical vertebral hemangioma.** The typical punctate hypertrophy of the trabeculae is clearly visualized on axial CT.

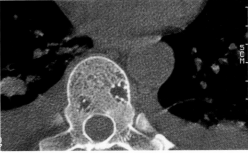

Fig. 13.**19** **Thoracic vertebral hemangioma.** While some hemangiomas involve the entire vertebral body, there are circumscribed forms that are not usually seen on conventional radiographs, like these two small hemangiomas in a thoracic vertebra.

lumbar spine. Hemangiomas are extremely rare in the cervical vertebrae.

Twenty-five percent of hemangiomas affect only the vertebral body, 25% affect only the vertebral arch, and the remaining 50% affect both structures. Purely extradural hemangiomas have been described but are very rare.

Histomorphologically, invasion of the normal medullary cavity by hemangioma vessels leads to a predominantly vertical hypertrophic sclerosis of the bony trabeculae. This creates the classic linear striation pattern seen on conventional radiography and CT scans.

Malignant transformation does not occur.

■ Frequency

Cavernous vertebral hemangiomas have an estimated incidence of approximately 9–12% in the general population. It has a higher prevalence in older age groups, and women predominate by a ratio of about 2 : 1. Most patients are asymptomatic, and most lesions are therefore detected incidentally in examinations carried out for other reasons.

■ Clinical Manifestations

Most hemangiomas are detected fortuitously or incidentally. Rarely, however, patients develop a progressive neurologic deficit that can have various causes:

- Subperiosteal intraspinal growth or expansion of the affected bone (e.g., the pedicles) leads to symptomatic spinal stenosis.
- Spontaneous hemorrhage can cause an acute spinal epidural hematoma.
- Compression fractures of the affected vertebral body are extremely rare.

■ CT Morphology

The hypertrophic trabeculae typically create a punctate ("polka-dot") pattern on axial CT scans. Contrast enhancement may occur but is not always seen. CT is the method of first choice for making a diagnosis.

Osteosarcoma

Frequency: the second most common malignant bone tumor in general, but extremely rare in the spine.

Suggestive morphologic findings: a destructive mass with an extensive soft-tissue component, necrotic foci, and hemorrhagic cysts; shows intense contrast enhancement.

Procedure: thin CT slices before and after contrast administration, bone-window views.

Other studies: MRI is most useful for follow-up. Conventional radiographs.

Checklist for scan interpretation:
▶ Location and extent?
▶ Instability and potential fracture risk?
▶ Cord compression?

■ Pathogenesis

Osteosarcoma is a malignant bone tumor in which malignant osteoblasts are differentiated from a sarcomatous stroma. Various histologic types of osteosarcoma have been identified. The most common forms are:

- Osteoblastic osteosarcoma
- Chondroblastic osteosarcoma
- Fibroblastic osteosarcoma

Less common forms are:

- Paget osteosarcoma
- Postirradiation osteosarcoma

Rare histologic subtypes occur mainly in the older population:

- Parosteal osteosarcoma
- Periosteal osteosarcoma
- Telangiectatic osteosarcoma

Except for parosteal sarcoma, all of the forms have a very poor prognosis.

Osteosarcomas typically arise in the metaphyseal portion of the long bones, but they may occur anywhere in the skeleton, including the spinal column.

■ Frequency

Osteosarcoma is the second most common malignant bone tumor after plasmacytoma. Spinal involvement is extremely rare, as it mainly affects long bones such as the femur and tibia in adolescents, and flat bones such as the pelvis and scapula in older patients. Osteosarcoma may arise anywhere in the skeleton, however, and can occur at multiple sites (Table 13.1).

■ Clinical Manifestations

The most common symptoms are listed below:

- Pain
- Swelling
- Fever
- Increased alkaline phosphatase

Up to 25 % of patients with central osteosarcoma have a paraneoplastic syndrome with diabetes mellitus.

■ CT Morphology

CT typically shows a destructive lesion that often has a large soft-tissue component. There may be a mixed pattern of bone destruction and new bone formation, combined with necrotic areas and hemorrhagic cysts. Osteosarcoma enhances strongly after contrast administration—especially the telangiectatic subtype.

Fibrous Dysplasia

Frequency: rare; approximately 1 % of cases occur in the spine.

Suggestive morphologic findings: variable presentation: cortical thinning, expansile growth, bone deformation, central calcification, cyst formation, sclerosis. Typically, there is no periosteal reaction, and most lesions do not enhance after contrast administration.

Procedure: thin CT slices, bone-window views.

Other studies: conventional radiographs and MRI are best for follow-up. Radionuclide bone scanning is a good screening study for the polyostotic form.

Checklist for scan interpretation:
▶ Location and extent?
▶ Instability and risk of fracture?
▶ Cord compression?

Table 13.1 Frequency distribution of osteosarcoma

	Age range (years)	Sex ratio (m : f)
Central osteosarcoma	10–25, > 60	3 : 2
Parosteal osteosarcoma	12–58	2 : 3
Periosteal osteosarcoma	10–20 (13–70)	2 : 3
Telangiectatic osteosarcoma	20–30	m > f

Pathogenesis

Fibrous dysplasia is a benign fibro-osseous disease, the cause of which is still unknown. Histologically, the disease consists of an interwoven mixture of fibromyxoid tissue, spindle cells, cysts, and bony trabeculae proliferating within the medullary cavity. The *monostotic form* (85% of cases) is distinguished from the less common *polyostotic form* (15%).

A special form, transmitted as an autosomal-dominant trait, is characterized by symmetrical involvement of the mandible and maxilla, which imparts a cherubic look to the child's face (cherubism). In another special form, called McCune–Albright syndrome, unilateral polyostotic fibrous dysplasia is accompanied by endocrine disturbances and café-au-lait spots.

Frequency

Fibrous dysplasia affects the spinal column in approximately 1% of cases. Spinal involvement is most common in the polyostotic form of the disease, which affects the lumbar spine about twice as frequently as the cervical spine. Other spinal segments are rarely affected.

The monostotic form of fibrous dysplasia shows a uniform age distribution, while the polyostotic form has a peak incidence between 3 and 15 years of age. In both forms, 75% of affected patients are younger than age 30.

Clinical Manifestations

Symptoms are often absent or scant and nonspecific. The occurrence of a pathologic fracture is marked by pain and possible neurologic deficits due to cord or nerve root compression.

CT Morphology

Fibrous dysplasia can have a broad spectrum of radiographic and CT appearances. It may be associated with significant cortical thinning, expansile growth, bone deformity, central calcifications, cystic changes, and areas of sclerosis. Typically, however, fibrous dysplasia is not as-

sociated with a periosteal reaction, and does not enhance after contrast administration—assuming that a pathologic fracture has not occurred.

Plasmacytoma (Multiple Myeloma, Kahler Disease)

> **Frequency:** the most common generalized malignant bone tumor; spinal involvement is found in 50% of cases.
>
> **Suggestive morphologic findings:** multiple osteolytic areas that do not have sclerotic margins (may occur in response to treatment). Periosteal reactions are seen only with pathologic fractures. Contrast enhancement may occur.
>
> **Procedure:** thin CT slices, bone-window views.
>
> **Checklist for scan interpretation:**
> ▶ Location and extent?
> ▶ Instability and risk of fracture?
> ▶ Cord compression?

Pathogenesis

Plasmacytoma (Figs. 13.**20**–13.**22**) is the most common disseminated malignant bone tumor.

It arises from a single plasma cell clone in the bone marrow and is therefore included in the category of B-cell lymphomas. Plasmacytoma may be localized or multicentric (multiple myeloma), and rarely it may occur outside the medullary cavity. It can arise at any site at which hematopoietic bone marrow is present, and sites of predilection are the vertebral bodies, ribs, calvarium, scapula, femur, and humerus.

Mature and immature plasma cells may infiltrate adjacent structures and form soft-tissue masses. Circulating myeloma precursor cells may form colonies in a histocompatible environment (typically the bone marrow), where they mature and form expansile metastatic deposits (Fig. 13.**20**). Morphologically, the lesions usually consist of focal cancellous bone defects and often crescent-shaped cortical defects with a "rat-eaten" appearance. These defects are filled with grayish-white tumor material composed of a dense aggregation of normal and atypical pleomorphic

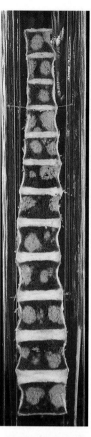

Fig. 13.**20 Diffuse involvement of the thoracic spine by foci of plasmacytoma.** This coronal section of a pathologic specimen clearly shows grayish-white lesions replacing the marrow and destroying the bony trabeculae (courtesy of the Department of Pathology, Charité Hospital, Berlin).

plasma cells. Calvarial defects in particular appear as punched-out lytic lesions with non-sclerotic margins.

Both the solitary and disseminated forms of plasmacytoma most commonly affect the vertebral bodies. In the classic pattern of involvement, the vertebral arches are spared because they do not contain hematopoietic marrow.

■ Frequency

The incidence among Europeans is approximately one to two per 100000 population. Males in the sixth and seventh decades are predominantly affected. Fewer than 2% of cases occur before age 40. Spinal involvement is present in at least 50% of cases.

■ Clinical Manifestations

Common symptoms are listed below:

- Immunodeficiency, with increased susceptibility to infections
- Anemia
- Thrombocytopenia
- Leukopenia
- Pathologic fractures
- Pain on motion
- Myeloid and monoclonal gammopathy leading to renal failure

Approximately 10% of patients develop intraspinal masses with cord or nerve root compression.

■ CT Morphology

CT usually demonstrates multiple osteolytic lesions, a coarse trabecular pattern, and sparing of the vertebral arches. Associated paraspinal or intraspinal soft-tissue masses may be seen. Generalized osteoporosis may be present. Periosteal reactions usually occur only in association with a pathologic fracture. Primary sclerosis is seen only in about 1–3% of plasmacytoma lesions, but sclerosis may develop in response to treatment (Figs. 13.**21**, 13.**22**).

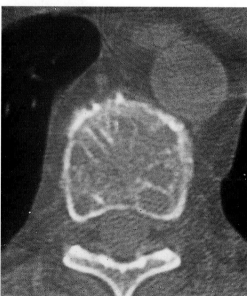

Fig. 13.**21 Plasmacytoma.** Typical CT appearance of a thoracic vertebra, with punched-out trabecular defects that do not have reactive or sclerotic margins.

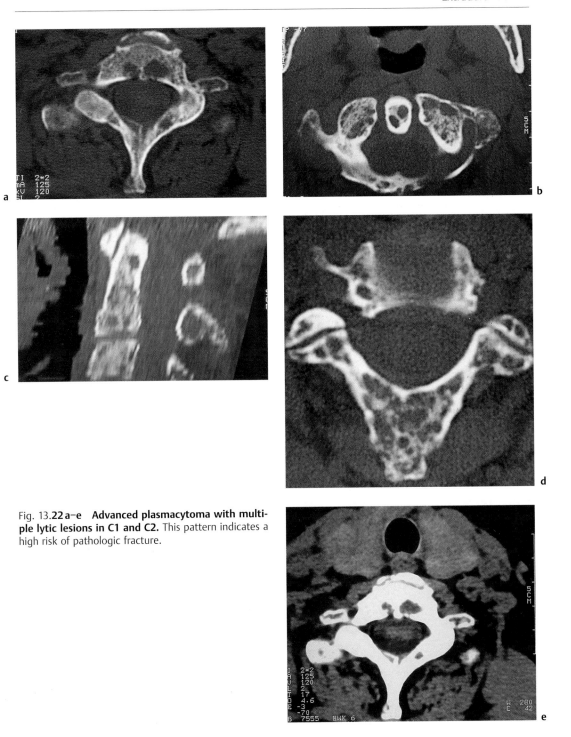

Fig. 13.**22 a–e   Advanced plasmacytoma with multiple lytic lesions in C1 and C2.** This pattern indicates a high risk of pathologic fracture.

Chondrosarcoma (Figs. 13.23–13.27)

> **Frequency:** the third most common bone tumor after plasmacytoma and osteosarcoma. Relatively rare in the spine.
>
> **Suggestive morphologic findings:** an expansile lytic bone lesion with a sharp transition to healthy bone. Irregular calcifications.
>
> **Procedure:** thin CT slices, contrast administration, bone-window views.
>
> **Other studies:** with intraspinal tumor, myelography and postmyelographic CT can help assess the degree of cord compression, so that the skin can be marked at the correct level for surgical decompression.
>
> **Checklist for scan interpretation:**
> ▶ Location and extent?
> ▶ Instability and risk of fracture?
> ▶ Cord compression?

■ Pathogenesis

Chondrosarcoma is a malignant tumor of cartilaginous origin that is composed of atypical cartilage tissue and scant connective tissue. *Primary* chondrosarcoma, which develops directly from local cartilaginous tissue, is distinguished from *secondary* chondrosarcoma, which results from the degeneration of a preexisting mass such as osteochondroma, enchondroma, or other chondrogenic tumor. The World Health Organization (WHO) has defined three grades of malignancy, based on the degree of anaplasia. Most chondrosarcomas grow slowly. They tend to invade blood vessels, forming intravascular extensions and seeding hematogenous metastases. Lymph-node metastases are rare. The tumor has a very high recurrence rate following partial excision and shows poor response to radiation and chemotherapy.

■ Frequency

Chondrosarcoma is the third most common malignant bone tumor after plasmacytoma and osteosarcoma. Spinal occurrence is relatively rare and usually results from secondary invasion of the spinal canal by tumor arising from cartilaginous structures of the costotransverse or costovertebral joints.

The peak age incidence is 45 years. Males are affected about twice as often as females.

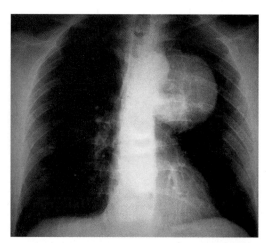

Fig. 13.**23 Chondrosarcoma.** Chest radiograph of a 44-year-old man who was admitted to the emergency department with left-sided chest pain and a 5-week history of slowly progressive weakness in both legs.

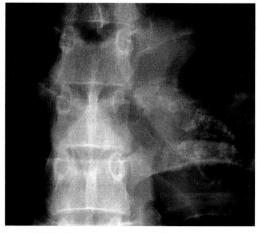

Fig. 13.**24 Chondrosarcoma.** The close-up view clearly shows destruction of the posteromedial sixth rib and flocculent calcifications projecting over the tumor mass.

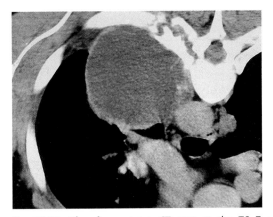

Fig. 13.**25** **Chondrosarcoma.** CT scan at the T6–7 level. The scan was performed with the patient in the prone position so that the tumor boundaries could be marked on the skin in the position that would be used at the subsequent operation. The intraspinal tumor component, identified by peripheral contrast enhancement, is already occupying three-quarters of the spinal canal.

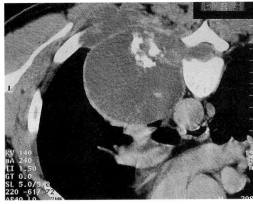

Fig. 13.**26** **Chondrosarcoma.** Tumor components of calcium density are seen. It is unclear whether these areas are intratumoral calcifications or portions of the eroded sixth rib that have been displaced by tumor growth. The tumor presumably arises from the costotransverse joint.

■ Clinical Manifestations

Spinal chondrosarcomas present with local pain and swelling, and intraspinal tumor causes cord compression symptoms that may be slowly or rapidly progressive.

■ CT Morphology

The typical radiographic appearance of chondrosarcoma is that of an expansile osteolytic lesion with a sharp transition to normal bone and containing irregular punctate or flocculent calcifications (Figs. 13.**23**–13.**26**).

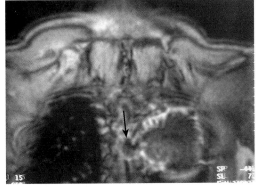

Fig. 13.**27** **Chondrosarcoma.** Coronal magnetic resonance imaging documents the nodular intraspinal extension of the tumor *(arrow)*.

Intradural Extramedullary Masses

Meningioma (Figs. 13.**28**–13.**31**)

Frequency: quite rare.

Suggestive morphologic findings: a sharply delineated mass arising from the meninges. Usually isodense on plain CT scans; shows intense, homogeneous contrast enhancement.

Procedure: contrast-enhanced scans; postmyelographic CT may be added.

Other studies: myelography and postmyelographic CT, MRI, angiography.

Checklist for scan interpretation:
▶ Determine location and precise extent (define tumor level in relation to vertebral bodies for surgical planning; the tumor location may be marked on the skin).
▶ Calcifications?
▶ Other sites of occurrence, especially in patients with known phakomatosis?
▶ Additional studies as needed (MRI, angiography).

■ Pathogenesis

Meningioma is a tumor arising from arachnoid meningothelial cells that have undergone neoplastic transformation. The following grades are distinguished in the WHO classification:

- Grade I: meningioma
- Grade II: atypical meningioma
- Grade III: anaplastic meningioma

Meningiomas are reported to represent 13–26% of primary intracranial and intraspinal tumors, depending on the source. A significant number of meningiomas, mostly intracranial, remain asymptomatic for life and are found incidentally at autopsy (1.44% of autopsies). Meningiomas have an estimated incidence of approximately six per 100 000.

Numerous histologic types have been identified:

- Meningotheliomatous meningioma
- Fibrous meningioma
- Mixed-cell meningioma
- Psammomatous meningioma
- Angiomatous meningioma
- Microcystic meningioma
- Secretory meningioma
- Clear-cell meningioma
- Lymphoplasmacyte-rich meningioma
- Metaplastic meningioma

The following classification, based on tumor growth pattern, is useful for CT evaluation:

- Solitary (globular) meningioma
- Meningioma en plaque
- Multicentric meningioma

The incidence of meningioma is increased with prior radiotherapy. Tumors are diagnosed an average of 19 years after high-dose radiation and 35 years after low-dose radiation. Given the marked female predominance, the frequent presence of estrogen and progesterone receptors detected by immunohistochemical assay may well play a role in tumor pathogenesis.

The treatment of choice for spinal meningioma is neurosurgical tumor removal to relieve pressure on the cord.

■ Frequency

Spinal meningiomas are most commonly located in the thoracic portion of the spinal canal. The peak age incidence is approximately 45 years (35–70). Women are affected about twice as often as men, and this female predominance is even more striking with spinal meningiomas than with intracranial tumors. It is noteworthy, however, that the atypical and anaplastic forms are more common in men than women and that even grade I meningiomas show a higher proliferation rate.

Meningioma has a marked association with neurofibromatosis type 2, in which a significant percentage of lesions are multifocal or occur as a diffuse meningiomatosis. Neither sex predominates in these cases. Approximately 50% of multiple and multicentric meningiomas occur in patients with neurofibromatosis type 2.

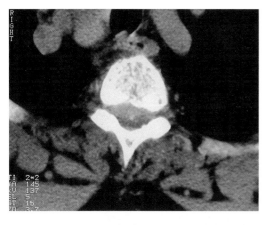

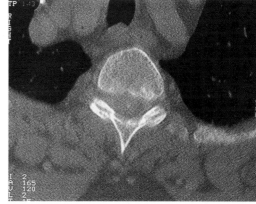

b

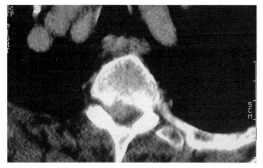

d

Fig. 13.28 a–d Meningioma.
a, b Plain CT scans demonstrate a broad-based, plaque-
like intraspinal mass that is hyperdense to the surrounding intraspinal structures. The small, circumscribed calcification is due to regressive change.
c A delayed scan after contrast administration shows
moderate enhancement.

d Sagittal CT reformatted image.
The patient was relatively asymptomatic, a finding consistent with the size and slow growth rate of the mass.
The lesion was identified histologically as meningotheliomatous meningioma *(arrow)*.

■ Clinical Manifestations

As with most intraspinal tumors, the clinical
presentation is dominated by symptoms of
cord compression and/or nerve root compression ranging to complete cord paralysis.

■ CT Morphology

CT demonstrates a mass with smooth, sharp
margins arising from the meninges. The tumor
is usually isodense on plain scans and shows
intense, homogeneous enhancement after
contrast administration. A frequent and highly
characteristic feature is an enhancing "dural
tail" that extends along the dura past the area

of tumor attachment. There is controversy
whether this feature represents dural infiltration. Plain CT often shows punctate calcifications, known as psammoma bodies (Fig.
13.28 a, b). Reactive hyperostosis of adjacent
bone may also be seen on plain CT and even on
conventional radiographs. This hyperostosis,
shown by histologic studies to result from bone
infiltration, is most common with meningiomas of the convexity or skull base. It is extremely rare with spinal meningiomas, due to
the predominantly intradural tumor growth,
the intervening epidural fat, and the tendency
for compression symptoms to develop earlier
within the confines of the spinal canal than in
the cranial cavity.

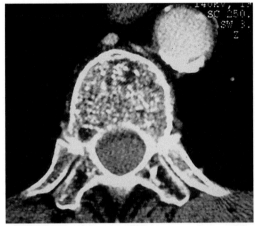

a

Fig. 13.**29 a, b Meningioma.** CT shows an intraspinal mass at the T11 level in an 86-year-old woman with a gradually progressive transverse cord lesion. The mass is located in the intradural–extramedullary compartment, has smooth margins, and shows slight, homogeneous contrast enhancement.

a The mass is faintly hyperdense in the initial phase after contrast administration (note the high density in the ascending aorta).
b Very little further density increase is noted on the delayed scan.

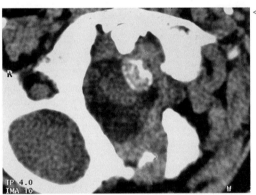

◁ Fig. 13.**30 A calcified intradural meningioma** at the craniocervical junction.

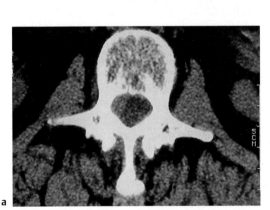
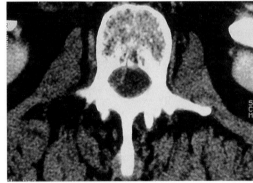

a

Fig. 13.**31 a, b A circumscribed intraspinal mass at the L2–3 level,** with no obvious relationship to the disk space. The lesion shows fine peripheral enhancement after intravenous contrast administration, prompting surgery for removal of a suspected meningioma. A sequestered disk herniation was found at surgery.

Schwannoma (Neurinoma, Neurilemoma), Neurofibroma
(Figs. 13.**32**–13.**45**)

- **Frequency:** approximately 30% of primary intraspinal tumors; there is an increased incidence in neurofibromatosis type 2.
- **Suggestive morphologic findings:** a sharply marginated mass on a spinal nerve, often with an intraspinal and extraforaminal component (hourglass tumor) expanding the neuroforamen. Typically shows intense contrast enhancement.
- **Procedure:** thin-slice spiral CT, if necessary with secondary reconstructions; contrast administration.
- **Other studies:** the tumor can be defined by myelography and postmyelographic CT, and its location can be marked on the skin if necessary. MRI can exclude other sites in patients diagnosed with neurofibromatosis type 2.

Checklist for scan interpretation:
- ▶ Location and extent (define tumor level in relation to vertebral bodies for surgical planning; the tumor location may be marked on the skin).
- ▶ Degree of cord compression?

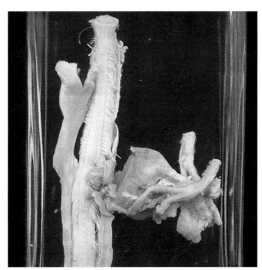

Fig. 13.**32** **Neurofibroma.** Pathologic specimen of a neurofibroma of the sixth cervical nerve (courtesy of the Department of Pathology, Charité Hospital, Berlin).

■ Pathogenesis

Schwannomas are benign tumors (WHO grade I) that arise from the Schwann cells of nerve sheaths and can occur anywhere in the peripheral nervous system. They can reach a remarkable size, and have a characteristic yellow cut surface, especially when they involve cranial nerve VIII.

Consistent with their benign behavior, schwannomas are not infiltrative or destructive. They have expansile margins, and produce a mass effect that can erode bone through pressure. Thus, extension through an intervertebral foramen can cause foraminal expansion with the development of an hourglass-shaped or dumbbell-shaped tumor (Fig. 13.**33**).

A special form is the *giant sacral schwannoma,* which can extensively erode the sacrum and produce a large tumor mass within the pelvis (Fig. 13.**40**).

■ Frequency

Schwannomas are common peripheral nerve tumors. They make up approximately 8% of intracranial tumors and 29% of primary intraspinal tumors. Their incidence is increased in the setting of neurofibromatosis type 2. Spinal schwannomas do not have a known age or predilection for either sex, but intracranial schwannomas are more common in women by a ratio of 2:1.

■ Clinical Manifestations

Clinical symptoms are radicular pain and signs of nerve-root and/or cord compression, ranging to a complete cord lesion.

■ CT Morphology

CT demonstrates a sharply marginated mass arising from a spinal nerve, often presenting as a transforaminal "hourglass tumor" with both an intraspinal and extraforaminal component. Foraminal expansion is often visible on conventional spinal radiographs (Fig. 13.**34**).

Intense contrast enhancement is a classic feature of schwannomas (Figs. 13.**33**–13.**35**).

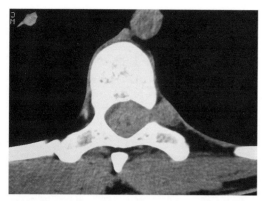

Fig. 13.**33** **Schwannoma** with the appearance of an intraforaminal hourglass-shaped tumor.

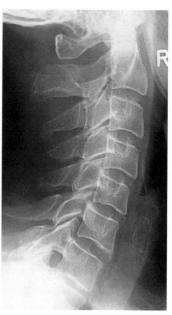

Fig. 13.**34** **Neurofibroma.** A conventional radiograph ▷ in a young patient with cervical spinal symptoms and predominantly right-sided occipital headaches. The film shows marked expansion of the atlantoaxial neuroforamen, raising a strong suspicion of an intraforaminal tumor.

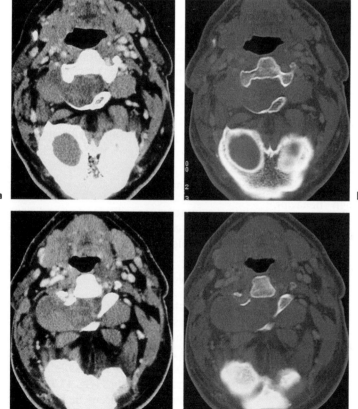

a

c

d

Fig. 13.**35 a–d** **Neurofibroma.** Contrast-enhanced scans with soft-tissue and bone-window settings demonstrate a large, dumbbell-shaped tumor in the right C1–2 intervertebral foramen, with an intraspinal component and an extraspinal component within the paravertebral muscles. The nonhomogeneous enhancement pattern is not typical of schwannoma, and raised the suspicion of a mixed neoplasm. The tumor was identified histologically as a neurofibroma.

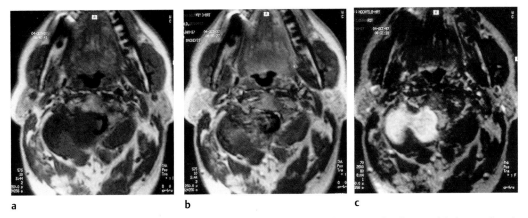

a   b   c

Fig. 13.**36 a–c** **Neurofibroma.** On postcontrast magnetic resonance imaging (**b**), the tumor shows a nonhomogeneous enhancement pattern similar to that seen on CT. Only the T2-weighted image (**c**) shows a largely homogeneous high signal intensity (same patient as in Fig. 13.**35**).

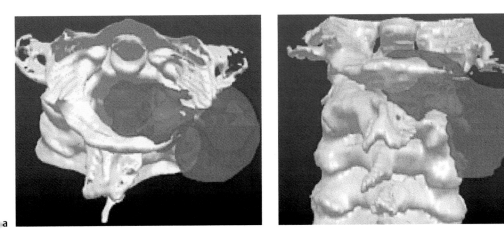

a

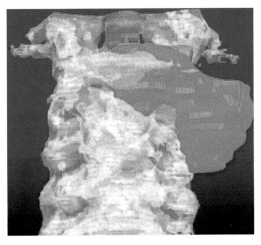

b

c

Fig. 13.**37 a–c** **Neurofibroma.** Color-coded shaded surface reconstructions of the region again demonstrate the relative position of the tumor and the thinning of the atlas arch caused by pressure erosion. The transparent view of the bone clearly demonstrates the dumbbell or hourglass shape of the tumor.

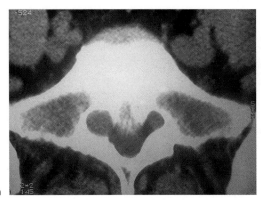 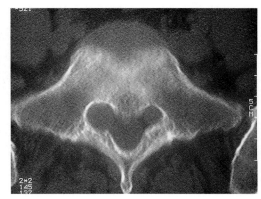

a

Fig. 13.38 a, b Schwannoma. All schwannomas do not have an hourglass shape. These scans show a schwannoma arising from the right S1 nerve root that has expanded the sacral neuroforamen.

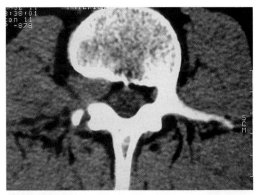 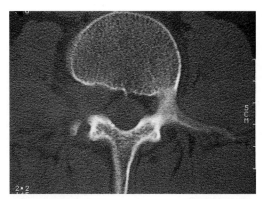

Fig. 13.39 a, b Schwannoma. Depending on the stage at which a schwannoma is detected, the tumor may be difficult to distinguish from a herniated disk clinically and by its CT features, as in this case. Contrast administration was not used, due to a presumptive clinical diag-

nosis of herniated disk. But the bone-window view already shows initial erosion of the posterior margin of the vertebral body and enlargement of the foramen, suggesting the correct diagnosis.

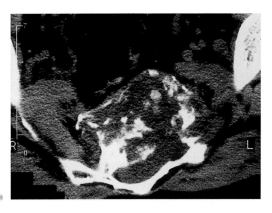

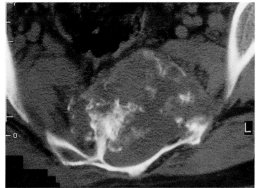

b

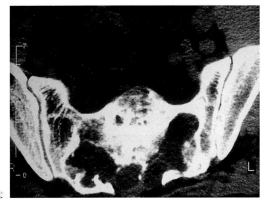

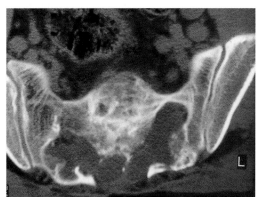

d

Fig. 13.**40 a–e Giant sacral schwannoma.** This patient was examined for nonspecific back pain 30 years after undergoing surgery for a "benign tumor" (his files were no longer available). CT revealed a large mass at the L5–S1 level that had almost completely eroded the sacrum. The patient was referred for CT-guided fine-needle biopsy, with a presumptive diagnosis of chordoma. The lesion was identified histologically as schwannoma. CT (**a–d**) demonstrates an extensive mass, the cranial portion of which still conforms to the anatomy of the sacral neuroforamina, despite their massive bilateral enlargement due to pressure erosion. The caudal portion of the tumor has grown along the spinal nerves, has destroyed much of the sacrum, and has formed a large presacral mass. The sagittal magnetic resonance image (**e**) clearly delineates the tumor.

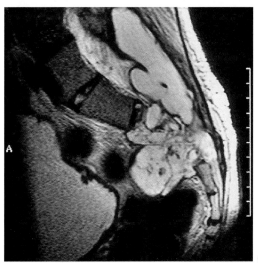

e

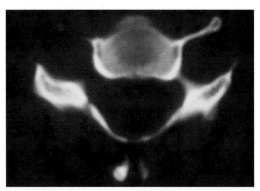
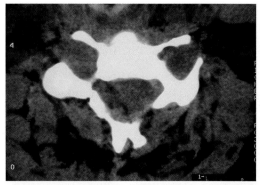

a

Fig. 13.**41 a, b** **Schwannoma.** Bone and soft-tissue window scans at the C3 level in a woman with known neurofibromatosis type 2 clearly show bilateral expansion of the neuroforamina by schwannomas.

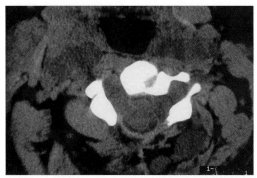

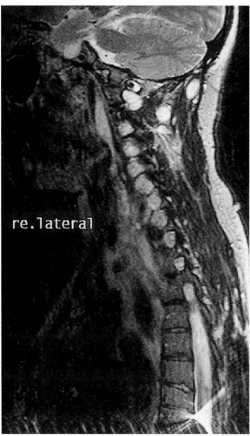

Fig. 13.**42** **Schwannoma/neurofibroma.** CT in a woman with known neurofibromatosis type 2 revealed multiple intraforaminal masses all along the spinal column, shown here at the C3 level. The lesions represent schwannomas or neurofibromas, which have caused marked expansion of the neuroforamina. In addition, the unenhanced scans showed numerous other neurofibromas on both sides of the pharynx and in the posterior neck muscles.

Fig. 13.**43** **Schwannoma/neurofibroma.** This T2- ▷ weighted parasagittal magnetic resonance image in the same patient clearly demonstrates a schwannoma or neurofibroma at the origin of the spinal nerves in each of the neuroforamina along the cervical spine.

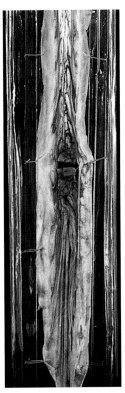

Fig. 13.**44 Intradural neurofibroma of the cauda equina** (specimen courtesy of the Department of Pathology, Charité Hospital, Berlin).

Paraganglioma

> **Frequency:** very rare.
>
> **Suggestive morphologic findings:** a nonspecific intradural mass that usually has well-defined margins. Isodense on plain CT scans; shows homogeneous enhancement after contrast administration. Most commonly located in the filum terminale or cauda equina.
>
> **Procedure:** thin CT slices, contrast administration.
>
> **Other studies:** MRI, myelography.
>
> **Checklist for scan interpretation:**
> ▶ Location and precise extent (define tumor level in relation to vertebral bodies for surgical planning; the tumor location may be marked on the skin).
> ▶ Cord or nerve root compression?

■ **Pathogenesis**

Paragangliomas are rare neuroendocrine tumors that are usually benign and encapsulated. They arise from highly specialized colonies of neural crest cells. They are distributed in association with segmental or collateral autonomic ganglia. Accordingly, the tumor may occur at extradural sites (e.g., retroperitoneal or mediastinal). This entity is also known by other location-specific terms, such as chemodectoma and glomus jugulare tumor.

■ **Frequency**

Paraganglioma is a generally rare tumor, but is significant in its tendency to involve the filum terminale and cauda equina. The peak age incidence is 45 years. Males predominate slightly, by a ratio of 3 : 2.

■ **Clinical Manifestations**

The symptoms are nonspecific, and usually start with radicular back pain. This may be followed by signs of cord compression or conus–cauda compression.

■ **CT Morphology**

There are no specific CT findings. Paraganglioma generally appears as a sharply marginated, intradural mass that is isodense on plain scans and shows homogeneous contrast enhancement.

Medulloblastoma

> **Frequency:** the most common brain tumor in children; has a strong propensity for leptomeningeal spread (drop metastases).
>
> **Suggestive morphologic findings:** leptomeningeal spread leads to multiple, partially confluent nodules that enhance intensely with intravenous contrast.
>
> **Procedure:** postcontrast examination is essential.
>
> **Other studies:** MRI is the study of choice for screening and follow-up.

■ Pathogenesis

Medulloblastoma is an invasive, high-grade embryonal tumor (WHO grade IV) that is most prevalent in childhood. It belongs to the group of primitive neuroectodermal tumors (PNETs), which also include:

- Retinoblastoma
- Pineoblastoma
- Neuroblastoma
- Esthesioneuroblastoma
- Ependymoblastoma
- Polar spongioblastoma

According to a controversial histogenetic concept, all of these tumors are derived from the same subependymal stem cells, and present histopathologically as undifferentiated round cells. Like their precursors, however, they have a capacity for neuronal, glial, or ependymal differentiation.

■ Frequency

Medulloblastoma is the most common brain tumor in the pediatric age group, accounting for 20–25% of cases. Its incidence is 0.5 per 100,000 children. Seventy percent of medulloblastomas are diagnosed in patients under age 16, and 80% of affected adults are 21–40 years of age. The peak age incidence is seven years. Approximately 65% of patients are male.

Seventy-five percent of medulloblastomas arise from the cerebellar vermis. The tumor is mentioned here due to its marked propensity for leptomeningeal spread along cerebrospinal fluid (CSF) pathways. Leptomeningeal spread has already occurred in approximately one-third of patients at the time of diagnosis.

■ Clinical Manifestations

The symptoms are usually caused by the primary tumor (ataxia, gait impairment, morning vomiting, signs of impaired CSF circulation). Leptomeningeal metastases generally do not cause symptoms.

■ CT Morphology

The metastatic deposits from leptomeningeal spread appear as solitary or multiple confluent nodules that enhance intensely after contrast administration, or produce a diffuse leptomeningeal enhancement. Postcontrast examination is essential for making a diagnosis.

Epidermoid, Dermoid, Teratoma
(Figs. 13.**45**–13.**47**)

■ Pathogenesis

These lesions constitute a group of relatively benign congenital tumors that develop from heterotopic tissue derived from one or more germ layers. Approximately two-thirds are extramedullary, and one-third are intramedullary. Combined forms with intramedullary and extramedullary components can occur in the setting of dysraphic anomalies.

The posterior lumbosacral area is a site of predilection, but these tumors may also occur at presacral sites where they can grow as large as 20 cm in diameter.

Epidermoids are unilocular or multilocular tumors, usually cystic, that consist entirely of epidermal cells. *Dermoids* additionally contain dermal appendages such as hair follicles, sebaceous glands, and fat. *Teratomas* by definition contain elements of all germ layers, and may also contain cartilage, bone, or teeth.

All three tumors may occur congenitally in the setting of a dysraphic anomaly, or they may occur in isolation. Approximately 25% of dermoids and epidermoids are associated with a dermal sinus. Dermoids and epidermoids may also be iatrogenic, developing from dermal elements that are implanted during open surgery or a percutaneous procedure (needle without a stylet).

Malignant degeneration is rare in dermoids and epidermoids, but common in teratomas (up to 40%).

■ Frequency

Dermoids and epidermoids are much more common at intracranial sites. The ratio of intracranial to intraspinal occurrence is approximately 6 : 1. Together, dermoids and epidermoids account for 1–2% of spinal tumors in children under 15 years of age. Solitary epidermoids are the most common form, followed by solitary dermoids and multiple lesions of both types.

The tumors are usually diagnosed in the first or second decade, but they may not become symptomatic until adulthood, in some cases as late as 50–60 years of age.

■ Clinical Manifestations

The clinical onset may be insidious and nonspecific, due to slow tumor growth. The symptoms are location-dependent, and relate to the

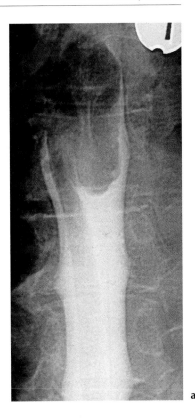

a

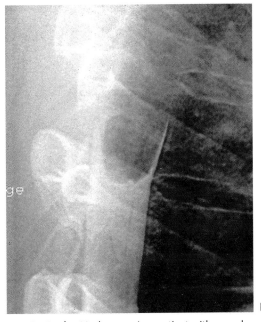

b

Fig. 13.**45 a, b** Myelograms in a patient with a gradually progressive incomplete cord lesion. The anteroposterior and lateral views clearly demonstrate an intradural–extramedullary mass with smooth margins.

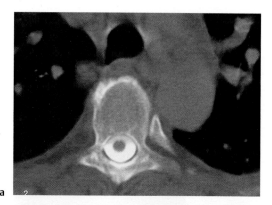

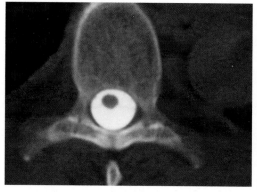

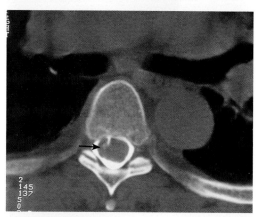

a

Fig. 13.**46 a–c   CT in a patient with a gradually progressive incomplete cord lesion.** The spinal cord is well delineated in postmyelographic CT scans cranial and caudal to the mass. At the level of the mass, the cord is displaced to the right and is markedly flattened *(arrow)*.

c

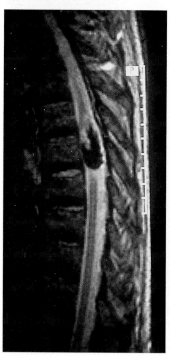

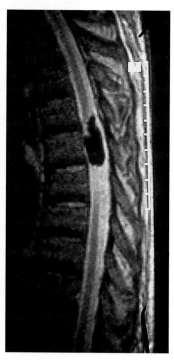

a

b

Fig. 13.**47   Marked hypointensity of the tumor** on T2-weighted magnetic resonance imaging may result from previous intralesional hemorrhage.

degree of cord or cauda equina compression. A complete cord lesion may develop in severe cases.

■ CT Morphology

Epidermoids are usually more homogeneous than dermoids and teratomas. All are isodense to hypodense on CT scans, depending on their fat or sebum content, usually appearing as an extramedullary mass displacing the spinal cord or cauda equina. Many lesions occupy the entire spinal canal at the time of diagnosis.

These cases are difficult to diagnose, because the tumor is often isodense after intravenous contrast administration, and is easily mistaken for the spinal cord. Postmyelographic CT is particularly helpful in these cases (Fig. 13.**46**).

Teratomas often contain calcium, and some may even contain teeth.

Contrast enhancement is unusual, and its occurrence in dermoids and epidermoids suggests infection of the cyst. Contrast enhancement in teratomas is suspicious for malignant transformation.

Intramedullary Masses

Ependymoma

■ **Frequency:** approximately 30% of intramedullary tumors.

Suggestive morphologic findings: sharply marginated, multilobular mass that may contain calcifications (50%) or cystic necrotic areas (50%). Enhances intensely after contrast administration.

Procedure: obtain scans after intravenous contrast administration. Postmyelographic CT may be of value. Use the bone window to detect calcifications.

Other studies: myelography may show blocking of the contrast column; can be used to help mark the tumor location on the skin. Sagittal MRI.

Checklist for scan interpretation:
▶ Determine location and precise extent (define tumor level in relation to vertebral bodies for surgical planning; the tumor location may be marked on the skin).
▶ Calcifications, cysts, contrast enhancement?
▶ Compression of nerve tissue?
▶ Need for MRI or angiography?

■ Pathogenesis

Ependymomas are mostly low-grade gliomas (WHO grade II) that can occur anywhere within the CNS and at any age. A higher-grade variant (WHO grade III) is anaplastic ependymoma. The most common site of occurrence is the posterior cranial fossa. The peak age incidences are 5 years for posterior fossa lesions and 30–40 years for spinal ependymomas. There is a slight female predilection (5:4).

The incidence of ependymomas is increased in patients with phakomatoses (neurofibromatosis type 2, Turcot syndrome). Fragments of simian virus 40 (SV40) DNA have been detected in the tumor genome, suggesting a viral etiology for ependymomas and plexus papillomas.

Tumor seeding along CSF pathways is described in 10–33% of cases.

Ependymomas have a good prognosis following complete surgical resection. Postoperative radiotherapy is advised only after an incomplete resection.

■ Frequency

Ependymomas make up approximately 30% of intramedullary tumors and 3–9% of neuroepithelial tumors. Thirty percent of all ependymomas, including intracranial lesions, affect children age 3 or under. Other small peaks occur in the third and sixth decades.

■ Clinical Manifestations

The intraspinal mass effect from ependymomas can produce a variety of compression symptoms that may include transverse cord symptoms or a conus–cauda compression syndrome. In a series of 101 cases described by Mork and Loken (1977), 82% of the patients were already symptomatic one year before their tumor was diagnosed.

■ CT Morphology

CT shows a sharply marginated mass that is isodense to slightly hyperdense on unenhanced scans, and may contain punctate calcifications (50%) or cystic areas of necrosis (50%). Solid portions of the tumor usually enhance intensely after contrast administration. Ependymomas most commonly involve the conus–cauda region or filum terminale.

Astrocytoma

Frequency: approximately 30% of intramedullary tumors.

Suggestive morphologic findings: a hypodense mass with ill-defined margins. Higher-grade lesions may enhance with intravenous contrast, but low-grade forms may not be detected by CT.

Procedure: thin CT slices, possibly as postmyelographic scans. Obtain secondary reconstructions to define the extent of the intramedullary mass.

Other studies: sagittal MRI is superior to CT, as it provides higher soft-tissue contrast, and is more sensitive in detecting contrast enhancement. Fluid-attenuated inversion recovery (FLAIR) sequences, proton-density images, and T2-weighted images are better for delineating low-grade, nonenhancing astrocytomas from the spinal cord.

Checklist for scan interpretation:
▶ Determine location and precise extent (define tumor level in relation to vertebral bodies for surgical planning; the tumor location may be marked on the skin).
▶ Contrast enhancement for tumor grading.
▶ Need for MRI or angiography?

■ Pathogenesis

Astrocytomas are tumors of glial origin that arise within the CNS. The WHO classification defines four grades of astrocytoma, based on the degree of anaplasia.

Table 13.**2** Stages in the progression of compression symptoms due to astrocytoma

Stage	Clinical symptoms
1	Pain (neuralgic)
2	Brown–Séquard syndrome (contralateral dissociated sensory loss and ipsilateral paralysis due to pyramidal tract and dorsal column lesion)
3	Incomplete cord lesion
4	Complete cord lesion

■ Frequency

Astrocytomas constitute about 30% of intramedullary tumors. Both higher-grade and lower-grade tumors are far more common in the cerebrum and cerebellum, but anaplastic astrocytoma and other forms may arise primarily in the spine. The peak age incidences are 25–45 years for low-grade astrocytomas and 45–55 years for higher-grade lesions. Females predominate by a ratio of about 3 : 2.

■ Clinical Manifestations

Cord compression symptoms depend on the location of the intramedullary mass. Usually there is an insidious progression of symptoms, ranging to complete cord paralysis. Other cases show rapid neurologic deterioration over a period of hours, especially in children. For this reason, the possible presence of spinal astrocytoma constitutes an emergency indication for sectional imaging.

The progression of compression symptoms can be divided into four stages (Table 13.**2**). It is common for patients to relate compression symptoms erroneously to an accident or injury that appears to coincide with the time of symptom onset.

CT Morphology

CT demonstrates a hypodense mass with ill-defined margins. Exophytic lesions lead to compression of the subarachnoid space. Higher-grade tumors may show partial enhancement after intravenous contrast administration.

Pilocytic Astrocytoma

Frequency: very rare.

Suggestive morphologic findings: a characteristic pattern is one or more mural nodules associated with a cystic mass. The nodules and cyst wall enhance after contrast administration.

Procedure: thin CT slices, contrast administration.

Other studies: MRI can demonstrate the entire spinal canal. Angiography may be necessary to differentiate from angioblastoma.

Checklist for scan interpretation:
▶ Determine the location and precise extent (define the tumor level in relation to vertebral bodies for surgical planning; the tumor location may be marked on the skin).
▶ Need for MRI or angiography?

Pathogenesis

Pilocytic astrocytoma is a low-grade glioma (WHO grade I). It is the most common glioma in children and affects both sexes equally. Most tumors are sharply marginated, with solid and spongy components, often taking the form of one or more nodules associated with a cyst.

The intense contrast enhancement is unusual for low-grade gliomas and results from the rich vascular supply, which is based mainly on microvascular proliferation in the cyst wall. The vessels in older lesions may undergo telangiectatic changes, or glomerular vascular structures may form, like those in glioblastoma multiforme.

Regressive changes in older lesions may also lead to calcifications or microcalcifications and hemosiderin deposits. Usually these changes are not visible on CT, however, and in any case they do not advance the differential diagnosis. Histopathologically, pilocytic astro-cytomas tend to expand toward the subarachnoid space. This explains the rare but definite seeding of CSF pathways. This spread does not indicate malignancy, however, as both the primary tumor and its deposits continue to grow very slowly or may even show spontaneous regression.

As a group, pilocytic astrocytomas have a remarkable tendency to maintain a low-grade status for years or even decades, and any morphologic changes are due mainly to regression. There are rare exceptions, however. Anaplastic forms and transformation to less differentiated forms, including glioblastoma, have been described. This potential has no practical relevance, however.

The incidence of pilocytic astrocytomas is increased in patients with neurofibromatosis type 2.

Frequency

Pilocytic astrocytoma makes up approximately 3 % of gliomas. Occurrence in the spinal canal is rare, but has been described by numerous authors. The tumor is usually diagnosed before 20 years of age and shows no predilection for either sex.

Clinical Manifestations

The clinical symptoms are nonspecific. Patients may develop signs of cord compression ranging to a complete cord lesion or conus–cauda compression symptoms.

CT Morphology

The most common and characteristic appearance of pilocytic astrocytoma is that of one or more mural nodules in direct association with a tumor cyst. The tumor is usually hypodense to isodense on plain CT scans. The nodules and cyst wall enhance intensely after contrast administration. In most cases, the cyst contents are approximately isodense to CSF.

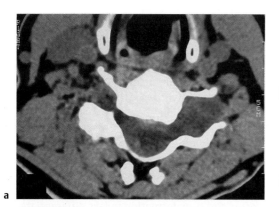

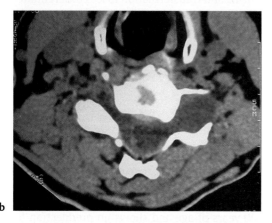

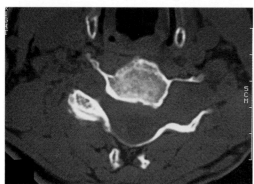

Fig. 13.**48**a–c **A large angioblastoma at the C5–6 level with an intramedullary and radicular intraforaminal/extraforaminal component.** Based on its CT appearance alone (especially without contrast medium), this hourglass-shaped tumor causing neuroforaminal expansion is indistinguishable from a schwannoma or neurofibroma.

Hemangioblastoma (Angioblastoma, Hippel–Lindau Tumor)
(Figs. 13.**48**–13.**50**)

Frequency: rare (approximately 1.5–2.5% of intramedullary tumors).

Suggestive morphologic findings: a very vascular mass, usually intramedullary and rarely affecting the nerve roots. Often has cystic components with a mural enhancing nidus.

Procedure: thin CT slices, contrast administration.

Other studies: angiography is the method of choice for detecting multifocal hemangiomatosis. MRI.
▶ Checklist for scan interpretation:
▶ Location (may be marked on the skin).
▶ Recommend further tests, especially angiography to detect additional hemangioblastomas.

■ Pathogenesis

Hemangioblastoma is a benign, slow-growing tumor that most commonly occurs in the posterior cranial fossa. The second most common location is the spinal canal, especially the cervical cord. To date, fewer than 100 cases of supratentorial occurrence have been described in the literature.

Approximately 20% of hemangioblastomas, whether solitary or multiple, occur in the setting of Hippel–Lindau syndrome, which has an autosomal-dominant inheritance. One or more of the following lesions may also be present in Hippel–Lindau syndrome:

- Retinal hemangioma
- Pheochromocytoma
- Syringomyelia
- Renal cysts
- Renal-cell carcinoma
- Pancreatic cysts

Malignant transformation does not occur, although the tumor may seed along CSF pathways following surgery. Like the primary tumor, the deposits are benign and grow by expansion rather than by infiltration.

Fig. 13.**49 a–d   A large angio-blastoma at the C5–6 level with an intramedullary and radicular intraforaminal/extraforaminal component.** Magnetic resonance imaging identifies the tumor as a scalloped, partly intramedullary mass that shows high T2-weighted signal intensity and intense contrast enhancement. There is a prominent vascular component with expansion of associated vessels.

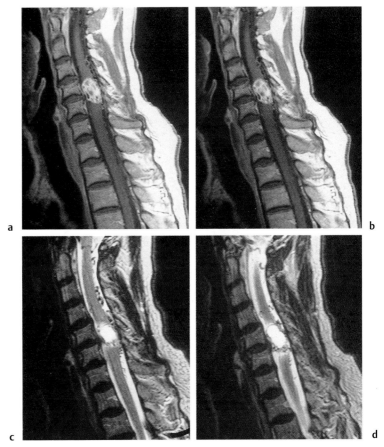

a

b

c

d

■ Frequency

While hemangioblastoma is the most common primary intra-axial tumor of the posterior cranial fossa in adults, spinal hemangioblastomas are rare neoplasms. Only about 3% of hemangioblastomas are intraspinal.

Hemangioblastomas make up approximately 1.5–2.5% of intramedullary tumors.

About one-fifth of cases are based on a familial incidence of hemangioblastoma in Hippel–Lindau syndrome. The average patient age is 33 years. Solitary hemangioblastomas affect males slightly more often than females, but a female predilection exists in the setting of Hippel–Lindau syndrome (one in 36,000 live births).

■ Clinical Manifestations

The main clinical features of spinal hemangioblastoma usually result from cord or nerve root compression. Erythropoietin secretion by the tumor can lead to polycythemia, which is found in up to 20% of hemangioblastoma patients. Intramedullary hemorrhage can develop as a complication.

■ CT Morphology

Approximately 75% of spinal hemangioblastomas are intramedullary, and 20% involve the nerve roots. A few lesions are intradural–extramedullary. The morphology and CT appearance of hemangioblastomas depend on the pattern of tumor growth.

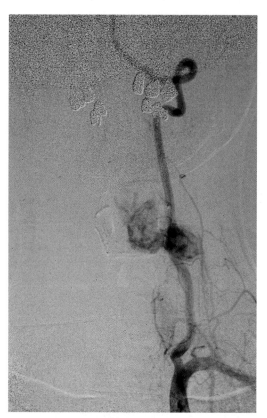

Fig. 13.**50 A large angioblastoma at the C5–6 level with an intramedullary and radicular intraforaminal/extraforaminal component.** The diagnosis of a vascular tumor suggested by magnetic resonance imaging is supported by digital subtraction angiography. The diagnosis of angioblastoma was confirmed at surgery.

Four basic growth patterns have been identified:

- Mural nodule or vascular nidus in association with an avascular cyst. This is the most common pattern, seen in about 50% of cases, and is the classic form encountered in the posterior cranial fossa.
- Hypervascular tumor wall with a central avascular cyst.
- Solid, hypervascular tumor nodule without a cyst.
- Multiple hypervascular tumor nodules.

The cyst contents may appear isodense or slightly hyperdense to the CSF, depending on the protein content. As a rule, marked en-

hancement is seen after intravenous contrast administration, owing to the rich vascularity of the tumor and cyst wall. It is common to find ectatic draining veins, which may form a kind of venous sinus on the dorsal side of the cord.

A morphologic variant is an elongated, hourglass-shaped tumor extending through an intervertebral foramen, similar to the typical appearance of schwannoma.

Hemangiopericytoma
(Figs. 13.**51**–13.**53**)

■ **Frequency:** rare.

Suggestive morphologic findings: a mass abutting the meninges. Contains no calcifications; shows nonhomogeneous contrast enhancement. Foci of bone destruction.

Procedure: thin-slice spiral CT with secondary reconstructions.

Other studies: MRI and angiography.

Checklist for scan interpretation:
- ▶ Location (may be marked on the skin).
- ▶ Recommend further tests, especially angiography and MRI.

■ Pathogenesis

Hemangiopericytomas are rare vascular tumors that arise from Zimmermann pericytes. They can occur at any age but are most common in the fourth and fifth decades. They may occur anywhere in the body but show a predilection for the trunk, retroperitoneum, and lower extremities. CNS lesions are often indistinguishable from meningeal tumors by CT, although they may be distinguished by the absence of calcifications and hyperostosis. Indeed, the adjacent bone often contains osteolytic areas caused by the tumor's aggressive growth. Hemangiopericytomas cannot be definitely classified as benign or malignant even by histologic examination, and therefore these tumors should always be considered potentially malignant.

Local recurrence almost always follows an incomplete resection (Fig. 13.**53**).

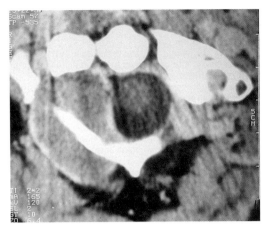

Fig. 13.**51 Hemangiopericytoma at the craniocervical junction.** The axial CT shows an extensive mass that is in broad contact with the meninges.

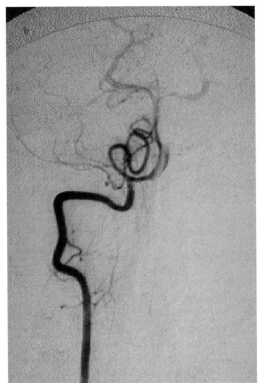

Fig. 13.**52 Hemangiopericytoma at the craniocervical junction.** The angiographic appearance of the lesion in Fig. 13.**51**.

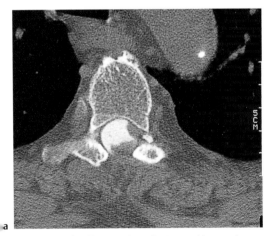

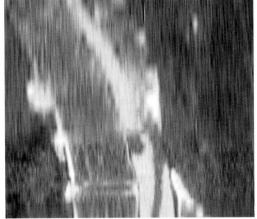

a   b

Fig. 13.**53 a, b Hemangiopericytoma.** Hemangiopericytomas usually recur, as in this patient who had a previous laminectomy at the T8 level. Postmyelographic CT. The sagittal reformatted image shows a mass impinging posteriorly on the spinal cord above, and more anteriorly below.

■ Frequency

Hemangiopericytoma is a very rare tumor that is far more common intracranially than in the spine.

■ Clinical Manifestations

The dominant clinical features are based on the mass effect of the tumor, which may cause compression of neural pathways or obstructive hydrocephalus due to impairment of CSF circulation.

■ CT Morphology

CT usually shows a mass abutting the meninges. The absence of calcifications can be helpful in distinguishing hemangiopericytoma from meningioma. The adjacent bones often show lytic changes with no reactive hyperostosis. Contrast administration generally produces an intense, sometimes nonhomogeneous pattern of enhancement (Fig. 13.**52**).

■ References

Recommended for further study

Metastases
Nakamura M, Toyama Y, Suzuki N, et al. Metastasis to the upper cervical spine. J Spinal Disord 1996; 9: 195–201.
• *Retrospective clinical study on surgical treatment methods for metastatic lesions of the cervical spine.*

Lymphoma
Stroszczynski C, Hosten N, Amthauer H, et al. [Dynamic computed tomography of the bone marrow of normal and pathologic vertebrae; in German]. RöFo Fortschr Geb Röntgenstr Neuen Bildgeb Verfahr 1997; 167: 240–6.

Chordoma
Manzone P, Fiore N, Forlino D, Alcala M, Cabrera CF. Chordoma of the lumbar L2 vertebra: case report and review of the literature. Eur Spine J 1998; 7: 252–6.
• *Describes a location that is extremely rare for chordomas.*
Wippold FJ, Koeller KK, Smirniotopoulos JG. Clinical and imaging features of cervical chordoma. AJR Am J Roentgenol 1999; 172: 1423–6.
• *Demonstrates the CT and MRI findings in 10 patients with cervical chordoma, includes aspects of differential diagnosis.*

Eosinophilic granuloma and giant-cell tumor/osteoclastoma
Helms CA. Fundamentals of skeletal radiology. Philadelphia: Saunders, 1995.

Osteoid osteoma, osteoblastoma
Assoun J, Richardi G, Railhac JJ, et al. Osteoid osteoma: MR imaging versus CT. Radiology 1994; 191: 217–23.
• *Comparative study, according to which CT is the modality of choice for this entity.*
Janin Y, Epstein JA, Carras R, et al. Osteoid osteomas and osteoblastomas of the spine. Neurosurgery 1981; 8: 31–8.
Sans N, Galy-Fourcade D, Assoun J, et al. Osteoid osteoma: CT-guided percutaneous resection and follow-up in 38 patients. Radiology 1999; 212: 687–92.
• *Describes a minimally invasive technique for removing (small) osteoid osteomas under CT guidance, but*

based on only two cases involving the spinal column and sacrum.

Aneurysmal bone cyst
Kransdorf MJ, Sweet DE. Aneurysmal bone cyst: concept, controversy, clinical presentation, and imaging. AJR Am J Roentgenol 1995; 164: 573–80.
• *Review that emphasizes the importance of identifying the primary underlying pathology of the bone cyst.*

Osteosarcoma
Baghaie M, Gillet P, Dondelinger RF, Flandroy P. Vertebra plana: benign or malignant lesion? Pediatr Radiol 1996; 26: 431–3.
• *Single case report of a vertebral osteosarcoma initially thought to be an eosinophilic granuloma/ giant-cell tumor.*
Korovessis P, Repanti M, Stamatakis M. Primary osteosarcoma of the L2 lamina presenting as "silent" paraplegia: case report and review of the literature. Eur Spine J 1995; 4: 375–8.
• *Single case report of rare laminar involvement by a tumor that is already rare in the spinal column.*

Fibrous dysplasia
Nishiura I, Koyama T, Takayama S. Fibrous dysplasia of the cervical spine with atlantoaxial dislocation. Neurochirurgia 1992; 35: 123–6.

Meningioma
Adams RD, Victor M. Intraspinal tumors. In: Adams RD, Victor M. Principles of neurology, 2nd ed. New York: McGraw-Hill, 1981: 638–41.

Schwannoma
Dominguez J, Lobato RD, Ramos A, et al. Giant intrasacral schwannomas: report of six cases. Acta Neurochir 1997; 39: 954–9.
• *Interesting collection of six cases of this entity, based largely on MR images.*

Paraganglioma
Abe H, Maeda M, Koshimoto Y, et al. Paraganglioma of the cauda equina: MR findings. Radiat Med 1999; 17: 235–7.
• *Case report demonstrating the MRI features of this tumor.*
Sonneland PR, Scheithauer BW, LeChago J, et al. Paraganglioma of the cauda equina region: clinicopathologic study of 31 cases with special reference to immunocytology and ultrastructure. Cancer 1986; 58: 1720–35.

Medulloblastoma
Kleihues P, Cavanee WK. Pathology and genetics of tumors of the nervous system. Lyons: International Agency for Research on Cancer, 1997.

Epidermoid, dermoid, teratoma
Lee VS, Provenzale JM, Fuchs HE, Osumi A, McLendon RE. Post-traumatic epidermoid cyst: CT appearance. J Comput Assist Tomogr 1995; 19: 153–5.
• *Case report on the traumatic etiology of an epidermoid (intracranial).*

Ependymoma
Dorwart RH, LaMasters DL, Watanabe TJ. Tumors. In: Newton TH, Potts DG, editors. Computed tomography of the spine and spinal cord. San Anselmo, CA: Clavadal Press, 1983: 115–31.
Mork SJ, Loken AC. Ependymoma: a follow-up study of 101 cases. Cancer 1977; 40: 907–15.

Pilocytic astrocytoma

Rauhut F, Reinhardt V, Budach V, et al. Intramedullary pilocytic astrocytomas: a clinical and morphological study after combined surgical and photon or neutron therapy. Neurosurg Rev 1989; 12: 309–13.

Hemangioblastoma

Ho VB, Smirniotopoulos JG, Murphy FM. Radiologic–pathologic correlation: hemangioblastoma. AJNR Am J Neuroradiol 1992; 13: 1343–52.

Hemangiopericytoma

Alpern MP, Thorsen MK, Keliman GM, Pojunas K, Lawson TL. CT appearance of hemangiopericytoma. J Comput Assist Tomogr 1986; 10: 264–7.
- *Morphologic study of this entity occurring at a site other than the posterior fossa.*

Recent and basic works

Metastases

Batson OV. The function of the vertebral veins and their role in the spread of metastasis. 1940. Clin Orthop 1995; 312: 4–9.
- *Classic study dating from 1940, reprinted in Clinical Orthopaedics.*

Chordoma

Anegawa T, Rai M, Hara K, et al. An unusual cervical chordoma: CT and MRI. Neuroradiology 1996; 38: 466–7.
Probst EN, Zanella FE, Vortmeyer AO. Congenital clivus chordoma. AJNR Am J Neuroradiol 1993; 14: 537–9.
- *Single case report includes CT, MRI, ultrasound, and histologic confirmation of the diagnosis.*

Eosinophilic granuloma

Mitnick JS, Pinto RS. CT in the diagnosis of eosinophilic granuloma. J Comput Assist Tomogr 1980; 4: 791–3.

Osteoid osteoma, osteoblastoma

Amacher AL, Eltomey A. Spinal osteoblastoma in children and adolescents. Child's Nerv Syst 1985; 1: 29–32.
Kroon HM, Schurmans J. Osteoblastoma: clinical and radiologic findings in 98 new cases. Radiology 1990; 175: 783–90.
- *Large study (including 98 patients) on the various imaging features of osteoblastoma at various sites on CT and MRI.*
Ozkal E, Erongun U, Cakir B, Acar O, Uygun A, Bitik M. CT and MR imaging of vertebral osteoblastoma: a report of two cases. Clin Imaging 1996; 20: 37–41.
- *Case reports based on CT and MR images.*

Aneurysmal bone cyst

Capanna R, Van Horn JR, Biagini R, Ruggieri P. Aneurysmal bone cyst of the sacrum. Skeletal Radiol 1989; 18: 109–13.
- *Small series of five cases at this location.*

Vertebral hemangioma

Fox MW, Onofrio BM. The natural history and management of symptomatic and asymptomatic vertebral hemangiomas. J Neurosurg 1993; 78: 36–45.
- *Clinical study (59 cases) on the spectrum of symptoms that may accompany vertebral hemangiomas.*
Healy M, Herz DA, Pearl L. Spinal hemangiomas. Neurosurgery 1983; 13: 689–91.
Richardson RR, Cerullo LJ. Spinal epidural cavernous hemangioma. Surg Neurol 1979; 12: 266–8.
Yamada K, Whitbeck MG Jr, Numaguchi Y, Shrier DA, Tanaka H. Symptomatic vertebral hemangioma: atypi-cal spoke-wheel trabeculation pattern. Radiat Med 1997; 15: 239–41.

Plasmacytoma

Laroche M, Assoun J, Sixou L, Attal M. Comparison of MRI and computed tomography in the various stages of plasma cell disorders: correlations with biological and histological findings. Clin Exp Rheumatol 1996; 14: 171–6.
- *Controlled study on the detection and staging of plasmacytoma with CT and MRI.*

Meningioma

Christopherson LA, Finelli DA, Wyatt-Ashmead J, Likavec MJ. Ectopic extraspinal meningioma: CT and MR appearance. AJNR Am J Neuroradiol 1997; 18: 1335–7.

Schwannoma

Ashkenazi E, Pomeranz S, Floman Y. Foraminal herniation of a lumbar disk mimicking neurinoma on CT and MR imaging. J Spinal Disord 1997; 10: 448–50.
- *Case report of an intraforaminal enhancing mass causing foraminal expansion (herniated disk).*

Paraganglioma

Wester DJ, Falcone S, Green BA, et al. Paraganglioma of the filum: MR appearance. J Comput Assist Tomogr 1993; 17: 967–9.

Medulloblastoma

Heinz R, Wiener D, Friedman H, Tien R. Detection of cerebrospinal fluid metastasis: CT myelography or MRI? AJNR Am J Neuroradiol 1995; 16: 1147–51.
- *Study on the superiority of MRI in detecting CSF metastases.*

Epidermoid, dermoid, teratoma

Roeder MB, Bazan C, Jinkins JR. Ruptured spinal dermoid cyst with chemical arachnoiditis and disseminated intracranial lipid droplets. Neuroradiology 1995; 37: 146–7.

Pilocytic astrocytoma

Minehan KJ, Shaw EG, Scheithauer BW, et al. Spinal cord astrocytoma: pathological and treatment considerations. J Neurosurg 1995; 83: 590–5.

Hemangioblastoma

Rohde V, Voigt K, Grote EH. Intra–extradural hemangioblastoma of the cauda equina. Zentralbl Neurochir 1995; 56: 78–82.

Hemangiopericytoma

Chiechi MV, Smirniotopoulos JG, Mena H. Intracranial hemangiopericytomas: MR and CT features. AJNR Am J Neuroradiol 1996; 17: 1365–71.
- *Systematic study of 34 cases.*

14 Inflammatory Diseases

Infections

Diskitis

Frequency: rare without involvement of the adjacent vertebral bodies; 0.2–4% following nucleotomy (depending on the series).

Suggestive morphologic findings: decreased density of the affected disk with a paravertebral soft-tissue reaction. Contrast enhancement is possible, but not obligatory.

Procedure: computed tomography (CT) scans parallel to the disk spaces, contrast administration.

Other studies: magnetic resonance imaging (MRI) is the method of choice for detecting edema and contrast enhancement, especially in children.

Checklist for scan interpretation:
▶ Determine the precise level of the affected disk.
▶ Extent of the surrounding reaction?
▶ Inflammatory soft-tissue tumor creating an intraspinal mass?

■ Pathogenesis

Diskitis is based on a rare primary infection of the nucleus pulposus with possible secondary involvement of the adjacent endplates and vertebral bodies. It may result from an invasive procedure such as herniated disk surgery, lumbar puncture, myelography, or chemonucleolysis, but spontaneous occurrence is more common.

Spontaneous bacterial diskitis is primarily a pediatric condition. The disk space becomes infected by the hematogenous route through vessels, still present in children, that penetrate the endplates to supply the nucleus pulposus. These vessels become obliterated with aging and usually disappear by age 20.

■ Frequency

Isolated spontaneous diskitis that does not involve the adjacent vertebral bodies and soft tissues is rare. It typically occurs in childhood, with peaks at 6 months to 4 years and at 10–14 years. The L3–4 and L4–5 levels are most commonly affected, and disk space infection above T8 is rare. Postoperative diskitis occurs in approximately 0.2–4% of patients who have undergone a nucleotomy, depending on the series.

■ Clinical Manifestations

Patients with spontaneous diskitis complain mostly of local pain that is aggravated by movement and often has a radicular distribution. In children too young to verbalize their symptoms, a refusal to walk and, later, to sit upright usually brings the child to the attention of a physician. Only about 30% of affected patients are febrile. Postinterventional diskitis usually presents clinically after a symptom-free interval of 1–4 weeks (3 days to 8 months). Typical features at that time are fever, localized pain in the affected segment, radicular pain, and laboratory signs of inflammation.

■ CT Morphology

CT sometimes shows decreased density at the affected level. Usually, there is an accompanying reaction of adjacent paravertebral soft tissues or even of intraspinal tissues, which may cause indentation of the dural sac. Contrast enhancement may occur but is not obligatory.

The following CT findings are pathognomonic for diskitis:

- Fragmentation of the endplates
- Paravertebral soft-tissue swelling that obliterates the intervening fat planes
- Paravertebral abscess

If only the first two criteria are present, the specificity is still 87%.

Spondylodiskitis

Frequency: a tuberculous etiology is rare but has been showing an upward trend. Postinterventional spondylodiskitis can occur in patients with a corresponding history and clinical presentation.

Suggestive morphologic findings: contiguous involvement of a disk space and the adjacent vertebral bodies with bone destruction, a paravertebral soft-tissue mass, disk space narrowing, and intense contrast enhancement.

Procedure: contiguous thin CT slices with secondary reconstructions after intravenous contrast administration.

Other studies: MRI is particularly useful for follow-up. Plain films, myelography, and postmyelographic CT can define the extent of dural sac compression by an intraspinal soft-tissue mass.

Checklist for scan interpretation:
- ▶ Determine the precise location of the affected level.
- ▶ Extent of the surrounding reaction?
- ▶ Inflammatory soft-tissue mass causing an intraspinal mass effect?

■ Pathogenesis

Spondylodiskitis refers to a combined infection of the disk space and one or both adjacent vertebrae. It is the most common form of inflammatory spinal disease encountered in adults. Two main types are distinguished based on etiology and causative agent:

- Spontaneous or postinterventional spondylodiskitis.
- Tuberculous (specific) and nontuberculous spondylodiskitis.

Spontaneous form. The spontaneous form of spondylodiskitis, like epidural abscess, most commonly results from the hematogenous spread of infection, often from pelvic organs. Infectious organisms can spread from that region to the spine through venous channels such as the ascending lumbar veins, which anastomose with draining veins from the vertebral bodies and from the epidural venous plexus. Infection is usually initiated in the anterior portions of the vertebral bodies near the endplates; from there it can spread to the intervertebral disk space and adjacent vertebral bodies by contiguous extension or by further hematogenous spread. The most common causative organism is *Staphylococcus aureus.*

Tuberculous spondylodiskitis (Figs. 14.1, 14.2). Ten percent of tuberculosis patients suffer bone and joint involvement. Fifty percent of these patients develop tuberculous spondylodiskitis, and half of these have a history of active pulmonary tuberculosis with hematogenous spread of infection to a disk space and the adjacent vertebral bodies. The resulting destruction most commonly involves the anterior two-thirds of the vertebral body and spares the posterior elements. There is a progressive loss of disk height over time, although the disk space usually remains intact for a longer period than in acute infections with *Staphylococcus aureus.* A conspicuous paraspinal soft-tissue mass frequently develops and is often associated with an abscess, usually sterile, that may show anterior or occasional posterior subligamentous extension over several segments.

■ Frequency

Tuberculous spondylodiskitis is a rare condition that has become more common in recent years, due to the rising worldwide incidence of tuberculous diseases and the growing prevalence of multiresistant mycobacterial strains. Moreover, recent publications show that the risk of contracting tuberculosis is approximately 80 times higher in patients with human

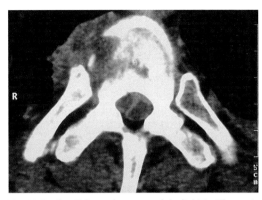

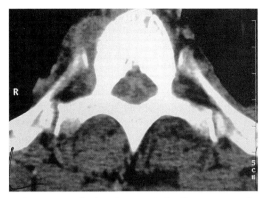

Fig. 14.**1 a, b** **Tuberculous spondylodiskitis.** The typical CT appearance of tuberculous spondylodiskitis, characterized by extensive vertebral body destruction and a paravertebral and intraspinal inflammatory soft-tissue mass with cord compression.

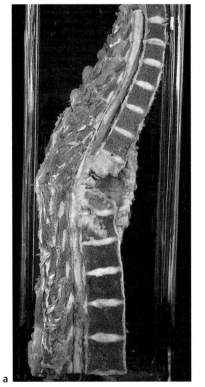

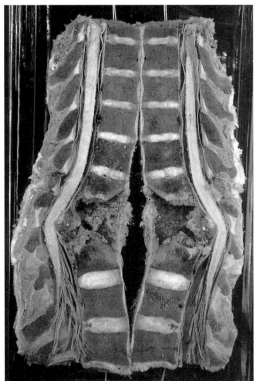

Fig. 14.**2 a, b** **Tuberculous spondylodiskitis.** Pathologic specimens (courtesy of the Department of Pathology, Charité Hospital, Berlin).

immunodeficiency virus (HIV) infection and 170 times higher in patients with acquired immune deficiency syndrome (AIDS) than in the uninfected population. This is another factor that may lead to increased case numbers of tuberculous spondylodiskitis.

The peak age incidence of the disease has been rising in recent decades from 20–30 years to 30–40 years in industrialized countries. The average latent period between bacterial colonization and overt clinical infection is 4.3 months in the cervical spine, 9.8 months in the upper thoracic spine, 17.3 months in the lower thoracic spine, and 20.7 months in the lumbar spine.

■ Clinical Manifestations

Most patients have local spontaneous pain, pain on percussion of the affected area, or pain on axial compression of the spine. The pain may be aggravated by movement, and may show a radicular distribution. Only about 30% of patients are febrile.

■ CT Morphology

CT shows contiguous involvement of a disk space and both adjacent vertebral bodies with bone destruction, a paravertebral soft-tissue mass, and a loss of disk height, which is less pronounced in tuberculous spondylodiskitis than in cases caused by *Staphylococcus aureus*. The affected level always shows intense enhancement after intravenous contrast administration.

Because of hematogenous spread from infected pulmonary foci, tuberculous spondylodiskitis more commonly affects the upper spinal segments, especially the thoracic spine, than the nontuberculous bacterial forms.

The inflammatory tissue usually enhances intensely after contrast administration, sparing areas of necrotic liquefaction.

Postinterventional spondylodiskitis usually presents clinically after an asymptomatic interval of 1–4 weeks (3 days to 8 months). Typi-

Table 14.**1** A tuberculous etiology is likely when the following criteria are satisfied.

- ESR < 50 mm/h
- History > 12 months
- Insidious course (usually afebrile or subfebrile)
- More than three vertebral bodies affected

Table 14.**2** A nontuberculous etiology is likely when the following criteria are satisfied

- ESR > 100 mm/h
- History < 3 months
- Rapid course with fever > 39 °C
- Patient less than 14 years of age
- Negative tuberculin skin test

cal features at that time are fever, localized pain in the affected segment, radicular pain, and laboratory signs of inflammation.

■ Differential Diagnosis

The differential diagnosis of tuberculous and nontuberculous spondylodiskitis is outlined in Tables 14.**1** and 14.**2**.

Spondylitis, Vertebral Osteomyelitis

Frequency: rarely seen in isolation; usually occurs in the setting of spondylodiskitis, or in association with an epidural abscess.

Suggestive morphologic findings: hypodensity of the affected portions of the vertebral body and/or adjacent disk space. Possible paravertebral soft-tissue mass with dural sac compression. Nonnecrotic areas enhance after contrast administration.

Procedure: thin contiguous CT slices, secondary reconstructions, contrast administration.

Other studies: MRI (high sensitivity and specificity, good spatial resolution) is particularly recommended for follow-up.

Checklist for scan interpretation:
▶ Intraspinal soft-tissue mass?
▶ Extent of vertebral body destruction? Potential instability?

■ Pathogenesis

Circumscribed osteomyelitis of a vertebral body is relatively rare, and occurs predominantly in the following high-risk groups:

- Intravenous drug abusers
- Patients with diabetes mellitus
- Patients on hemodialysis
- Elderly patients with no other apparent risk factors

Vertebral osteomyelitis may be complicated by a compression fracture, with retropulsion of necrotic bone fragments into the spinal canal. The source of infection is similar to that in spondylodiskitis—i.e., a urinary or respiratory tract infection, or an infected surgical site. *Staphylococcus aureus* is the causative organism most frequently identified. An important variant is tuberculous spondylitis (Pott's disease), which usually affects more than one level, usually in the lower thoracic and upper lumbar spine. Typically, the vertebral arches are spared. Over time, there is progressive compression of the vertebral body, leading to vertebra plana with kyphotic angulation of the spinal column in the affected segment.

■ Frequency

Circumscribed vertebral osteomyelitis makes up about 2–4% of osteomyelitis cases. It is rarely seen in isolation, and usually occurs in the setting of an extensive inflammation involving multiple compartments (e.g., spondylodiskitis) or in association with an epidural abscess.

■ Clinical Manifestations

The following clinical symptoms are characteristic:

- Fever
- Back pain
- Weight loss
- Radicular pain
- Signs of myelopathy

Circumscribed spondylitis is often associated with only a few systemic signs of inflammation. Leukocytosis, an elevated sedimentation rate, and neurologic symptoms may be absent, especially initially—often causing a delay in diagnosis.

■ CT Morphology

CT shows decreased density of the affected portions of the vertebral body and/or adjacent disk space. There may be an associated paravertebral soft-tissue mass, which may have an intraspinal component that compresses the dural sac. Intense enhancement of the inflammatory tissue usually occurs after contrast administration, sparing foci of necrotic liquefaction.

Epidural Abscess (Figs. 14.3–14.5)

Frequency: relatively common; rising incidence.

Suggestive morphologic findings: elongated, encapsulated epidural mass with a cystic center. The capsule is often hyperdense on plain scans, and is clearly demarcated after contrast administration. Usually located on the dorsal side of the spinal canal.

Procedure: contiguous CT slices with secondary reconstructions after contrast administration.

Other studies: sagittal MRI can define the full extent of the abscess.

Checklist for scan interpretation:
▶ Craniocaudal extent of the lesion?
▶ Degree of dural sac compression?
▶ Signs of accompanying spondylitis or diskitis?

■ Pathogenesis

Spinal epidural abscess rarely occurs in isolation, and it is usually associated with diskitis or spondylitis. This particularly applies to abscesses located anterior to the dural sac or encircling the sac. By contrast, an abscess located posterior to the dural sac is almost always unrelated to diskitis or spondylitis. Epidural ab-

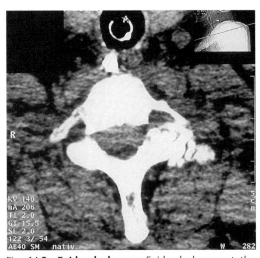

Fig. 14.**3 Epidural abscess.** Epidural abscess at the C7–T1 level in a patient with bacterial spondylodiskitis at the T5–6 level caused by infection with *Staphylococcus aureus*. CT clearly defines a crescent-shaped mass located anterior to the dural sac and encroaching on the spinal canal.

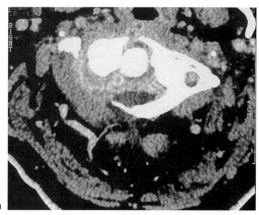 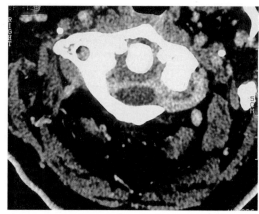

a

Fig. 14.**4a, b** **Epidural abscess.** A patient who previously had a retropharyngeal injection for pain relief was evaluated for progressive weakness in both arms and very severe, motion-dependent posterior neck pain. The symptoms were caused by the contiguous spread of a retropharyngeal infection with *Staphylococcus aureus* to the spine, inciting a suppurative inflammation that

has completely encompassed the dens and caused significant spinal stenosis. The inflammation is clearly demarcated after intravenous contrast administration. In particular, the bilateral pus-filled abscess cavities bordering the lateral mass of C2 are better demonstrated by CT than magnetic resonance imaging.

scess should be suspected in a patient with high fever, back pain, and spinal tenderness to percussion. Risk factors are diabetes mellitus, chronic renal failure, alcoholism, and intravenous drug abuse. The most common mode of infection, seen in 25–50% of cases, is hematogenous spread directly to the epidural space or to a vertebral body with subsequent spread to the epidural space. Possible sources

of infection include skin lesions such as furuncles; bacterial endocarditis; urinary tract infection; respiratory tract infections, including sinusitis; parapharyngeal abscesses; and dental infections.

Infection can reach the spine by contiguous extension from a decubital ulcer, psoas abscess, open injury, parapharyngeal abscess, or mediastinitis.

A third etiologic group consists of operative and therapeutic procedures on the spine, including open procedures, such as disk operations, and percutaneous procedures, such as epidural catheter insertion.

■ Frequency

The incidence of spinal epidural abscess in the early 1970s was 0.2–1.2 cases per 10,000 hospitalizations per year. Recent publications suggest that the incidence has been rising. The peak age of occurrence is 58 ± 16 years. As the longest spinal region, the thoracic spine is most commonly affected (approximately 50% of cases), followed by the lumbar spine (35%) and cervical spine (15%). In one series of 39 patients, 82% of the abscesses were located posterior to the dural sac, and 18% were anterior.

Fig. 14.**5** **Epidural abscess.** T1-weighted coronal magnetic resonance image of the patient in Fig. 14.**4** clearly demonstrates an inflammatory soft-tissue mass encompassing C1 and C2.

■ Clinical Manifestations

A classic symptom is very severe pain over the affected spinal segment, which is dramatically increased by light percussion. Patients often have a high fever and display meningeal signs. Within a few days, the clinical picture expands to include bowel and bladder symptoms and lower extremity palsy, extending to complete cord paralysis. With a postoperative epidural abscess, these findings may be considerably milder, or even absent.

■ CT Morphology

CT typically shows an elongated, encapsulated extradural mass of low density with a cystic center. The capsule may be slightly hyperdense on unenhanced scans, and is clearly demarcated after contrast administration. The craniocaudal extent of the mass can be considerable and may span the entire thoracic spine, for example (Fig. 14.**3**).

Spinal Arachnoiditis, Arachnopathy
(Figs. 14.**6**, 14.**7**)

■ **Frequency:** relatively rare; develops after multiple spinal interventions (surgery, myelography).

Suggestive morphologic findings: postmyelographic CT demonstrates intraspinal adhesions and nonvisualization of root sleeves. Block of the contrast column is seen in advanced cases.

Procedure: postmyelographic CT in the prone position (to opacify the root sleeves).

Other studies: MRI. Contrast injection for myelography and postmyelographic CT can prove difficult in advanced stages. MRI is also better for defining lesions that extend over multiple segments.

Checklist for scan interpretation:
▶ Degree and craniocaudal extent of the changes?
▶ Differential diagnosis should include a tumor or cerebrospinal fluid (CSF) metastasis as the cause of the changes.

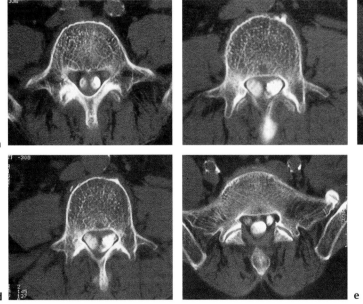

Fig.   14.**6 a–e Arachnoiditis/arachnopathy.**   This patient had undergone several prior disk operations and was admitted with suspicion of a new herniated disk. Clinically, however, the patient manifested polyradicular pain and neurologic deficits. Postmyelographic CT clearly shows multiple septations and filling defects in the subarachnoid space. For example, the S1 root sleeve on the right side is poorly opacified while the opposite side is well visualized. At surgery, the roots at several levels were found to be embedded in extradural scar tissue, which was causing radicular compression.

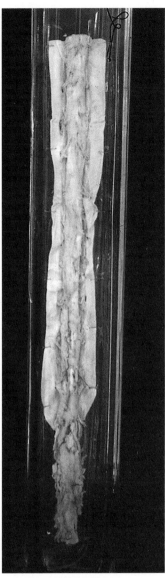

Fig. 14.**7** **Arachnopathy.** Pathologic specimen shows pronounced arachnopathy secondary to purulent meningitis (courtesy of the Department of Pathology, Charité Hospital, Berlin).

■ Pathogenesis

Arachnoiditis is an inflammatory process that affects the arachnoid lining of the dural sac and root sleeves. Older synonyms were circumscribed serous spinal meningitis and adhesive spinal arachnoiditis.

Etiologies include numerous causes of syphilis, tuberculosis, and other infections, traumatic or spontaneous subarachnoid hemorrhage, and the injection of oily or aqueous contrast media, local anesthetics, and chemotherapeutic agents. Infectious etiologies have become less common since the introduction of antibiotics.

Arachnoiditis is caused by an immune reaction of the arachnoid membrane that leads to adhesions and consequent impairment of CSF circulation. It has been known since Rydevik et al. (1984) that the nerve roots derive approximately 50 % of their nutrition from the CSF. As a result, the web-like structure of the arachnoid is essential for maintaining a healthy metabolic exchange. Progressive fibrosis and collagen deposition can also impair the microcirculation, causing damage to the nerve roots. The clinical manifestations of these changes are nonspecific and range from back pain and/or radicular pain to sensorimotor deficits (usually affecting the L5 and S1 roots) or bowel and bladder dysfunction.

■ Frequency

Arachnoiditis is often underestimated in terms of its effects on individual quality of life and public health. A 1994 publication estimates the worldwide case numbers at approximately a million, occurring mainly in patients who have undergone Pantopaque myelography. The economic impact of the resulting occupational disability, chronic drug and alcohol abuse, and suicidal tendencies is correspondingly great. A follow-up study in 50 patients found that the average lifespan was shortened by 12 years (Guyer et al. 1989).

■ Clinical Manifestations

The clinical symptoms are nonspecific. They can range from diffuse back pain, radicular pain, causalgia, and sensorimotor deficits to autonomic disturbances of bowel and bladder function and impotence.

■ **CT Morphology**

The most rewarding CT technique is postmyelographic scanning. Adhesions in the caudal dural sac can be detected at an early stage as filling defects in the root sleeves (prone examination may be helpful). Over time, the root sleeves become adherent to one another and to the dural sac, creating the appearance of a featureless ("empty") dural sac. Finally, progressive transmeningeal fibrosis leads to a conglomerate mass that produces a complete block in myelography and postmyelographic CT.

A single axial scan is inadequate for diagnosis, which requires visualizing and evaluating the process over multiple levels.

■ **Differential Diagnosis**

The differential diagnosis should include an intrathecal tumor or intrathecal seeding, especially if there is a history of factors predisposing to arachnopathy.

Rheumatoid Arthritis (Fig. 14.8)

Frequency: atlantoaxial joint involvement is present in 44–88 % of patients with rheumatoid arthritis.

Suggestive morphologic findings: atlantoaxial subluxation, pannus formation, basilar impression. CT function views may show spinal instability.

Procedure: contrast administration. Next to MRI, postmyelographic CT is best for demonstrating narrowing of the spinal canal. Obtain axial CT function views in maximum flexion and coronal views in maximum extension.

Other studies: MRI is the method of choice for demonstrating pannus and especially for detecting possible cervical myelopathy. Postmyelographic CT can demonstrate bony changes and the degree of spinal stenosis.

Checklist for scan interpretation:
▶ Degree of atlantoaxial subluxation and basilar impression, if present?
▶ Degree of compression of the medulla oblongata?

■ **Pathogenesis**

Involvement of the upper cervical spine by rheumatoid arthritis is common, occurring in 44–88 % of patients in different series. Synovial proliferation in these cases leads to the destruction of bone and of the ligaments that bind the vertebrae together. The resulting instability can range from a mild, asymptomatic atlantoaxial subluxation to a severe dislocation of the dens with compression of the spinal cord and brain stem.

The inflammatory degenerative changes that affect the cervical spine in rheumatoid arthritis typically lead to atlantoaxial subluxation, found in approximately 25 % of patients, and to basilar impression, found in about 8 % of patients.

Atlantoaxial subluxation is the result of erosive changes in the dens based on inflammatory disease of the synovial atlantoaxial joint. The resulting destruction of the dens and laxness of the transverse ligament attachment to the atlas can eventually lead to anterior dislocation of the atlas arch with cord impingement. Inflammatory pannus formation leads to further narrowing of the residual spinal canal. On CT these changes cause a widening of the joint space, which normally does not exceed 2–3 mm. The pannus itself appears as a soft-tissue mass that enhances after contrast administration.

The degree of subluxation tends to progress steadily over time. In a long-term study published in 1972 and covering an average of four and a half years, the initial atlantoaxial subluxation of 3.5–5 mm increased to 5–8 mm in 45 % of the patients and to more than 8 mm in 10 %. Subluxation of 9 mm or more is almost invariably associated with cervical myelopathy.

Basilar impression is the result of erosive changes in the lateral mass of the atlas arch combined with laxness of the transverse ligament. This leads to an upward herniation of the dens, anterior displacement of the atlas arch,

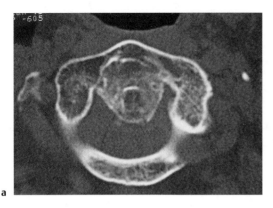

a

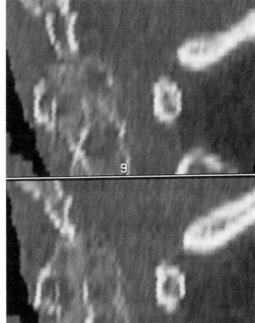

Fig. 14.**8 a, b Rheumatoid arthritis.** Much of the atlantoaxial joint has been destroyed. The pannus is heavily calcified, and the atlantoaxial distance is approximately 1 cm. The sagittal reformatted images clearly demonstrate the overall extent of the changes and the cortical destruction of the dens.

and frequent protrusion of the atlas posterior arch into the foramen magnum. The results are narrowing of the spinal canal and brain-stem compression.

■ Frequency

The upper cervical spine, particularly the atlantoaxial joint, is involved in approximately 44–88 % of patients with rheumatoid arthritis. Atlantoaxial subluxation is found in about 25 % of cases and basilar impression in about 8 %.

■ Clinical Manifestations

The most common symptom is pain, both local and radiating to the mastoid or to the frontal, temporal, or occipital region. Cervical cord compression may occur, leading to signs of cervical myelopathy with hyperactive reflexes, ataxia, spasticity, palsies, and sensory loss.

■ CT Morphology

Atlantoaxial subluxation is diagnosed by CT if the distance between the posterior border of the atlas anterior arch and the anterior surface of the dens is more than 3 mm (Fig. 14.**8**). In addition, reactive granulation tissue (pannus) is often visible as a soft-tissue mass surrounding the dens. Frequently this tissue enhances after contrast administration. MRI and postmyelographic CT are best for demonstrating osseous changes and the degree of spinal canal narrowing.

Atlantoaxial instability can be detected by obtaining CT function views of the cervical spine. Coronal scans are taken with the head in maximum extension, and axial scans are obtained in maximum flexion.

Paget Disease (Osteitis Deformans)

Frequency: relatively rare in the spinal column.

Suggestive morphologic findings: osteolytic lesions predominate in the initial phase. Later, zones of resorption coexist with reparative ossification. The lesions are nonenhancing.

Procedure: contiguous thin CT slices, secondary reconstructions, bone-window views.

Other studies: plain radiographs of other potentially affected body regions.

Checklist for scan interpretation:
▶ Monostotic or polyostotic involvement?
▶ Have the changes caused narrowing of the spinal canal and neuroforamina?

Pathogenesis

Paget disease is a disease of osteoclasts, presumably of viral origin, that leads to an acceleration of bone resorption with reactive osteoblast hyperactivity. The newly formed bone has a soft, disordered structure instead of a normal lamellar architecture. The initial phase is dominated by osteoclasts in a vascular stroma, which later regresses. Reactive osteoblast hyperactivity in the reparative phase leads to the formation of very dense, sclerotic bone. In about 1% of cases the reactive osteoblasts undergo malignant transformation, forming an osteosarcoma, fibrosarcoma, or chondrosarcoma. Degeneration is less common in spinal lesions that at other sites, however.

Compression myelopathy occurs almost exclusively when several adjacent segments are involved. It does not occur with the monostotic form.

Frequency

The prevalence of the disease is approximately 3%, but most cases take an asymptomatic course. A familial pattern of occurrence is seen in about 15% of cases. Males predominate by a 3:2 ratio.

Clinical Manifestations

Spinal involvement by Paget disease is asymptomatic in most cases. If symptoms arise, they usually result from narrowing of the spinal canal or neuroforamina by reactive hyperostosis or from the pathologic fracture of a vertebral body.

CT Morphology

Osteolytic lesions are predominant in the acute phase. Later, cotton-wool areas of bone resorption coexist with sites of reactive bone formation, accompanied by cortical thickening. Contrast enhancement is unusual.

Multiple Sclerosis

Frequency: rarely a primary CT diagnosis.

Suggestive morphologic findings: rarely detected by CT, but scans may be positive when the diagnosis is known. Acute inflammatory foci may show contrast enhancement.

Procedure: contrast administration.

Other studies: contrast-enhanced MRI is the method of choice for visualizing the entire central nervous system (CNS).

Checklist for scan interpretation:

In *positive* cases (IE, an enhancing mass detected in a young patient), supplement CT with MRI or compare the findings with other studies.

In *negative* cases, CT is insufficient to exclude the disease. If clinical suspicion exists, recommend further studies.

■ Pathogenesis

Multiple sclerosis is an acquired, inflammatory, demyelinating disease affecting the white matter of the CNS. In principle, it may occur anywhere within the CNS.

Multiple sclerosis often presents initially with signs of myelopathy, particularly motor and sensory disturbances.

A clinical distinction is drawn between acute and chronic forms, but in both cases MRI is the method of choice for demonstrating the associated changes. The lesions of multiple sclerosis are rarely detectable by CT, particularly in an acute inflammatory form associated with a disruption of the blood–brain barrier leading to contrast enhancement on CT. In this case as well, MRI is far superior to CT owing to its higher sensitivity to contrast enhancement.

■ Frequency

Epidemiologic studies suggest that multiple sclerosis is an autoimmune disorder in which genetic predisposition and environmental factors also play an important role. Concordance is present in 25% of affected monozygotic twins, and the risk of contracting the disease is 20–50 times higher in siblings or offspring of affected patients. Regional differences in the prevalence of multiple sclerosis suggest that environmental factors play a role. Persons who move from a higher-prevalence region to a lower-prevalence region still have an increased risk, while persons who move into an endemic region maintain their normal low risk. This is true only if the move takes place before about age 15, however.

■ Clinical Manifestations

Multiple sclerosis can present with a variety of sensory, motor, and mixed sensorimotor deficits. Asymmetric spastic paraparesis is the most common motor symptom. The most common sensory symptom in multiple sclerosis of the spinal cord is atactic paraparesis with asymmetric proprioceptive deficits. Motor disturbances are somewhat more common in males, sensory disturbances in females. Like the disease itself, the clinical manifestations can take an undulating course with periods of complete remission.

■ CT Morphology

As noted above, multiple sclerosis is rarely detectable by CT. Scanning in acute cases may demonstrate multiple sclerosis lesions as enhancing intraspinal masses. This finding is nonspecific when the diagnosis is unknown, and warrants immediate further investigation by MRI and comparison with clinical and laboratory parameters.

A negative CT examination is of no value in excluding an inflammatory, demyelinating disease of the CNS.

■ References

Recommended for further study

Diskitis

Boden SD, Davis DO, Dina TS, et al. Postoperative discitis distinguishing early MR imaging findings from normal postoperative disc space changes. Radiology 1992; 184: 765–71.

Spondylodiskitis

Fam AG, Rubenstein J. Another look at spinal tuberculosis. J Rheumatol 1993; 20: 1731–40.

Jain R, Sawhney S, Berry M. Computed tomography of vertebral tuberculosis: patterns of bone destruction. Clin Radiol 1983; 47: 196–9.

Epidural abscess

Siegelmann R, Findler G, Faibel M, et al. Postoperative spinal epidural empyema: clinical and computed tomography features. Spine 1991; 16: 1146–9.

Spinal arachnoiditis, arachnopathy

Guyer DW, Wiltse LL, Eskay ML, Guyer BH. The long-range prognosis of arachnoiditis. Spine 1989; 14: 1332–41.

Kumar A, Montanera W, Willinsky R, TerBrugge KG, Aggarwal S. MR features of tuberculous arachnoiditis. J Comput Assist Tomogr 1993; 17: 127–30.

Ross JS, Masaryk TJ, Modic MT, et al. MR imaging of lumbar arachnoiditis. AJNR Am J Neuroradiol 1987; 8: 885–92.

Rydevik B, Brown MD, Lundborg G. Pathoanatomy and pathophysiology of nerve root compression. Spine 1984; 9: 7–15.

Rheumatoid arthritis

Ostensen H, Gudmundsen TE, Haakonsen M, Lagerqvist H, Kaufmann C, Ostensen M. Three-dimensional CT evaluation of occipito-atlanto-axial dislocation in rheumatoid arthritis. Scand J Rheumatol 1998; 27: 352–6.

Paget disease

Zlatkin MB, Lander PH, Hadjipavlou AG, Levine JS. Paget disease of the spine: CT with clinical correlation. Radiology 1986; 160: 155–9.

Recent and basic works

Diskitis

Kopecki KK, Gilmor RL, Scott JA, et al. Pitfalls of CT in diagnosis of discitis. Neuroradiology 1985; 27: 57–66.

Spondylodiskitis

Allali F, Benomar A, El Yahyaoui M, Chkili T, Hajjaj-Hassouni N. Atlantoaxial tuberculosis: three cases. Joint Bone Spine 2000; 67(5): 481–4.

Lmejjati M, Maaqili M, El Abbadi N, Bellakhdar F. Tumor-like tuberculosis of the sacrum. Joint Bone Spine 2000; 67(5): 468–70.

Schellinger D. Patterns of anterior spinal canal involvement by neoplasms and infections. AJNR Am J Neuroradiol 1996; 17: 953–9.

Epidural abscess

Baker AS, Ojemann RG, Swartz MN, Richardson EP. Spinal epidural abscess. N Engl J Med 1975; 293: 463–8.

Rheumatoid arthritis

Czerny C, Grampp S, Henk CB, Neuhold A, Stiskal M, Smolen J. Rheumatoid arthritis of the craniocervical region: assessment and characterization of inflammatory soft tissue proliferations with unenhanced and contrast-enhanced CT. Eur Radiol 2000; 10(9): 1416–22.

Index